EVALUATION OF PSYCHOLOGICAL THERAPIES

EVALUATION OF PSYCHOLOGICAL THERAPIES

Psychotherapies, Behavior Therapies, Drug Therapies, and Their Interactions

Edited by Robert L. Spitzer and Donald F. Klein

Proceedings of the Sixty-fourth Annual Meeting of the American Psychopathological Association

The Johns Hopkins University Press
Baltimore and London

The Johns Hopkins University Press, Baltimore, Maryland 21218
The Johns Hopkins University Press Ltd., London

Library of Congress Catalog Card Number 75-11360
ISBN 0-8018-1721-8

Library of Congress Cataloging in Publication data will be found on the last printed page
of this book.

CONTENTS

American Psychopathological Association

Officers for 1973-1974

Max Fink, M.D., President   Stony Brook, N.Y.
Charles Shagass, M.D., President-Elect   Philadelphia, Pa.
Arnold Friedhoff, M.D. Vice-President   New York, N.Y.
Jonathan O. Cole, M.D., Secretary   Philadelphia, Pa.
Donald F. Klein, M.D., Treasurer   Glen Oaks, N.Y.
Henry Brill, M.D., Councillor   West Brentwood, N.Y.
Gerald Klerman, M.D., Councillor   Boston, Mass.

Committee on Program

Donald F. Klein, M.D.   Glen Oaks, N.Y.
Robert L. Spitzer, M.D.   New York, N.Y.

Arrangements

Jonathan O. Cole, M.D.   Philadelphia, Pa.

Publicity

David L. Dunner, M.D.   New York, N.Y.

FOREWORD

Despite a popular acceptance of psychiatric therapy, there remains a gnawing professional suspicion that treatment methods leave much to be desired, with neither the process well defined nor the outcome assured. For decades, we have been concerned with the therapeutic process as much as with the methods of evaluation, and yet the methods of classification, the processes of remediation, and the criteria and methods of evaluation of outcome for many psychiatric disorders are matters of concern and argument. Ten years ago, the American Psychopathological Association reflected on "The Evaluation of Psychiatric Treatment," assessing the range of therapies in treating the varieties of the mentally ill.

For the psychological therapies, the observers noted that little outcome data were available, much of it uncontrolled. They found an emphasis on process rather than outcome, for the definition of outcome criteria was seen as complex, reflecting intraindividual, family, and social factors. For outcome criteria, they suggested standardized histories, patient questionnaires, projective tests, and the recording and analysis of psychotherapeutic sessions at milestones in the therapeutic career (Wolberg, 1964; Burdock & Hardesty, 1964; Greenhouse, 1964).

As the editors stated in 1964, periodic audit is necessary not only in commerce but in the sciences as well. Such an audit in therapy must include the selection of subjects, criteria of evaluation, and comparisons with such alternate modes of intervention as may be available. It is on such data that the scientific community will ultimately have to rest its judgments, and through their evaluations, the public may be offered the best return for their therapeutic dollar. The professions of psychiatry and psychology are increasingly called upon to support their recommendations for interventions as worth the charges and the time involved. Considering the widespread use of psychological therapies, the Association drew together those scientists who have endeavored to evaluate the therapies, looking more to an assessment of outcome than to the processes of evaluation.

In contrast to the breadth of psychiatric therapies reviewed a decade ago, this evaluation is focused on three of the more widely used psychological therapies: individual psychoanalysis and psychotherapy, behavior therapy, and the combined use of pharmacological agents and psychotherapy. The data of the presentations should provide a basis for the intelligent application of these complex modes of interaction, as well as for the cost-benefit analyses which have become so popular in social management operations, both governmental and private.

Max Fink

REFERENCES

Wolberg, Lewis R. The evaluation of psychotherapy. In P. Hoch and J. Zubin (Eds.), *The Evaluation of Psychiatric Treatment*. New York: Grune & Stratton, 1964, pp. 1–13.

Burdock, Eugene I., & Hardesty, Anne S. Quantitative techniques for the evaluation of psychiatric treatment. In P. Hoch and J. Zubin (Eds.), *The Evaluation of Psychiatric Treatment*. New York: Grune & Stratton, 1964, pp. 58–74.

Greenhouse, Samuel W. Principles in the evaluation of therapies for mental disorders. In P. Hoch and J. Zubin (Eds.), *The Evaluation of Psychiatric Treatment*. New York: Grune & Stratton, 1964, pp. 94–105.

PREFACE

For several decades, society has had laws requiring manufacturers of drugs to offer data proving the safety and the efficacy of their products before they can be used in treating patients. For a host of reasons, society is apparently unable and/or unwilling to make similar demands of practitioners and proponents of psychological therapies. In the absence of legal requirements, the responsibility for demonstrating the value of the psychological therapies falls to the mental health professions.

We believe that there is a continuing and urgent need for data from carefully designed studies of the efficacy of the psychological therapies. For this reason, the participants in the Sixty-fourth Annual Meeting of the American Psychopathological Association, on the "Evaluation of Psychological Therapies," were required to present data, not mere speculation.

This book contains the papers presented at that meeting. The first day was devoted to the evaluation of psychoanalysis, psychotherapy, and behavior therapy. The second day was devoted to the combined use of drug and psychological therapies.

We express our appreciation to Dr. David Rimm for providing us with a discussion of the papers presented in the session devoted to "Aspects of Behavior Therapy," in lieu of a paper by a formal discussant who at the last moment was unable to be at the meeting. We also express our thanks for the thoughtful editorial work of Mr. David Zubin and the excellent secretarial help provided by Mrs. Jennie Gilliland.

R. L. S.
D. F. K.

PART I:
PSYCHOANALYSIS
AND PSYCHOTHERAPY

1   COMPARATIVE STUDIES OF PSYCHOTHERAPIES: Is It True That "Everybody Has Won and All Must Have Prizes"?

LESTER LUBORSKY, BARTON SINGER, and LISE LUBORSKY

The quotation in the title of this article you will recognize since it is from *Alice in Wonderland*—it was the dodo-bird who handed down this happy verdict after judging the race. It was also the subtitle of that classical paper by Saul Rosenzweig (1936), "Some Implicit Common Factors in Diverse Methods of Psychotherapy." Our title implies what I think many of us believe—that all the psychotherapies produce some benefits for some patients. What we do not know is whether there are psychotherapies which produce significantly better results and whether certain psychotherapies are especially well suited to certain patients. Here, when we use the word "know," we are not using it in the clinical sense, where we believe a great deal is known, but in the controlled research sense, where we believe we are just beginning. We "know," for example, that psychoanalysis works better with patients who have high ego strength, but we can find no research evidence for this of the kind considered in this review.

Lester Luborsky, Ph.D., Professor of Psychology in Psychiatry, University of Pennsylvania; research staff member, Eastern Pennsylvania Psychiatric Institute.

Barton Singer, Ph.D., Assistant Professor of Psychology in Psychiatry, University of Pennsylvania; Senior Staff Psychologist, Philadelphia Veterans Administration Hospital.

Lise Luborsky, Villanova University.

A version of a panel presented at the third annual meeting of the Society for Psychotherapy Research, Nashville, Tenn., June 16, 1972, entitled "The Essence of What We Know from Controlled Comparative Studies of Psychotherapies—Is It True That 'Everybody Has Won and *All* Must Have Prizes'?" Panel participants: Charles P. O'Brien, M.D., Ph.D., University of Pennsylvania, "Comparisons of Individual Psychotherapy and Group Psychotherapy"; Bruce Sloane, M.D., and Fred Staples, Ph.D., Temple University, "Comparisons of Psychoanalytically Oriented Psychotherapy and Behavior Therapy"; Karl Rickels, M.D., University of Pennsylvania, "Comparisons of Psychotherapy and Pharmacotherapy"; Lester Luborsky, Ph.D., University of Pennsylvania, moderator. A larger version of this paper appears in *Archives of General Psychiatry*, 1975, **32**, 995–1008.

The work was supported in part by United States Public Health Service Research Grant MH-15442 and Research Scientist Award MH-40710.

With thanks to Drs. Hans Strupp and John Paul Brady for their suggestions on the manuscript and, for their assistance, to Mrs. Marjorie Cohen and Mrs. Freda Greene.

Comparative studies of psychotherapies are not an area where one or two decisive experiments can be telling—one must rely on the verdict of a series of at least passably well-controlled studies. Ideally, one would want to have an impeccable, definitive study that would settle the question of comparative worth once and for all, but that is not possible since *every* study has some uniqueness of sample characteristics, measuring instruments, and other less easily defined aspects. A consensus of many studies is what we must hope for.

The best way to summarize the studies is to consider them separately for each of the main types of comparisons that have been done, e.g., group versus individual psychotherapy, time-limited versus unlimited psychotherapy, and client-centered versus other traditional psychotherapies. For each type of comparison, a convenient "box score" is given with the number of studies in which the treatments were better or worse, or "tie score." There can be no mistake about how each "score" is determined since the specific studies are noted in the tables of results.

Only studies in which some attention was paid to the main requirements of controlled comparative research were included. All such studies were graded according to how well they fit the desirable principles of controlled comparative studies on a scale from A to E: $A =$ the main principles of research design were satisfied; $B =$ one or two were partially deficient; $C =$ three or four were partially deficient; $D =$ three or four were partially deficient and one was seriously deficient; $E =$ the deficiencies were so serious that the results were not worth considering and the study therefore was not included. The criteria which were applied in evaluating each study were derived from further elaboration of those listed in Fiske, Hunt, Luborsky, Orne, Parloff, Reiser, and Tuma (1970). The primary purpose of our grading system was not to provide highly reliable subdivisions of grading as much as it was to weed out the worst studies. Nevertheless, it was reassuring to find that independent grading judgments by two of us (L. L. and B. S.) on 16 randomly selected studies yielded a correlation of .84.

All studies included dealt with adults or young adults and the majority of them were nonpsychotic patients. Since studies of patients seem more likely to have relevance to the problems of practitioners than studies of non-patients, this review will consider only research in which bona fide *patients* were in bona fide treatment—excluded were role-playing studies and studies using student volunteers.

Within these limits, the present review is more complete than any other. It combines many of the studies of the two most complete reviews, Meltzoff and Kornreich (1970) and Luborsky, Chandler, Auerbach, Cohen, and Bachrach (1971), with additional types of comparisons which have not been reviewed before. The difficulties encountered in locating and evaluating the relevant research are impressive. Therefore, it is not surprising that some previous reviewers have presented biased conclusions about the verdict of this research literature as to the relative value of certain forms of psychotherapy (see two replies to some of these: Luborsky, 1954, 1972).

Since we tried to do a complete review—within the limits noted—we can now complete our introduction with a historical perspective. From a tabulation of the publication dates of the studies we learn that the entire field of controlled comparative treatment research got its start only in the middle and late 1950's: the bulk of the studies were done in the last two decades. Within this period each type of comparison had its special era. Group versus individual treatment comparisons started as far back as 1949 and continued up to the present, but most of them were done in the decade of the 1950's. The time-limited versus time-unlimited comparison was done mostly in the late 1950's and early 1960's. The client-centered versus other psychotherapy comparisons began in the 1950's and extended to the first half of the 1960's. The psychotherapy versus behavior therapy comparisons only began in 1960; most studies were done in the late 1960's and some continue to the present. The psychotherapy versus pharmacotherapy comparisons were represented by three studies done in the late fifties, with most of them being done in the sixties and continuing on until the present. The psychotherapy versus medical regimen for psychosomatic illnesses covers the longest time span, beginning in 1936, although studies are sparse in the entire period. The psychotherapy versus no-psychotherapy comparison started in the fifties and was well represented then, but the vogue was over by the first half of the sixties.

Finally, it is satisfying to note that the research quality of the studies, in terms of our quality ratings, for most types of comparisons, has improved some in the last few decades. The simplest way to demonstrate this was to divide all studies into quality ratings A and B versus C and D, and then note the mean publication date in each category—the C's and D's tend to be somewhat older.

PSYCHOTHERAPY VERSUS GROUP PSYCHOTHERAPY

For 13 comparative studies of individual versus group psychotherapy, the gains for each treatment were usually reported to be similar—in 9 comparisons. Only 2 comparisons showed a slight advantage for individual treatment, and 2 an advantage for group treatment (but 1 of these only in terms of improvement in ethnocentrism). The only study with schizophrenic patients (O'Brien, Hamm, Ray, Pierce, Luborsky, & Mintz, 1972) showed an advantage for group treatment. A box score summarizes these results and makes plain that most of the 13 comparisons[1] showed no

Table 1. Box Score: Comparison of Individual and Group Psychotherapy

Group was better	2[a]
Tie	9[b]
Individual was better	2[c]

[a] 69, 74 (numbers refer to the reference section).
[b] 4, 5, 14, 34, 39, 69, 75, 91, 95.
[c] 2, 26.

significant difference between these treatments. In view of the general opinion that group psychotherapy is less intensive, the results are a surprise.

TIME-LIMITED VERSUS TIME-UNLIMITED PSYCHOTHERAPY

Since Otto Rank, treatments which are structured at the outset as time-limited have been thought by some practitioners to be as good as the more usual time-unlimited treatment. The eight available controlled comparative studies are mostly (5 out of 8) consistent with this view in that there is no significant difference between the two. Only in Henry and Shlien (1958) was time-limited psychotherapy shown to be inferior in one criterion; that is, patients showed a decline in affect differentiation on the TAT. In two studies time-limited psychotherapy was shown to be better (Muench, 1965; Reid & Schyne, 1969). Our conclusion, therefore, is that usually differences in this treatment dimension seemed to make no significant difference in treatment results.

CLIENT-CENTERED VERSUS OTHER TRADITIONAL PSYCHOTHERAPIES

Of 11 studies comparing results of different schools of treatment (client-centered, psychoanalytic, Adlerian, etc.), only 4 of the 11 found a

Table 2. Box Score: Comparison of Time-Limited and Time-Unlimited Psychotherapy

Time-limited was better	2[a]
Tie	5[b]
Time-unlimited was better	1[c]

[a] 68, 79.
[b] 24, 36, 72, 88, 89.
[c] 36.

significant difference between one school's treatment and another. However, except for 5 studies of client-centered psychotherapy, there are not enough comparative studies in any one category to draw conclusions about a specific school of treatment. Furthermore, some studies were not acceptably controlled (and not included among the 11); for example, Ellis (1957), with only one therapist practicing two different treatments, reported that rational emotive therapy yielded better results than psychoanalytically oriented therapy!

The comparisons of client-centered with other psychotherapies revealed a similar phenomenon—most (4 out of 5) showed "ties," regardless of what other school it was compared with (i.e., psychoanalytic, neo-Freudian, or Adlerian).

Table 3. Box Score: Comparison of Client-Centered and Other Traditional Psychotherapies

Client-centered (i.e., "nondirective") was better	0
Tie	4[a]
Other traditional psychotherapies were better	1[b]

[a]3, 9, 35, 89.
[b]1.

BEHAVIOR THERAPY VERSUS PSYCHOTHERAPY[2]

There are 18 controlled comparisons in 11 studies dealing with patients (although there are many more with student volunteers).[3] Of these, behavior therapy emerged as superior to the other psychotherapies in 6 comparisons, and as no different in 12. Those which showed some form of behavior therapy to be superior include Gelder, Marks, and Wolff (1967); Cooper, Gelder, and Marks (1965); King, Armitage, and Tilton (1960); Lazarus (1961); Levis and Carrera (1967); and Patterson, Levene, and Breger (1971). The 12 comparisons in which they were not significantly different include Gelder et al. (1967) (in patients with more complex symptoms); Cooper et al. (1965) (general change measures as opposed to specific improvement in phobias); Gelder and Marks (1966): Lazarus (1961); Marks and Gelder (1965); McReynolds (1969); and Sloane, Wolpe, Cristol, Yorkston, Freed, Whipple, and Staples.[4]

Thus we see that in most of the comparisons of behavior therapy with other psychotherapies (i.e., 12 out of 18) the differences in the amount of benefits they provide for patients are not significant.

All six treatment comparisons in which a form of behavior therapy was superior utilized very brief therapies (5 out of 6 of these comparisons are based upon studies of relatively poor research quality; i.e., with a rating of

Table 4. Box Score: Comparison of Behavior Therapy and Psychotherapy

Behavior therapy (usually desensitization) was better	6[a]
Tie	12[b]
Psychotherapy was better	0

[a] 13 (enlargement of 12), 26, 42, 48, 49, 73.
[b] 13, 13, 16, 25, 25, 26, 48, 59, 64, 73, n.4, n.4.

C or D). There is a trend for behavior therapy to achieve benefits earlier while more traditional psychotherapies move at a slower rate. The more rapid initial gains of behavior therapy may appear because it is more directive and/or because it is more often structured as time-limited treatment. According to Shlien, Mosak, and Dreikurs (1962), time-limited treatment yielded earlier onset of improvement.

In the two studies with patients with circumscribed and mild phobias there was a tendency for desensitization to do better (Gelder et al., 1967; Cooper et al., 1965). More studies are needed in which behavior therapies are applied to patients who have generalized maladjustments (as in Sloane et al.)

Most of the behavior therapy studies we have listed deal only with one form of behavior therapy, systematic desensitization. More comparative studies within the behavior therapies need to be done with other specific behavioral techniques such as, for example, a study by Boulougouris, Marks, and Marset (1971) comparing desensitization and flooding for phobias which showed a significant advantage for flooding.[5]

PSYCHOPHARMACOTHERAPY VERSUS PSYCHOTHERAPY[6]

Most of these controlled comparisons have been surveyed in the reviews by May (1968), and by Uhlenhuth, Lipman, and Covi (1969); our own review includes those which fit our criteria. The studies fall into three main types of comparisons: psychotherapy versus pharmacotherapy, psychotherapy plus pharmacotherapy versus psychotherapy alone, and psychotherapy plus pharmacotherapy versus pharmacotherapy alone, with box scores for each below.

Table 5. Box Score: Comparison of Psychotherapy and Pharmacotherapy

Psychopharmacological agent was better	7[a]
Tie	1[b]
Psychotherapy was better	0

[a] 21, 29, 38, 45, 51, 62, 71.
[b] 47.

Table 6. Box Score: Comparison of Psychotherapy plus Pharmacotherapy and Pharmacotherapy Alone

Psychotherapy plus pharmacotherapy was better	6[a]
Tie	5[b]
Pharmacotherapy alone was better	0

[a] 15, 29, 38, 43, 45, 51.
[b] 21, 44, 45, 62, 71.

1. Psychotherapy versus pharmacotherapy: pharmacotherapy alone is usually superior to psychotherapy (7 comparisons versus 1).

2. Combined treatment versus pharmacotherapy alone: the combined treatment, however, is often better than pharmacotherapy alone (6 comparisons better versus 5 the same). The probable implication is that something is added by the combination.

3. Combined treatment versus psychotherapy alone: again, the combined treatment is usually better than the single treatment; i.e., than psychotherapy alone (13 better versus 3 the same). (This result for combined treatment is the same as in the review by Uhlenhuth et al., 1969.)

The studies in these three comparisons include many more inpatients (of whom the majority are schizophrenic) than is true for our other comparisons. Of course we wondered whether a division into inpatient versus outpatient or a diagnostic categorization would make a difference in these results. Table 8 suggests there is no obvious difference. However, it is likely that for many, if not most, of these studies the selection of the patients, even for the outpatient groups, favored those who would benefit from pharmacotherapy; i.e., patients who would expect to be given medication rather than psychotherapy.

One other conclusion is noteworthy: a few studies reported that pharmacotherapy effects occur earlier and may decline in time, while psychotherapy effects are slower to develop but may increase in time (e.g., Shlien et al., 1962).

Table 7. Box Score: Comparison of Psychotherapy plus Pharmacotherapy and Psychotherapy Alone

Psychotherapy plus pharmacotherapy was better	13[a]
Tie	3[b]
Psychotherapy alone was better	0

[a] 15, 17, 21, 29, 31 (also reported in 32, 85), 37, 41, 45, 51, 62 (also reported in 63), 71, 78, 80.
[b] 27, 41, 50.

Table 8. Box Score: Psychotherapy vs. Pharmacotherapy Comparative Studies, Subdivided According to Diagnosis and In- vs. Outpatient Status

| | Combined Therapy vs. Psychotherapy Alone | | | | Combined Therapy vs. Drugs Alone | | | | Drug Therapy (Alone) vs. Psychotherapy (Alone) | | | |
| | Better | | Same | | Better | | Same | | Better | | Same | |
	N	Study #[a]	N	Study #	N	Study #	N	Study #	N	Study #	N	Study #
Schizophrenic inpatients	5	62, 15, 31, 41, 29	2	27, 41	4	15, 43, 29, 38	2	44, 62	3	29, 62, 38	0	
Mixed inpatients	2	21, 71	0		0		2	21, 71	2	21, 71	0	
Subtotal	7		2		4		4		5		0	
Mixed outpatients	1	51	1	50	1	51	0		1	51	0	
Depressed outpatients	1	45	0		1	45	1	45	1	45	0	
Neurotic (anxious) outpatients	4	80, 17, 37, 78	0		0		0		0		1	47
Subtotal	6		1		2		1		2		1	
Total	13		3		6		5		7		1	

[a]Numbers refer to the reference section.

PSYCHOTHERAPY PLUS A MEDICAL REGIMEN
VERSUS A MEDICAL REGIMEN ALONE
(FOR PSYCHOSOMATIC CONDITIONS)

For a variety of psychosomatic symptoms, the comparisons are over-whelmingly in favor of combined treatment—psychotherapy plus a medical regimen. Of 11 studies where the target of treatment was change in a psychosomatic symptom, 9 showed a significant advantage for psychotherapy plus a medical regimen,[7] or psychotherapy as opposed to a medical regimen alone.

Why do the results for comparative studies of psychosomatic symptoms favor psychotherapy so strongly? Aside from the fact that combined treatment is being compared with a single treatment, most likely the reassurance and support provided by psychotherapy are especially useful for the patients with psychosomatic symptoms. The results may also derive from the greater ease of evaluating the benefits of psychotherapy for patients with a clearcut target psychosomatic symptom.

Table 9. Box Score: Comparison of Psychotherapy plus Medical Regimen
and Medical Regimen Alone

Psychotherapy plus medical regimen was better	9[a]
Tie	1[b]
Medical regimen was better	1[c]

[a]8, 10, 30, 33, 57, 70, 90, 101, n. 13.
[b]28.
[c]96.

PSYCHOTHERAPY VERSUS "CONTROL" GROUPS
(INCLUDING "NO-PSYCHOTHERAPY,"
"WAIT-FOR-PSYCHOTHERAPY,"
MINIMAL PSYCHOTHERAPY, OR HOSPITAL CARE)

A final special comparison is between psychotherapy and its absence. "Absence of psychotherapy" is typically measured in these studies by arranging for a more or less matched group of patients to be assessed before and after an interval without treatment. Such groups, by virtue of their contacts and relationship with the researchers, or because they were sometimes maintained by general hospital care, were provided with some of the nonspecific ingredients of treatment but without formal psychotherapy. Such studies tend to be shaky in meeting design criteria, particularly because of the inequality in how the patients and staff value what is provided to each group of patients. Of course there is also an inequality in the patient's motivation and level of expectation of benefiting—if the "control" group patients achieve any benefits, they might well be surprised and pleased; if the treated patients do not achieve commensurate benefits, they might well be surprised and disappointed. Both conditions might well affect the outcome judgments so as to increase their incomparability.

Many of the 33 comparisons in the box score below were among the much larger number surveyed in Meltzoff and Kornreich (1970). Many of those listed by them, however, were not used by us because of research design inadequacies, or because they were not usual patient populations (e.g., prisoners).

Table 10. Box Score: Comparison of Psychotherapy and Control Groups

Psychotherapy was better	20[a]
Tie	13[b]
Control group was better	0

[a] 7, 11, 20, 30, 40, 41, 42, 49, 67, 77, 77, 81, 82, 86, 87, 89, 89, 92, 97, n. 4.
[b] 4, 7, 38, 42, 49, 56, 63, 63, 82, 92, 99, 100, n. 4.

Twenty, (or about 60 percent), of the comparisons significantly favored psychotherapy, but 13 showed a tie, meaning that the psychotherapy was not significantly better than the nonpsychotherapy. None of the comparisons favored the control group. We considered, in searching for explanations, whether the 13 comparisons showing a tie might have included more chronic inpatients—no evidence was found for this. Two likely explanations might be (1) that the nonspecific ingredients are often powerful for both the psychotherapy and the "control groups" (Frank, 1965), and (2) that the treatment effects often are not powerful enough to produce significant advantage over the beneficial forces activated by nonspecific factors.

CONCLUSIONS AND IMPLICATIONS

Conclusion 1:

Most comparative studies of different forms of psychotherapy found insignificant differences in proportions of patients who improved by the end of psychotherapy. It is both because of this and because all psychotherapies produce a high percentage of benefit (see Conclusion 2) that we can reach a "dodo-bird verdict"—it *is* usually true that "everybody has won and all must have prizes." This predominance of tie scores appears when different forms of psychotherapy are compared with each other; that is, it applies to the first four comparisons: group versus individual psychotherapy, time-limited versus time-unlimited psychotherapy, client-centered versus other traditional psychotherapies, and behavior therapy versus other psychotherapies. Only the last two comparisons involved "schools" of psychotherapy. It is noteworthy that in the 25 years of comparative treatment studies only two schools of treatment have sufficient numbers of comparative studies to permit a conclusion about the comparison with other psychotherapies: client-centered psychotherapy and behavior therapies. The preponderance of nonsignificant differences between treatments may be an even more impressive finding because many of these comparisons are studied by partisans of one treatment or the other. Also, researchers as well as editors of journals may tend to hesitate about publishing results of studies with nonsignificant differences.

Conclusion 2:

The controlled comparative studies indicate that a high percentage of patients who go through any of these psychotherapies gain from them. Meltzoff and Kornreich (1970, p. 178), for example, basing their conclusions on the controlled comparative studies, estimate that for both individual and group therapy about 80 percent of the studies show mainly positive results. The same can be said for the other kinds of treatment which were compared. This fact may contribute to the high frequency of tie scores—if a very high percentage of all patients receive benefits, it is more difficult to achieve a significant difference between different forms of treatment.

Conclusion 3:

The "dodo-bird verdict" does not apply when one ventures beyond comparisons of psychotherapies with each other; i.e., to comparisons of psychotherapy with other forms of treatment. (1) a preponderance of tie scores does not apply when psychotherapy versus other types of treatment such as pharmacotherapy are compared *singly*—in the available studies, pharmacotherapy produces significantly higher numbers of patients judged as benefiting. (2) it does not apply to combined treatments versus single treatments. The advantage for combined treatment is striking in that it appears for all three of the box scores dealing with combinations: for psychotherapy plus pharmacotherapy versus psychotherapy alone; for psychotherapy plus pharmacotherapy versus pharmacotherapy alone; for psychotherapy plus a medical regimen versus a medical regimen alone (for psychosomatic illnesses). A combination of treatments may represent more than an additive effect of two treatments—a "getting more for one's money"—there may also be some mutually facilitative interactive benefits for the combined treatments. (3) it does not apply to psychotherapy versus "control groups" (e.g., no psychotherapy) comparisons—more than half of these comparisons favor psychotherapy.

Conclusion 4:

There are only a few especially beneficial matches of type of treatment and type of patient—which is to be expected since Conclusion 1 is the dominant trend: (1) the most impressive match for the alleviation of a variety of psychosomatic symptoms is psychotherapy (and related psychological treatments) added to appropriate medical treatment in comparison with a medical regimen alone; (2) behavior therapy may be especially suited for circumscribed phobias (but not for severe phobias).

But it is, nevertheless, amazing in view of the large clinical literature on matching patient and treatment that in our review we have come upon only two especially beneficial matches between type of treatment and type of patient. There are some other good candidates but these are supported only by single studies rather than by the massing of studies which we require for our present review.[8]

Could the conclusions be artifacts of poor research? Deficiencies in the research designs and other artifactual problems described in Fiske et al., (1970) and Rosenthal and Rosnow (1969) probably do *not* account for our main conclusion concerning similar improvement rates for the different forms of psychotherapy, because: (1) the criterion in the majority of these studies is the usual criterion—that is, therapist's judgment of improvement.[9] Although this criterion (like any criterion) has its own vantage point (the therapist's opinion), studies using other criteria show a trend which is similar (in terms of comparative percentages of patients benefiting) to those using only the therapist's judgment as a criterion; (2) compared to many studies of psychotherapeutic results, especially those of three or four decades ago, those in our review are relatively well controlled—although only a few of them fulfill *all* of the recommendations for comparisons of treatment listed by Fiske et al. (1970). Furthermore, despite deficiencies in the quality of the research in the studies selected for the box scores, *the best-designed do not show a very different trend from those that are less well designed.*[10]

What are the main ways of improving these comparative treatment studies? Through the experience of evaluating the quality of these studies, we have evolved a system for judging them according to a list of criteria partly based on Fiske et al. (1970). We will here highlight only a few of the criteria on which most of the research is in need of improvement.

With regard to Criterion 1, the patients should be described, especially on certain crucial dimensions. This will permit something better than random assignment of patients to treatment. Composing groups by matching pairs of patients on crucial dimensions, such as severity of illness, is highly desirable, but only a few of the studies did this. Adequate description of the sample will also permit further exploration of specific interactions of type of treatment with type of patient. This last recommendation for improving experimental designs could lead to the confirmation of special patient-treatment matches and the discovery of new ones. Also, the lead provided in the O'Brien et al. (1972) study that group therapy may be especially suitable for schizophrenics should be explored in new studies; similarly more replications of Penick, Filion, Fox, and Stunkard (1971) and Stunkard (1972) should be done.

With regard to Criterion 5, in many studies there was insufficient effort made to present the treatments to the patients as equally valued. Then, in addition, the patients in some studies may have known which therapies were most valued by the therapists or by the experimenters.

With regard to Criterion 7, this criterion emphasizes the importance of evaluating the treatment outcome by independent measures. Since treatments have a variety of impacts, it is also important to include the main types in the outcome criteria. The two main types of outcomes that must be evaluated are those related to *specific symptoms* and those related to *general adjustment*. Different therapies may produce different proportions of these. For example, the behavior therapies and the pharmacotherapies may have more influence on the symptom-outcome measures while the long-term, intensive psychoanalytically oriented psychotherapies may have more influence on the general adjustment measures.

With regard to Criterion 9, usually there is no evidence offered that the treatment given actually fits the intended form of treatment. The simplest and most direct way of doing this—rarely done in practice—is to take samples of the administered treatment and have them judged independently. Judging samples in this way will also do much to permit comparisons across treatments in different studies since there are so many varieties of treatment designated "psychotherapy"—e.g., the psychotherapy provided for schizophrenia may be quite different from the psychotherapy provided for neurosis.

Another aspect of Criterion 9 is equally important: the length of the treatment and the length of the followup must be such as to be considered reasonable examples of the designated form of treatment. Some forms of treatment exert their effects early (probably behavior therapy, pharmacotherapy, time-limited therapy, and directive therapies); some have a slower course and more long-lasting effects (probably the insight-oriented psychotherapies, and particularly psychoanalysis). The insight-oriented psychotherapies are poorly represented in most of these comparative studies—treatment lengths are rarely more than one year and usually much, much less, and followups are either absent or too brief to catch the long-term benefits of the insight-oriented psychotherapies.

Is there a practical application of our conclusions in terms of the assignment of patients to different forms of treatment? Taken at face value, our conclusions seem to dictate that from now on we should stop paying attention to the form of the treatment in referring patients for psychotherapy. Yet there are several reasons why we should hesitate to recommend such a drastic setting aside of all the clinical wisdom.

1. One most compelling reason for hesitation is the following. Similarities in numbers of patients benefiting from various forms of psychotherapy probably should not be taken to imply that the quality of the improvement is necessarily the same. The patient who has improved via group therapy or individual therapy may have gained something different in his conception of himself or in his capacity for reflecting from that gained by the patient who has improved via behavior therapy or Librium. There is some fair evidence for this supposition: e.g., Heine (1953), Klerman, Paykel, and Prusoff (1973), and Dudek (1970). Much more research needs to be done on this.[11]

2. As noted earlier, the studies we reviewed are almost entirely limited to a relatively short-term treatment, that is, about two months to twelve months. This is a glaring omission in the research literature. We do not know enough about what conclusions we would reach for long-term, intensive treatment.

3. Our conclusions apply to the results of comparative studies of *designated* forms of treatment; as indicated above, usually no step is taken to show how well the designation fits. Even beyond this problem, it is very likely that certain ingredients of the treatment which cut across treatment labels are the main influencers of outcome. The therapist, for example, can be supportive, warm, and empathic in a variety of designated forms of treatment, and this may be a powerful influence on the outcome of treatment.

4. As we have noted in Conclusion 4, there are a couple of especially promising matches between type of patient and type of treatment, and others may be soon established.

In sum, for these reasons (and for other more general ones noted in Luborsky, 1969) we should not yet consider ourselves ready to make assignments on a random basis.

How do we interpret the main finding in Conclusion 1? Essentially, three factors are involved in accounting for the main finding that the studies do not produce any clearcut winners *when psychotherapies are compared with each other*. To start with the least of the three first: (1) since all forms of psychotherapy tend to achieve a high percentage of improved patients (our Conclusion 2), it is difficult (statistically) for any single form of psychotherapy to show a significant advantage over any other form—the higher these percentages, the less room at the top for significant differences between treatments. (A survey by Mintz and Luborsky[12] of the distribution of improvement rates reported by different studies supports this.) (2) although each psychotherapeutic system differs in some elements of its philosophy, each system attempts to provide the patient with a plausible explanatory system for his difficulties and also with principles which may guide his future behavior. Such an organized explanatory and guidance system may be one of the common elements which facilitates the benefits from any psychotherapeutic system (as is suggested by Rosenzweig, 1936, and others). (3) the most potent explanatory factor is that the different forms of psychotherapeutic treatment have a major common element—a helping relationship with a therapist is present in all of them, along with the other related nonspecific effects such as suggestion and abreaction. This explanation is stressed by Rosenzweig (1936) and many others, and especially persuasively by Frank (1965) and Strupp (1974). This is exactly where more research needs to be done—on the components of a helping relationship. These components ought to be evaluated in the comparative studies; then, when differences among treatments do appear in some studies, they might be explicable in terms of the helping relationship.

NOTES

1. One study provided two comparisons.

2. Our thanks for the assistance of Dr. Bruce Sloane, Dr. John Paul Brady, and Dr. Peter E. Nathan in this section.

3. Also not reviewed is the large literature on treatment comparisons for people who have *specific* "habit" disturbances, e.g., smoking, bed-wetting, drug-taking, overeating, etc. (rather than pervasive personality and adjustment disorders which lead them to seek psychotherapy).

4. Sloane, R. B., Wolpe, N., Cristol, A., Yorkston, N., Freed, H., Whipple, K., & Staples, F. Short-term psychoanalytically oriented psychotherapy vs. behavior therapy. In preparation, 1974.

5. The brief review by Dr. Peter Nathan (at the 1973 Society for Psychotherapy Research meeting) suggests that the trend for results of comparisons of behavior therapies with each other will also be "tie scores." Similarly, the typical result for the comparison of behavior therapy vs. other psychological treatments (other than psychotherapy) is probably consistent with Marks, Gelder, and Edwards (1968), who compared behavior therapy with hypnosis and found no significant difference.

6. Our thanks for the invaluable assistance of Dr. Karl Rickels in preparing this section.

7. Two of these studies use primarily some form of psychotherapeutic treatment alone.

8. A symposium at the 1973 Society for Psychotherapy Research meeting was focused on these, evaluating two matches and attempting to locate others. This symposium, titled "Therapeutic Technology: Effects of Specific Techniques on Specific Disorders," included Dr. Lester Luborsky, the chairman, discussing the advantage for psychosomatic symptoms of psychotherapy plus a medical regimen vs. a medical regimen alone; Dr. Arnold Goldstein presenting research on modifications of psychotherapy for patients of a lower socioeconomic class with special focus on prescriptive and modeling techniques; Dr. Peter E. Nathan reviewing behavior therapy in the treatment of phobias both circumscribed and generalized; and Dr. Albert Stunkard discussing his research with Dr. Sydnor Penick on group behavior therapy for obesity. Some other candidates as special patient-treatment matches were

considered briefly; one of them was a special form of conditioning for enuresis provided in the context of complete environmental control (particularly the work of Dr. John Atthowe), and another was a special kind of conditioning for delinquency developed by Dr. Gerald Patterson.

9. Some rely upon independent clinical judges, and some—especially those using inpatients—utilize discharge and readmission rates.

10. One direct way to illustrate this is to divide the studies into two groups; those receiving a quality rating of *A* or *B* and those receiving a rating of *C* or *D*. In general, the subgroups show the same main trends.

It may also be of interest to note the overall research quality for each type of comparative study. Here the largest number of poor studies are to be found in the comparison of psychotherapy plus psychopharmacological agents with psychopharmacological agents alone. Also, for psychological treatment plus a medical regimen versus a medical regimen alone, 5 of the 9 studies have *D* or *D*- ratings.

11. Malan (1973) makes this the centerpiece in the conclusions to his review of outcome research problems, i.e., "the failure to design outcome criteria and do justice to the complexity of the human personality." Malan has in mind developing better measures that rely upon clinical judgment to estimate the quality of the outcome. Comparative studies of educational treatments (Messick, 1970) are also becoming more concerned with learning the *possible* outcomes, not just the *intended* outcomes, and with the interaction of the treatment conditions and individual differences in the students.

12. Mintz, J., and Luborsky, L. The distribution of therapists' and patients' ratings of improvement in psychotherapy (in preparation).

REFERENCES

References are numbered to facilitate their use in the tables.

1. Ashby, J. D., Ford, D. G., Guerney, B. G., Jr., & Guerney, L. F. Effects on clients of a reflective and a leading type of psychotherapy. *Psychological Monographs*, 1957, **71** (24, Whole No. 453).
2. Baehr, G. O. The comparative effectiveness of individual psychotherapy, group psychotherapy and a combination of these methods. *Journal of Consulting Psychology*, 1954, **18**, 179–183.
3. Baker, E. The differential effects of two psychotherapeutic approaches on client perceptions. *Journal of Counseling Psychology*, 1960, 7, 46–50.
4. Barron, F., & Leary, T. F. Changes in psychoneurotic patients with and without psychotherapy. *Journal of Consulting Psychology*, 1955, **19**, 239–245.
5. Boe, E., Gocka, E. F., & Kogan, W. S. The effect of group psychotherapy on interpersonal perceptions of psychiatric patients. *Multivariate Behavior Research*, 1966, **1**, 177–187.
6. Boulougouris, J. C., Marks, I. M., & Marset, P. Superiority of flooding (implosion) to desensitization for reducing pathological fear. *Behavior Research & Therapy*, 1971, **9**(1), 7–16.
7. Brill, N. Q., Koegler, R. R., Epstein, L. J., & Forgy, E. W. Controlled study of psychiatric outpatient treatment. *Archives of General Psychiatry*, 1964, **10**, 581–595.
8. Brown, D. G., & Bettley, F. R. Psychiatric treatment of eczema: a controlled trial. *British Medical Journal*, 1971, **2**, 729–734.
9. Cartwright, R. D. A comparison of the response to psychoanalytic and client centered psychotherapy. In L. Gottschalk & A. Auerbach (Eds.), *Methods of research in psychotherapy*. New York: Appleton-Century-Crofts, 1966, p. 654.
10. Chappell, M. N., & Stevenson, T. I. Group psychological training in some organic conditions. *Mental Hygiene*, 1936, **20**, 588–597.

11. Coons, W. H. Interaction and insight in group psychotherapy. *Canadian Journal of Psychology*, 1957, **11**, 1–8.
12. Cooper, J. E. A study of behaviour therapy in thirty psychiatric patients. *Lancet*, 1963, **1**, 411–415.
13. Cooper, J. E., Gelder, M. G., & Marks, I. M. Results of behaviour therapy in seventy-seven psychiatric patients. *British Medical Journal*, 1965, **1**, 1222–1225.
14. Covi, L., Lipman, R. S., Derogatis, L. R., et al. Drugs and group psychotherapy in neurotic depression. *American Journal of Psychiatry*, 1974, **131**, 191–198.
15. Cowden, R. C., Zax, M., & Sproles, J. A. Reserpine alone and as an adjunct to psychotherapy in the treatment of schizophrenia. *Archives of Neurological Psychiatry*, 1955, **74**, 518–522.
16. Crighton, J., & Jehu, D. Treatment of examination anxiety by systematic desensitization or psychotherapy in groups. *Behaviour Research & Therapy*, 1969, **7**, 245–248.
17. Daneman, E. A. Imipramine in office management of depressive reactions (a double blind clinical study). *Diseases of the Nervous System*, 1961, **22**, 213–217.
18. Dudek, S. Z. Effects of different types of therapy on the personality as a whole. *Journal of Nervous and Mental Disease*, 1970, **150**, 329–345.
19. Ellis, A. E. Outcome of employing three techniques of psychotherapy. *Journal of Clinical Psychology*, 1957, **13**, 344–350.
20. Endicott, N. A., & Endicott, J. Prediction of improvement in treated and untreated patients using the Rorschach Prognostic Rating Scale. *Journal of Consulting Psychology*, 1964, **28**, 342–348.
21. Evangelakis, M. G. De-institutionalization of patients (the triad of trifluoperazine-group-adjunctive therapy). *Diseases of the Nervous System*, 1961, **22**, 26–32.
22. Fiske, D. W., Hunt, H. F., Luborsky, L., Orne, M. T., Parloff, M. B., Reiser, M. F., & Tuma, A. H. The planning of research on effectiveness of psychotherapy. (Report on workshop sponsored and supported by the Clinical Projects Research Review Committee, National Institute of Mental Health.) *Archives of General Psychiatry*, 1970, **22**, 22–32; also *American Psychologist*, 1970, **25**, 727–737.
23. Frank, J. D. *Persuasion and healing: a comparative study of psychotherapy.* Baltimore: Johns Hopkins Press, 1965.
24. Frank, J. D., Gliedman, L. H., Imber, S. D., Stone, A. R., & Nash, E. G., Jr. Patients' expectancies and relearning as factors determining improvement in psychotherapy. *American Journal of Psychiatry*, 1959, **115**, 961–968.
25. Gelder, M. G., & Marks, I. M. Severe agoraphobia: a controlled prospective trial of behaviour therapy. *British Journal of Psychiatry*, 1966, **112**, 309–319.
26. Gelder, M. G., Marks, I. M., & Wolff, H. H. Desensitization and psychotherapy in the treatment of phobic states: a controlled inquiry. *British Journal of Psychiatry*, 1967, **113**, 53–73.
27. Gibbs, J. J., Wilkins, B., & Lauterbach, C. G. A controlled clinical psychiatric study of chlorpromazine. *Journal of Clinical & Experimental Psychopathology: Quarterly Review of Psychiatry & Neurology*, 1957, **18**, 269–283.
28. Glen, A. I. M. Psychotherapy and medical treatment for duodenal ulcer compared using the augmented histamine test. *Journal of Psychosomatic Research*, 1968, **12**, 163–169.
29. Gorham, D. R., Pokorny, A. D., Moseley, E. C., McReynolds, P., & Kogan, W. S. Effects of a phenothiazine and/or group psychotherapy with schizophrenics. *Diseases of the Nervous System*, 1964, **25**, 77–86.
30. Grace, W. J., Pinsky, R. H., & Wolff, H. G. The treatment of ulcerative colitis: II. *Gastroenterology*, 1954, **26**, 462–468.
31. Grinspoon, L., Ewalt, J. R., & Shader, R. Long term treatment of chronic schizophrenia: a preliminary report. *International Journal of Psychiatry*, 1967, **4**, 116–128.
32. Grinspoon, L., Ewalt, J. R., & Shader, R. Psychotherapy and pharmacotherapy in chronic schizophrenia. *American Journal of Psychiatry*, 1968, **124**, 1645–1652.
33. Groen, J., & Pelser, H. E. Experiences with, and results of group psychotherapy in patients with bronchial asthma. *Journal of Psychosomatic Research*, 1960, **4**, 191–205.

34. Haimowitz, N. R., & Haimowitz, M. L. Personality changes in client-centered therapy. In W. Wolff & J. A. Precher (Eds.), *Success in psychotherapy*. New York: Grune and Stratton, 1952, pp. 63–93.
35. Heine, R. W. A comparison of patients' reports on psychotherapeutic experience with psychoanalytic, nondirective and Adlerian therapists. *American Journal of Psychotherapy*, 1953, 7, 16–25.
36. Henry, W. E., & Shlien, J. M. Affective complexity and psychotherapy: some comparisons of time-limited and unlimited treatment. *Journal of Projective Techniques*, 1958, 22, 153–162.
37. Hesbacher, P. T., Rickels, K., Hutchison, J., Raab, E., Sablosky, L., Whalen, E. M., & Phillips, F. I. Setting, patient, and doctor effects on drug response in neurotic patients. II. Differential improvement. *Psychopharmacologia*, 1970, 18, 209–226.
38. Hogarty, G. E., & Goldberg, S. C. Drug and sociotherapy in the aftercare of schizophrenic patients. *Archives of General Psychiatry*, 1973, 28, 54–64.
39. Imber, S. D., Frank, J. D., Nash, E. H., Jr., Stone, A. R., & Gliedman, L. H. Improvement and amount of therapeutic contact: an alternative to the use of no-treatment controls in psychotherapy. *Journal of Consulting Psychology*, 1957, 21, 308–315.
40. Jensen, M. B. Consultation vs. therapy in the psychological treatment of NP hospital patients. *Journal of Clinical Psychology*, 1961, 17, 265–268.
41. Karon, B. P., & Vandenbos, G. R. Experience, medication, and the effectiveness of psychotherapy with schizophrenics. *British Journal of Psychiatry*, 1970, 116, 427–428.
42. King, G. F., Armitage, S. G., & Tilton, J. R. A therapeutic approach to schizophrenics of extreme pathology: an operant-interpersonal method. *Journal of Abnormal & Social Psychology*, 1960, 61, 276–286.
43. King, P. D. Regressive ECT, chlorpromazine and group therapy in treatment of hospitalized chronic schizophrenics. *American Journal of Psychiatry*, 1958, 115, 354–357.
44. King, P. D. Controlled study of group psychotherapy in schizophrenics receiving chlorpromazine. *Psychiatry Digest*, 1963, 24, 21–26.
45. Klerman, G. L., DiMascio, A., Weissman, M., Prusoff, B., & Paykel, E. S. Treatment of depression by drugs and psychotherapy. *American Journal of Psychiatry*, 1974, 131, 186–191.
46. Klerman, G. L. Paykel, E. S., & Prusoff, B. A. Antidepressant drugs and clinical psychopathology. In J. Cole, A. Freeman, & A. Friedhoff (Eds.), *Psychopathology and psychopharmacology*. Baltimore: Johns Hopkins Press, 1973, pp. 177–189.
47. Koegler, R. R., & Brill, N. Q. *Treatment of psychiatric outpatients*. New York: Appleton-Century-Crofts, 1967.
48. Lazarus, A. A. Group therapy of phobic disorders by systematic desensitization. *Journal of Abnormal & Social Psychology*, 1961, 63, 504–510.
49. Levis, D. J., & Carrera, R. Effects of ten hours of implosive therapy in the treatment of outpatients: a preliminary report. *Journal of Abnormal Psychology*, 1967, 72, 504–508.
50. Lorr, M., McNair, D. M., Weinstein, G. J., Michaux, W. W., & Raskin, A. Meprobamate and chlorpromazine in psychotherapy: some effects on anxiety and hostility of outpatients. *Archives of General Psychiatry*, 1961, 4, 381–389.
51. Lorr, M., McNair, D. M., & Weinstein, G. J. Early effects of chlordiazepoxide (Librium) used with psychotherapy. *Journal of Psychiatric Research*, 1963, 1, 257–270.
52. Luborsky, L. A note on Eysenck's article: the effects of psychotherapy: an evaluation. *British Journal of Psychology*, 1954, 45, 129–131.
53. Luborsky, L. Research cannot yet influence clinical practice. (An evaluation of Strupp and Bergin's "Some empirical and conceptual bases for coordinated research in psychotherapy: critical review of issues, trends, and evidence.") *International Journal of Psychiatry*, 1969, 7, 135–140. Also in A. Bergin & H. Strupp (Eds.), *Changing frontiers in the science of psychotherapy*. Chicago: Aldine-Atherton, 1972, pp. 120–127.
54. Luborsky, L. Another reply to Eysenck. *Psychological Bulletin*, 1972, 78, 406–408.

55. Luborsky, L., Chandler, M., Auerbach, A. H., Cohen, J., & Bachrach, H. M. Factors influencing the outcome of psychotherapy: a review of quantitative research. *Psychological Bulletin*, 1971, **75**, 145–185.
56. MacDonald, W. S., Blochberger, C. W., & Maynard, H. M. Group therapy: a comparison of patient-led and staff-led groups in an open hospital ward. *Psychiatric Quarterly Supplement*, 1964, **38**, 290–303.
57. Maher-Loughnan, G. P., MacDonald, N., Mason, A. A., & Fry, L. Controlled trial of hypnosis in the symptomatic treatment of asthma. *British Medical Journal*, 1962, **2**, 371–376.
58. Malan, D. The outcome problem in psychotherapy research. *Archives of General Psychiatry*, 1973, **29**, 719–729.
59. Marks, I. M., & Gelder, H. G. A controlled retrospective study of behaviour therapy in phobic patients. *British Journal of Psychiatry*, 1965, **111**, 561–573.
60. Marks, I. M., Gelder, M. G., & Edwards, G. Hypnosis and desensitization for phobias: A controlled prospective trial. *British Journal of Psychiatry*, 1968, **114**, 1263–1274.
61. May, P. R. A. *Treatment of schizophrenia*. New York: Science House, 1968.
62. May, P. R. A. & Tuma, A. H. The effect of psychotherapy and stelazine on length of hospital stay, release rate and supplemental treatment of schizophrenic patients. *Journal of Nervous and Mental Disease*, 1964, **139**, 362–369.
63. May, P. R. A., & Tuma, A. H. Treatment of schizophrenia. *British Journal of Psychiatry*, 1965, **3**, 503–510.
64. McReynolds, W. T. Systematic desensitization, insight-oriented psychotherapy and relaxation therapy in a psychiatric population. Unpublished Ph.D. dissertation, University of Texas at Austin, 1969.
65. Meltzoff, J., & Kornreich, M. *Research in psychotherapy*. New York: Atherton Press, 1970.
66. Messick, S. The criterion problem in the evaluation of instruction: assessing possible, not just intended, outcomes. In M. C. Wittrock & D. Wiley (Eds.), *The evaluation of instruction: issues and problems*. New York: Holt, Rinehart and Winston, 1970.
67. Morton, R. B. An experiment in brief psychotherapy. *Psychological Monographs*, 1955, **69** (Whole No. 386).
68. Muench, G. A. An investigation of the efficacy of time-limited psychotherapy. *Journal of Counseling Psychology*, 1965, **12**, 294–298.
69. O'Brien, C., Hamm, K., Ray, B., Pierce, J., Luborsky, L., & Mintz, J. Group versus individual psychotherapy with schizophrenics: a controlled outcome study. *Archives of General Psychiatry*, 1972, **27**, 474–478.
70. O'Conner, J. F., Daniels, G., Flood, C., Karush, A., Moses, L., & Stern, L. O. An evaluation of the effectiveness of psychotherapy in the treatment of ulcerative colitis. *Annals of Internal Medicine*, 1964, **60**, 587–602.
71. Overall, J. E., & Tupin, J. P. Investigation of clinical outcome in a doctor's choice treatment setting. *Diseases of the Nervous System*, 1969, **30**, 305–313.
72. Pascal, G. R., & Zax, M. Psychotherapeutics: success or failure? *Journal of Consulting Psychology*, 1956, **20**, 325–331.
73. Patterson, V., Levene, H., & Breger, L. Treatment and training outcomes with two time-limited therapies. *Archives of General Psychiatry*, 1971, **25**, 161–167.
74. Pearl, D. Psychotherapy and ethnocentrism. *Journal of Abnormal and Social Psychology*, 1955, **50**, 227–229.
75. Peck, R. E., Comparison of adjunct group therapy with individual psychotherapy. *Archives of Neurology and Psychiatry*, 1949, **62**, 173–177.
76. Penick, S. B., Filion, R., Fox, S., & Stunkard, A. J. Behavior modification in the treatment of obesity. *Psychosomatic Medicine*, 1971, **39**, 49–55.
77. Peyman, D. A. R. An investigation of the effects of group psychotherapy on chronic schizophrenic patients. *Group Psychotherapy*, 1956, **9**, 35–39.
78. Podobnikar, I. G. Implementation of psychotherapy by Librium in a pioneering rural-industrial psychiatric practice. *Psychosomatics*, 1971, **12**, 205–209.

79. Reid, W. J., & Schyne, A. W. *Brief and extended casework.* New York: Columbia University Press, 1969.
80. Rickels, K., Cattell, R. B., Weise, C., Gray, B., Yee, R., Mallin, A., & Aaronson, H. G. Controlled psychopharmacological research in private psychiatric practice. *Psychopharmacologia,* 1966, **9,** 288–306.
81. Rogers, C. R., & Dymond, R. F. (Eds.), *Psychotherapy and personality change.* Chicago: University of Chicago Press, 1954.
82. Rogers, C. R., Gendlin, E., Kiesler, D., & Truax, C. (Eds.), *The therapeutic relationship and its impact: a study of psychotherapy with schizophrenics.* Madison: University of Wisconsin Press, 1967.
83. Rosenthal, R., & Rosnow, R. (Eds.), *Artifact in behavioral research.* New York: Academic Press, 1969.
84. Rosenzweig, S. Some implicit common factors in diverse methods of psychotherapy. *American Journal of Ortho-psychiatry,* 1936, **6,** 412–415.
85. Shader, R. I., Grinspoon, L., Ewalt, J. R., & Zahn, D. A. Drug responses in acute schizophrenia. In D. V. S. Sankar, (Eds.), *Schizophrenia: current concepts and research.* Hicksville, N.Y.: PJD Publications, 1969, pp. 161–173.
86. Shattan, S. P., Dcamp, L., Fujii, E., Fross, G. G., & Wolff, R. J. Group treatment of conditionally discharged patients in a mental health clinic. *American Journal of Psychiatry,* 1966, **122,** 798–805.
87. Sheldon, A. An evaluation of psychiatric after-care. *British Journal of Psychiatry,* 1964, **110,** 662–667.
88. Shlien, J. M. Time-limited psychotherapy: an experimental investigation of practical values and theoretical implications. *Journal of Counseling Psychology,* 1957, **4,** 318–322.
89. Shlien, J. M., Mosak, H. H., & Dreikurs, R. Effects of time limits: a comparison of two psychotherapies. *Journal of Counseling Psychology,* 1962, **9,** 31–34.
90. Sinclair-Gieben, A. G. C., & Chalmers, D. Evaluation of treatment of warts by hypnosis. *Lancet,* 1959, **2,** 480–482.
91. Slawson, P. F. Psychodrama as a treatment for hospitalized patients: a controlled study. *American Journal of Psychiatry,* 1965, **122,** 530–533.
92. Stotsky, B. A., Daston, P. G., & Vardack, C. N. An evaluation of the counseling of chronic schizophrenics. *Journal of Counseling Psychology,* 1955, **2,** 248–255.
93. Strupp, Hans H. Toward a reformulation of the psychotherapeutic influence. *International Journal of Psychiatry,* 1974, in press.
94. Stunkard, A. New therapies for the eating disorders: behavior modification of obesity and anorexia nervosa. *Archives of General Psychiatry,* 1972, **26,** 391–398.
95. Thorley, A. S., & Craske, N. Comparisons and estimate of group and individual methods of treatment. *British Medical Journal,* 1950, **1,** 100.
96. Titchener, J. L., Sheldon, M. B., & Rose, W. D. Changes in blood pressure of hypertensive patients with and without group therapy. *Journal of Psychosomatic Research,* 1959, **4,** 10–12.
97. Tucker, J. E. Group psychotherapy with chronic psychotic soiling patients. *Journal of Consulting Psychology,* 1956, **20,** 430.
98. Uhlenhuth, E. H., Lipman, R., & Covi, L. Combined pharmacotherapy and psychotherapy: controlled studies. *Journal of Nervous and Mental Disease,* 1969, **148,** 52–64.
99. Volsky, T., Jr., Magoon, T. M., Norman, W. T., & Hoyt, D. P. *The outcomes of counseling and psychotherapy. Theory and research.* Minneapolis: University of Minnesota Press, 1965.
100. Walker, R. G., & Kelley, F. E. Short term psychotherapy with hospitalized schizophrenic patients. *Acta Psychiatrica et Neurologica Scandinavica,* 1960, **35,** 34–55.
101. Zhukov, I. A. Hypnotherapy of dermatoses in resort treatment. In R. B. Winn (Ed.), *Psychotherapy in the Soviet Union.* New York: Philosophical Library, 1961, pp. 178–181.

2 SOME METHODOLOGICAL AND STRATEGIC ISSUES IN PSYCHOTHERAPY RESEARCH: Research Implications of the Menninger Foundation's Psychotherapy Research Project

OTTO F. KERNBERG

The sample of the Psychotherapy Research Project consisted of 42 adult hospital patients and outpatients treated at the Menninger Foundation. Diagnosed as suffering from neurotic conditions, borderline conditions, latent psychosis, or characterological disturbances, the 42 patients underwent treatment designed within the framework of psychoanalytic theory ranging from supportive psychotherapy to psychoanalysis.

Three areas were chosen as primary foci: (1) the patient, (2) the treatment and therapist, and (3) the environment. These areas were studied at three different points in time: (1) at the beginning of the treatment (Initial), (2) at the end of the treatment (Termination), and (3) two years after the end of the treatment (Followup).

The material obtained was organized in each of the three areas (patient, treatment, environment) at the three points in time (Initial, Termination, Followup) according to the basic assumptions of psychoanalytic theory and to factors believed most relevant, practically and theoretically, to treatment conducted at the Menninger Foundation. These assumptions and factors were conceptualized according to variables designated as Patient, Treatment, and Situational (Environmental).

Otto F. Kernberg, M. D., Director, General Clinical Service, New York State Psychiatric Institute; Professor of Clinical Psychiatry, College of Physicians and Surgeons, Columbia University.

Sections 1 and 2 of this paper outline the design and findings detailed in Psychotherapy and psychoanalysis: final report of the Menninger Foundation's Psychotherapy Research Project, by Otto F. Kernberg, M.D., Esther D. Burstein, Ph.D., Lolafaye Coyne, Ph.D., Ann Appelbaum, M.D., Leonard Horwitz, Ph.D., and Harold Voth, M.D., published in *Bulletin of the Menninger Clinic*, 1972, 36(1/2).

While ways of organizing the material were being devised, a method which would allow statistical analysis while preserving the clinical nature of those variables was sought. The method found to fit such requirements was a modification of the Fechnerian Method of Paired Comparison (Sargent, 1956a and b, 1967; Wallerstein, Luborsky, Robbins & Sargent, 1956). The application of this method constituted the basis of the Quantitative Study. Some additional measures were developed, primarily the Health-Sickness Rating Scale—an absolute anchored rating scale assessing overall health-sickness (Luborsky, Fabian, Hall, Ticho, & Ticho, 1958).

For the method of Paired Comparisons, the data for variables were compiled and summarized in special forms designated as Form B for Patient Variables, Form T for Treatment Variables, and Form S for Situational Variables. Thus, as a final organization of the material for each of the 42 patients, there was a Form B and a Form S for each of the three points in time (Initial, Termination, and Followup); and a Form T for Termination and Followup. These forms were filled out by teams of senior clinicians who had participated in the collection of the data.

The Paired Comparisons were made by teams of two clinicians. Their task was to compare, for each variable in Form B (Patient), T (Treatment), and S (Situational) and at the three points in time (Initial, Termination, and Followup), each patient with every other patient in a group of 12 patients. Independently, the clinicians read the writeup for the variable under consideration for every pair of patients they compared. Then, also independently, they stated which of the two patients had "more" of the variable, using a special sheet to mark their choice.

Difficulties arose from several sources. The method is time-consuming and the work repetitious: an average of 1.5 hours was consumed in reading the writeups and making the judgments about *one* variable for *one* group of patients; the 66 judgments made on each group necessitated reading 66 pairs of paragraphs; to complete the whole task, over 30,000 comparisons had to be made. Much time was also required to collect the data: we waited for several years until the treatments were completed and then two more years to obtain the followup information. Despite the differences in background, experience, and investment in the project, with very few exceptions the judges were consistent in their judgments and the teams achieved adequate reliability between judges.

In addition to the quantitative studies, based largely upon the method of Paired Comparisons, we also applied facet theory and the technique of Multidimensional Scalogram Analysis to a comprehensive study of all the quantitative data of the Psychotherapy Research Project. The general method of research was developed by Professor Louis Guttman, Scientific Director of the Israel Institute of Applied Social Research in Jerusalem. The application of Guttman's method to our data seemed of particular interest because we had a large number of variables for a relatively small sample of patients, making statistical methods such as correlation and multiple correlation of limited use for our data. In addition, all of these variables were implicitly linked in a common definitional system which seemed to warrant the application of facet theory.

Under the title of facet analysis are subsumed two distinct methods: facet theory and nonmetric analysis. Each method is distinct and can be used independently.

Facet theory, in its most general sense, can be thought of as a conceptual analysis of the content of the research; i.e., a system by which complex concepts or variables are broken down into simple sets of elements called facets (Foa, 1965; Guttman, 1954–1955, 1959a and b, and 1965a and b). Facet theory itself can be subdivided into two parts: facet design and test of the facet design.

Facet design seeks to define the universe of content of whatever is being studied. It is, in a sense, similar to Fisher's factorial design of experiments. Facet design starts with a Mapping Sentence which incorporates a definition of what is to be studied according to a number of sets, or facets, consisting of two or more basic elements. Following the construction of the Mapping Sentence, the variables to be used are defined in terms of the facets of the Mapping Sentence.

A second aspect of facet theory is the nonstatistical *test of the facet design* by means of a geometric representation. Whether one uses a factor analysis or one of the nonmetric analyses, one is dealing with relationships or similarities by means of a geometric representation. The test of the facet design is achieved by looking at the empirical results obtained by nonmetric or other analyses to see whether the patterns or configurations predicted by the facet design do exist. If they do exist, the facet design is considered to be confirmed, although not in a statistical sense.

Nonmetric analysis (Kruskal, 1964a and b; Shepard, 1962) is the second method represented by facet analysis. There are two kinds of Guttman-Lingoes nonmetric analyses: Smallest Space Analysis and Multidimensional Scalogram Analysis (MSA) (Lingoes, 1966a, b, and c, 1968). MSA starts with a set of profiles of subjects' scores on a number of variables. The scores do not represent continuous data but rather discrete categories. A variable can be measured crudely as "presence" or "absence" and still be included in a MSA, or it can have up to 20 categories. Since some of our data, quite important to a study of change, were in the form of "presence-absence" or other kinds of category data, MSA was the nonmetric analysis we chose.

Since these nonmetric analyses are geometric in their approach, the set of subject's profiles must be represented geometrically. In MSA, each subject's profile of scores is plotted as a point in a space with the same number of dimensions as there are variables. The object of the MSA is to take the points standing for subjects and to represent all the relationships among them in a considerably smaller space, that is, a space with considerably fewer dimensions.

To interpret a space diagram, one considers how each of the separate variables contributes to it. If all the subjects belonging to each category of the variable under consideration are represented by points which all fall together in the same region, the variable is said to "partition" the space. This means that the variable divides the space diagram into a number of nonoverlapping regions, one for each category of the variable. Thus, it is demonstrated graphically that this variable contributed to the arrangement of the points on the space diagram.

There are many advantages of the nonmetric method of Multidimensional Scalogram Analysis for our kind of research. It permits including in the same analysis variables that represent purely categorical data (with no a priori assumptions at all about order among the categories) and variables that represent continuous data. A related advantage is that no assumptions whatsoever are required about the nature of the underlying distributions of the variable. All that is required for MSA is for the categories of each variable to be mutually exclusive and exhaustive; that is, every subject must be tallied in one and only one category for each variable.

Perhaps most important of all, the results of an MSA (in terms of clusters on a diagram representing groups of subjects or, more generally, typologies) are more than just a tallying of the number of cases in the cells of a multidimensional contingency table. The emergence of such clusters of points as a result of an MSA is strengthened because (1) this particular two-dimensional space or projection into a two-dimensional space came from a large number of variables, not just those involved in the statement of a particular hypothesis; (2) the variables chosen for the analysis were not chosen arbitrarily but were grouped and linked by common facet elements; (3) replications of this space with different numbers of variables and different choices of variables are possible; and (4) such relationships were hypothesized in advance based on a statement of the theory in terms of facets.

The major disadvantage of the Guttman-Lingoes nonmetric analyses, in general, and of MSA, in particular, is shared with factor analysis. These approaches are mathematical rather than statistical, which means that significance tests are not made and conclusions cannot be stated in probability terms.

SUMMARY OF THE INTEGRATED FINDINGS OF THE STATISTICAL ANALYSIS AND THE MULTIDIMENSIONAL SCALOGRAM ANALYSIS (MSA)

Major Findings from Both Studies Reinforcing or Complementing Each Other. The statistical analysis revealed that a high level of initial *Ego Strength* of the patient indicates a good prognosis for the entire spectrum of treatments conducted within the framework of psychoanalytic theory, that is, psychoanalysis, expressive psychotherapy, expressive-supportive psychotherapy, and supportive psychotherapy. As a result of the factor analysis of our Patient Variables, *Ego Strength* was defined as a combination of three intimately linked characteristics: (1) the degree of integration, stability, and flexibility of the intrapsychic structures (including variables such as *Patterning of Defenses* and *Anxiety Tolerance*, and, implicitly, the concepts of impulse control, thought organization, and sublimatory channeling capacity); (2) the degree to which relationships with others are adaptive, deep, and gratifying of normal instinctual needs (corresponding to the variable *Quality of Interpersonal Relationships*); (3) the degree to which the malfunctioning of the intrapsychic structures is manifested directly by symptoms (corresponding to the variable *Severity of Symptoms*).

The MSA similarly led us to conclude that there exists an overriding relationship between overall outcome (change) and *Ego Strength*, especially regarding those aspects of *Ego Strength* related to the *Quality of Interpersonal Relationships*: patients with high initial *Ego Strength* showed most improvement, and patients with low initial *Ego Strength* (particularly low initial *Quality of Interpersonal Relationships*) showed least improvement. The MSA differentiated one modality of treatment from another and concluded that while supportive treatment of patients with high initial *Ego Strength* was related to a good outcome, the greatest improvement was evidenced by patients with high initial *Ego Strength* who had undergone psychoanalysis. The MSA also concluded that patients with high *Ego Strength* improved less with supportive psychotherapy than with psychoanalysis, supportive-expressive psychotherapy, or expressive psychotherapy.

Our general conclusion was that while high initial *Ego Strength* implies a good prognosis for all modalities of treatment within a psychoanalytic frame of reference, psychoanalysis may bring about the highest degree of improvement in such patients. This overall finding, supported by both quantitative studies, raises the question of whether psychoanalysis may be considered the ideal treatment for patients who need it least, that is, for those with high initial *Ego Strength*. High *Ego Strength* is not to be confused, however, with freedom from *Severe Symptoms*. High initial

Ego Strength in these studies refers to one extreme of a continuum within our patient population and not to an ideal, or optimum, of normal psychological functioning.

The combined statistical analysis of the relationship between outcome, on the one hand, and focus on the transference, *Therapist's Skill*, and initial *Ego Strength*, on the other, revealed that patients with low initial *Ego Strength* treated by therapists with high skill improved to a significantly greater extent when the focus on the transference (as assessed by the variable *Transference Resolution*, considered as a process variable rather than an outcome variable) was high. Therefore, we concluded that the lower the initial *Ego Strength* of the patient, the more important is the work with the transference in determining the outcome of the treatment. The Multidimensional Scalogram Analysis revealed that patients with low *Ego Strength* who had been given supportive treatment, as well as patients with low *Ego Strength* who had been treated by psychoanalysis, belonged to the group of patients with the least degree of improvement. In contrast, patients with low *Ego Strength* tended to improve when treated with an expressive-supportive approach, and a group of patients with low initial *Ego Strength* who underwent supportive-expressive psychotherapy belonged to the region of high or highest degree of improvement.

The MSA showed that patients with low *Ego Strength* who received supportive-expressive psychotherapy with concomitant hospitalization belonged to the group showing a high increase in *Ego Strength* as measured at the followup point. In contrast, *Ego Strength* was not highly increased at followup among patients with low initial *Ego Strength* who were treated with supportive psychotherapy in which the therapist actively structured the patient's daily life. These findings support the conclusion that the best treatment for such patients may be the combination of an expressive approach (with little structure during the treatment hours) and as much concomitant hospitalization as the patient needs. This approach is in contrast to a purely supportive treatment, in which a good deal of structure is provided during the treatment hours and there is no hospital support.

In more general terms, both quantitative studies concluded that patients with ego weakness (which in our studies was mainly found in patients suffering from borderline conditions) require a special modality of treatment which could be described as a modified expressive or supportive-expressive approach. This approach focuses especially on work with the transference phenomena in the treatment hours.

Other clinical studies derived from the Psychotherapy Research Project suggest that patients with low *Ego Strength* (especially those with borderline personality organization) do indeed require a special modality of treatment, a modality best described as an expressive approach which is neither standard psychoanalysis nor supportive psychotherapy (Kernberg, 1968).

The particular form of expressive, psychoanalytically oriented psychotherapy suggested for patients with borderline personality organization on the basis of these findings is characterized by a consistent focus upon the transference (particularly the negative transference insofar as it blocks the psychotherapeutic relationship), and by consistent interpretation in the "here and now" of the pathological defenses of these patients. Parameters of technique or modification of technique and/or concomitant hospitalization would be used when necessary to control transference acting out; it would not necessarily be possible or desirable for all of these parameters or modifications to be resolved during the course of treatment.

We concluded on the basis of the MSA that patients with low initial *Quality of Interpersonal Relationships*, low initial *Anxiety Tolerance*, and low initial *Motivation* did poorly in psychoanalysis and in supportive psychotherapy. In the light of the statistical analyses, all these patient variables are intimately related to *Ego Strength*. It may well be that the *Quality of Interpersonal Relationships* is of particular importance in determining the prognosis for psychotherapeutic treatment, especially in the case of patients with low *Ego Strength* and low *Quality of Interpersonal Relations* who belonged to the group which showed least improvement with psychotherapy or psychoanalysis.

Low initial *Quality of Interpersonal Relationships* is a poor prognostic sign for all types of psychological treatment. The poor quality of object relationships needs to be compensated for by the special focus on the transference as part of the optimal treatment modality recommended for borderline conditions.

In using the MSA technique, one major question for which no positive answers emerged was that of whether environmental factors (other than hospitalization or its absence) influenced the treatment outcome in patients with low *Ego Strength*. In fact, throughout all the MSA runs we found no relationship between outcome and the environmental variables. The statistical analysis also revealed that the initial characteristics of the environment (as conceptualized and assessed within the context of our project) have no significant value as predictors of the outcome of treatments conducted within the framework of psychoanalytic theory, a negative and important finding.

Major Findings Derived from One of the Two Quantitative Studies Only. The statistical analyses revealed that a high level of manifest anxiety (independent of high or low *Ego Strength*) is a good prognostic sign for treatments conducted within the framework of psychoanalytic theory. The statistical analysis also suggested that the decrease in the level of manifest anxiety has a relatively weak relationship to improvement in other areas of the patient's functioning. We interpreted this combination of findings as suggesting that the painful experience of anxiety is an important aspect of motivation for treatment during its initial stages.

Another finding derived from the statistical analysis was that a highly skilled therapist contributes significantly to the improvement of patients regardless of whether the treatment is expressive or supportive. A less skilled therapist contributes more effectively to the improvement of patients if the modality of treatment is expressive. The implication is that expressive modalities include built-in safeguards for an optimal psycho-therapeutic procedure: they imply a rather standardized technique stem-ming from psychoanalytic theory and a relatively "neutral" stand on the therapist's part, combined with an ongoing focus on the transference. In contrast, a purely supportive approach requires additional special skills on the therapist's part because, in this modality, the psychotherapist has less control over the influence his personality and countertransference have on the treatment process, and he operates within a less clearly de-fined technical framework.

Another finding in the statistical analysis was that the skill of the therapist is of particular significance for the improvement of very sick patients, but it is not greatly related to the improvement of the "stronger" patients.

SOME MAJOR IMPLICATIONS FOR FUTURE RESEARCH

In general, the statistical analysis contributed toward clearer conceptuali-zations of our variables, while the Multidimensional Scalogram Analysis contributed to the flexibility of our investigation by permitting the study of smaller subsamples with more variables. The great advantage of the statistical analysis was that we could obtain statistically significant findings confirming or disconfirming our hypotheses. The main disadvantage of this method was the small sample size of 42 cases and the fact that a number of hypotheses were applicable to only a part of the sample, thus reducing the chances of obtaining significant results.

In more general terms, the MSA technique permitted us to single out the more relevant variables determining the overall clusters on a diagram which represented groups or subjects or, more generally, typologies. It allowed an evaluation of the overriding variables while considering the simultaneous influence of a larger number of variables (up to 50 with the computer program used here). The major disadvantage of this method (and of the Guttman-Lingoes nonmetric analyses in general) is shared with factor analysis; namely, these approaches do not allow a testing of statistical significance, and conclusions cannot be stated in probability terms. The findings derived from the MSA indicated what group of variables had overriding relationships throughout our patient population and permitted an overall approach to the study of outcomes, which could then be compared with the more specific hypothesis testing completed in the statistical analysis.

The method of Paired Comparisons permitted the study of a large number of variables from a point of view close to the ordinary clinical level. We found that the feasibility of quantifying clinical variables was closely linked with the clinical relevance of the variable. Quantification in itself was not the problem: the problem lay in the conceptualization of what was to be quantified. Usually, what is clinically most relevant is most amenable to clear conceptualization, the most significant requirement for successful quantification. The method of Paired Comparisons was, in short, helpful in translating naturalistic clinical data into variables which could be studied statistically. Its major disadvantage is the enormously time-consuming nature of the work.

The emergence of fewer, more precise, and clinically more relevant variables regarding the patient, the treatment, and the outcome was an important product of the factor analysis, and should be the first step in establishing scales permitting a less time-consuming quantitative assessment of these variables in future psychotherapy research. In this regard, the Health-Sickness Rating Scale, an anchored rating scale of proved reliability and validity (Luborsky, 1962), may indicate the general interest that clinically anchored rating scales may have for future research in this area.

The major findings of outcome in relation to *Ego Strength*, the therapist's skill, and the modality of treatment as summarized here should permit establishing selected groups of patients, an important step forward in comparing the effectiveness of various psychotherapeutic approaches. In the past, the lack of differentiation of type of patients, quality of therapists, and modality of treatment within the range of the psychoanalytic framework has hindered research.

The clinical implications of the findings of the Psychotherapy Research Project have been or are being incorporated into the clinical practice of the Menninger Clinic. I believe that our findings in regard to the diagnosis, prognosis, and treatment of patients with low *Ego Strength* (the borderline conditions) may have a particularly broad impact within the psychiatric field.

Quantification of Major Clinical Variables. One rather unexpected finding of the Menninger Foundation's Psychotherapy Research Project was that a relatively simple, quantitative measure of outcome, namely, the

Health-Sickness Rating Scale, was as accurate as the major qualitative writeups of change (involving multiple, individualized criteria) that were evaluated in terms of paired comparisons of change. In contrast to our earlier theoretical thinking that psychotherapy outcome implied change along various dimensions which could not be integrated into one global measure of improvement, our findings convinced us that an integrated and quantified measure of improvement was possible, and indeed, simple.

Another major finding of the project was the possibility of quantifying relatively complex clinical variables such as "ego strength," "interpretative techniques," etc., if and when such variables meet certain criteria. These criteria reflect our experience in applying paired comparisons to all the quantifiable variables of the Psychotherapy Research Project, and they were elaborated in a working document of the Menninger Foundation's Research Team on Personality and Change Assessment (Burstein, 1971). These criteria are listed below.

1. *Essentiality.* It is indispensable, for a research project which attempts to tease out the main factors related to treatment outcome in terms of a certain theory of treatment, that only essential variables be selected. This may seen trivial; however, when sophisticated clinicians participate in psychotherapy research they are tempted to include an ever-growing number of variables which have clinical relevance. "Essentiality" means that (within the theory underlying the research endeavor) the variable selected has a central function in accounting for the relationship between the patient, the treatment, and the outcome.

2. *Conceptual Clarity.* The variable must be clearly defined in terms of its basic characteristics, its differentiation from other basic concepts at the same theoretical level, and its hypothesized relationship to the overall theory which attempts to explain change in patients undergoing treatment. The advantages of a clear conceptualization of the variable are that it decreases the amount of overlap between concepts and variables, that it helps in the quantitative differentiation of the variable from patient to patient, and that it protects the concept from distortion when its phenomenological or behavioral characteristics are specified in order to do actual quantification. We found that all crucial variables involved in our research were stretched, so to say, between a theoretical pull, on one side, which could be so distant from phenomenological and behavioral manifestations that measurement became impossible, and, on the other side, a pragmatic, empirical, or observational pull in which the need for precise behavior manifestations threatened at times to make a variable trivial or to sever its connection with the basic concepts from which it derived.

3. *Observability.* The counterpart to conceptual clarity, observability refers to the need to define clinical manifestations which can be observed by staff and which permit quantification in comparing individual patients on

this criterion. The relationship between the conceptual formulation and the behavioral characteristics of the variables should be clear, and there should not be too much of a span between the concept and the actual behavior. An excessive distance between concept and behavior usually indicates either that the concept is unclear or that the behavioral characteristics have been accommodated to the observational skills of unsophisticated raters of a project. Variables whose operational definition captures only a minor part of the concept involved may become trivial. In other words, there should not be too many inferential steps from what can be observed to the concept, nor an excessive disproportion between the limited nature of the observable behavior and the broad nature of the concept.

4. *Presence throughout the Entire Sample.* The variable to be quantified must be evaluated in all the members of the sample and must be differentiated quantitatively from member to member.

5. *Clinical Relevance.* However clear and precise the concept and its observational implications may be in the mind of the researchers, a different set of assumptions and clinical considerations on the part of the clinicians actually carrying out the treatment will interfere with the gathering of data and the interpretations of observations. The implication is that there exists a dynamic interaction between treatment and research on treatment. The more closely the operation of the research project is integrated within the treatment situation, the greater the opportunity for rich, detailed, accurate observations of what goes on. However, the closer such integration, the greater the danger that conceptual clashes between what seems clinically relevant and what seems relevant for theory and research will distort the communication processes between researchers and clinicians. It may also decrease and even invalidate the gathering and interpretation of the material. A further implication is that in order to do significant research on psychotherapy one must make the research philosophy, design, and procedures acceptable to those actually carrying out clinical operations.

In broader terms, the integration of research with clinical operations should go a long way toward fostering the interaction of researchers and clinicians in the long run. Much criticism and concern has been expressed regarding the lack of relevance and clinical impact of much psychotherapy research in the last 20 years (Malan, 1973). Researchers have felt that clinicians have been reluctant to accept study findings because these threaten the clinicians' basic identity; clinicians have felt that a good part of psychotherapy research is irrelevant to their actual clinical problems and is even naive or uninformed. It has been a source of great satisfaction to the members of the Psychotherapy Research Project that the findings of the project made a significant impact on clinical operations throughout the Menninger Foundation, and perhaps also within the larger community of psychoanalytically oriented psychotherapists. An important reason for this impact was the intimate relationship between the research team and clinical operations, and of particular importance was the direction of research operations by senior clinicians who were recognized and respected as such by their clinical peers.

The Emergence of Clinically Anchored Rating Scales as a Major Research Instrument. A major conclusion stemming from the Psychotherapy Research Project is that "quantification in itself is not a problem and that the problem is really in the area of selecting what is going to be quantified" (Burstein, 1971). One problem in the development of quantitative measures has been that objective rating scales and questionnaires are often focused on limited aspects of phenomenological or behavioral characteristics of the variables under scrutiny, that they require a lengthy time for their application, and that they are difficult to construct in a way which does justice to higher conceptual levels of a variable. The method of Paired Comparisons was an ideal instrument for evaluating complex variables related to levels of conceptualization quite distant from actual observations, and permitted a degree of freedom in selecting the theoretically most crucial variables which would have been seriously constricted by ordinary rating scales. However, the shortcomings of the method of Paired Comparisons, particularly the enormous amount of time consumed, convinced us that although Paired Comparisons is an excellent first approach to teasing out the overall range of a quantifiable variable, it should be replaced eventually by more simple and less time-consuming instruments.

The clinically anchored Health-Sickness Rating Scale (Luborsky, 1962) provided us with an ideal transfer from the method of Paired Comparisons to a simple, more manageable rating scale. Although the construction of clinically anchored rating scales is time-consuming, the actual application time of this instrument is brief, and it is possible for an expert to carry out the rating of an individual patient in a few minutes, sometimes in less than a minute. Theoretically, if a set of less than 50 variables could be selected as reflecting the crucial body of hypotheses involved in a psychotherapy research project, each patient could be evaluated in less than two hours. It was impressive that senior clinicians with very little or no experience in clinical research who were asked to pinpoint a patient's overall level of health-sickness along a 100-point rating scale anchored with clinical examples were able to do so with very little instruction at a high level of reliability (and without the clinician's often-heard protest that the information required did not do justice to the actual reality of the patient).

One major apparent disadvantage of the use of clinically anchored rating scales is that the clinical evidence for the ratings will be lost because the entire clinical material available has become the basis for the inferential nature of the decision-making process involved. In other words, the more sophisticated the clinically anchored rating scale, the more the inferential judgment of experienced observers becomes the main underlying evidence. In my opinion, far from being a disadvantage, this has several additional advantages. There is less danger of distortions of the ratings in terms of social pressures operating on the researchers: for example, the ratings of the therapist's skill and the overall judgment of treatment effectiveness or failure can be made with more freedom. Certain confidential material that at times enters powerfully into patient assessment and treatment development may be included freely in the rater's judgment. In addition, I think that to employ highly experienced raters for evaluating highly sophisticated material is a more direct and efficient research method in the field of psychotherapy than is the construction of simplified, behaviorally oriented rating scales geared to be understood and rated by relatively unsophisticated observers or research assistants.

It might be argued that the construction of clinically anchored rating scales fulfilling all the criteria for quantification mentioned above may be possible in areas previously explored by other quantitative methods but is not feasible as a first approach to new fields of inquiry. For example, the patient variables and treatment variables of the psychotherapy research project may lend themselves easily to a new generation of outcome research based entirely upon clinically anchored rating scales, but this may be much more difficult to achieve in unexplored areas, such as the measurement of the influence of the hospital milieu or of the family situation on the treatment.

Patient and Treatment Variables Related to Outcome. Some patient and treatment variables emerged as major factors related to the treatment outcome of the Psychotherapy Research Project. Among the patient variables these were, *Ego Strength*, *Quality of Interpersonal Relationships*, *Anxiety Tolerance*, *Motivation*, and initial level of *Anxiety*; the treatment variables included the various modalities of psychoanalytically oriented treatments (ranging from psychoanalysis through expressive and expressive-supportive to supportive psychotherapy), expressive techniques and supportive techniques, skill of the therapist, and focus on the transference. Clinical studies from the project, particularly my work with patients presenting borderline personality organization (Kernberg, 1967, 1968, and 1972), focused on some of these same variables as major determinants of treatment outcome.

For future research on long-term psychoanalytic psychotherapy, a design focusing upon the combined impact of patient and treatment variables should include measures of *Ego Strength*, particularly in three areas: the severity of symptoms, including the initial level of anxiety; the quality of object-relations, including here a special dimension of antisocial features (which reflect an extreme polarity of poverty of object-relations); and nonspecific aspects of ego strength such as anxiety tolerance, impulse control, and sublimatory effectiveness. As noted earlier, the Health-Sickness Rating Scale seems an excellent overall quantitative measure of severity of illness which lends itself well to evaluating change and improvement. As far as treatment variables are concerned, future research on long-term psychoanalytic psychotherapy and psychoanalysis should include, as a minimum, a measure of the therapist's skill and evaluations of the extent to which interpretive techniques (including the focus on the transference) and supportive techniques (including structuring of the treatment during the treatment hours and in the life situation of the patient at large) are utilized. The patient variables of motivation and insight are intimately linked to the treatment process, and it is debatable to what extent they can be considered as pure "patient variables" rather than "process variables" which may be important in the evaluation of outcome. In this connection, the "negative therapeutic reaction," representing a polarity opposite to that of motivation and insight, may be an important measure to be included.

Some Final Thoughts about the Strategy of Psychotherapy Research in a Clinical Setting. While there is a great advantage to having people from different theoretical backgrounds and expertise working together as a psychotherapy research team, one requirement of that work is an integrative theoretical frame for the overall research design and procedures; otherwise, a great danger exists of fuzzy design, methods, and interpretation of data.

Another important aspect of research work in a clinical setting is the need for acceptance of that research effort on all levels of the administrative hierarchy. As always, when top management is opposed or is not favorably inclined to a certain research project, subtle but important distortions in the communication between researchers and clinicians will develop and seriously threaten research procedures. When top management of an institution is in agreement with the research project but the clinicians in charge of the actual operation feel "forced" to participate in the research, similar distortions will occur and reduce the availability of the material and the openness of communication. Because issues of confidentiality are so often involved in long-term treatment of patients, lack of open communication between clinicians and researchers may seriously inhibit the gathering and interpretation of crucial aspects of individual cases.

Another related issue is the need for a functional, rather than an authoritarian, institutional environment, particularly if the psychotherapy research will include the analysis of environmental factors such as the hospital milieu on the treatment process. The study of the hospital milieu as a social system influencing treatment brings about even greater stress between clinicians and researchers than is the case when patients are treated in relative isolation from the overall social environment of the psychiatric institution.

Finally, there is an advantage in having within a major research team a sophisticated member who is rather skeptical of the research philosophy, the research measures, and the hypotheses formulated. Such a sophisticated and questioning attitude within the team may go a long way toward avoiding a gradual narrowing of the research team's perceptions and a lack of self-criticism at crucial stages of its work. This does not mean, however, that such a natural skeptic should carry out these functions in terms of an incompatible theoretical frame of reference.

This paper reflects my conviction that the Menninger Foundation's Psychotherapy Research Project was able to point to crucial variables influencing long-term psychoanalytically oriented treatment, and that its conceptual as well as practical implications are of great significance for the understanding and carrying out of intensive psychotherapy, particularly that of patients with serious characterological problems and borderline conditions, and for the development of the forthcoming new generation of psychotherapy research.

REFERENCES

Burstein, D. Some thoughts about the quantitative research project on the assessment of personality and change. 1971, unpublished.

Foa, U. G. New developments in facet design and analysis. *Psychological Review*, 1965, 72: 262–274.

Guttman, L. An outline of some new methodology for social research. *Public Opinion Quarterly*, 1954–1955, **18**, 395–404.

Guttman, L. A structural theory for intergroup beliefs and action. *American Sociological Review*, 1959, **24**, 318–328. (a)

Guttman, L. Introduction to facet design and analysis. In *Proceedings of the fifteenth international congress of psychology, Brussels, 1957*. Amsterdam: North-Holland, 1959. (b)

Guttman, L. The structure of interrelations among intelligence tests. In *Proceedings of the 1964 invitational conference on testing problems*. Princeton: Educational Testing Service, 1965, pp. 25–36. (a)

Guttman, L. A faceted definition of intelligence. In *Scripta hierosolymitana*. Jerusalem: Magnes Press, 1965, pp. 166–181. (b)

Kernberg, O. Borderline personality organization. *Journal of the American Psychoanalytical Association*, 1967, **15**, 641–685.

Kernberg, O. The treatment of patients with borderline personality organization. *International Journal of Psycho-Analysis*, 1968, **49**, 600–619.

Kernberg, O., Burstein, E. D., Coyne, L., Appelbaum, A., Horwitz, L., & Voth, H. Psychotherapy and psychoanalysis: final report of the Menninger Foundation's psychotherapy research project. *Bulletin of the Menninger Clinic*, 1972, **36** (1/2).

Kruskal, J. B. Multidimensional scaling by optimizing goodness of fit to a nonmetric hypothesis. *Psychometrika*, 1964, **29**, 1–27. (a)

Kruskal, J. B. Nonmetric multidimensional scaling: a numerical method. *Psychometrika*, 1964, **29**, 115–129. (b)

Lingoes, J. C. An IBM-7090 program for Guttman-Lingoes multidimensional scalogram analysis. *Journal of the Behavioral Sciences*, 1966, **11**, 76–78 (Abstract). (a)

Lingoes, J. C. Recent computational advances in nonmetric methodology for the behavioral sciences. In *Proceedings of the international symposium: mathematical and computational methods in social sciences.* Rome: International Computation Centre, 1966, pp. 1–38. (b)

Lingoes, J. C. New computer developments in pattern analysis and nonmetric techniques. In *Uses of computers in psychological research—the 1964 IBM symposium of statistics.* Paris: Gauthier-Villars, 1966, pp. 1–22. (c)

Lingoes, J. C. The multivariate analysis of qualitative data. *Multivariate Behavioral Research*, 1968, **3**, 61–94.

Luborsky, L. Clinicians' judgments of mental health: a proposed scale. *Archives of General Psychiatry*, 1962, **7**, 407–417.

Luborsky, E., Fabian, M., Hall, B. H., Ticho, E., & Ticho, G. R. The psychotherapy research project of the Menninger Foundation, second report: II. Treatment variables. *Bulletin of the Menninger Clinic*, 1958, **22**, 126–147.

Malan, D. H. The outcome problem in psychotherapy research. *Archives of General Psychiatry*, 1973, **29**, 719–729.

Sargent, H. D. The psychotherapy research project of the Menninger Foundation: II. Rationale. *Bulletin of the Menninger Clinic*, 1956, **20**, 226–233. (a)

Sargent, H. D. The psychotherapy research project of the Menninger Foundation: III. Design. *Bulletin of the Menninger Clinic*, 1956, **20**, 234–238. (b)

Sargent, H. D., Coyne, L., Wallerstein, R. S., & Holtzman, W. H. An approach to quantitative problems of psychoanalytic research. *Journal of Clinical Psychology*, 1967, **23**, 243–291.

Shepard, R. N. The analysis of proximities: multidimensional scaling with an unknown distance function: I and II. *Psychometrika*, 1962, **27**, 125–140.

Wallerstein, R. S., Luborsky, L., Robbins, L.L., & Sargent, H. D. The psychotherapy research project of the Menninger Foundation: rationale, method and sample use: first report. *Bulletin of the Menninger Clinic*, 1956, **20**, 221–278.

3
THE SPECIFICITY OF PSYCHOANALYTIC CONCEPTS FOR UNDERSTANDING PSYCHOTHERAPY

LEWIS L. ROBBINS

Although psychotherapy of many varieties has been helpful to many people, it is more of an art than a science. Psychoanalysis has played a major role by providing a theoretical framework within which a range of treatment methods were developed, but its theories and techniques have evolved almost exclusively through case reports and metapsychological writings in the manner so brilliantly used by Freud. However, methodologies for the systematic study of psychotherapy have not yet developed sufficiently to deal adequately with the multiplicity of factors involved, the subtleties of the intimate dyadic relationships, the different goals of psychotherapy, and the lack of agreement on criteria of improvement.

Bergin and Strupp (1972) formulated the problems of psychotherapy research as follows: "What specific therapeutic interventions produce specific changes in specific patients under specific conditions? [p. 8]." These authors also point out that "thus far, research in psychotherapy has failed to make a deep impact on practice and technique [p. 6]."

Wallerstein and Sampson (1971) in their extensive discussion of the issues involved in psychoanalytic research raise questions regarding the necessity for, as well as the possibility of, conducting research on psychoanalytic therapy. They conclude that it is time to proceed beyond the limitations of the informal case study method to more formalized investigations. Questions of therapeutic effectiveness, regardless of the mode of treatment, confront all of psychiatry.

One of the problems in psychotherapy research concerns the differing goals of different types of psychotherapy. Oberndorf (1950) differentiated psychoanalysis from other forms of psychotherapy "in that it attempts a reconstruction of the personality rather than the limited goal of symptom relief [p. 395]." Wallerstein (1965) refers to psychoanalysis as "the most

Lewis L. Robbins, M.D., Psychiatrist-in-Chief, Long Island Jewish-Hillside Medical Center, Hillside Division, Glen Oaks, N.Y.

ambitious of therapies in its overall outcome goals [but one which] often achieves no more than other less ambitious therapeutic approaches [p. 752]."

This paper, like Dr. Kernberg's, is based upon the Psychotherapy Research Project of the Menninger Foundation, the methodology of which has been described in numerous publications. The final report by Kernberg, Burstein, Coyne, Appelbaum, Horwitz, and Voth (1972) concerns itself with quantitative findings. The prediction study findings, which will be focused on here, are from a forthcoming publication by Horwitz (1974) (the author is greatly indebted to Dr. Horwitz for having made the manuscript of his book available and for permission to quote from it freely).

The aim of this project was to "study the process and course of psychotherapy in order to increase our understanding of how psychotherapy contributes to changes in patients" and to find and refine a series of hypotheses contained within psychoanalytic theory which "implicitly guide our regular clinical treatment planning and treatment practice."

The assumptions, stated in simple form, without the inclusion of other contributory propositions such as the roles of constitutional capacities and environment pressures, are as follows.

1. Mental illness derives from otherwise insoluble intrapsychic conflicts.
2. These conflicts are in large part unconscious.
3. Intrapsychic conflicts are related to early childhood experiences and represent inadequately resolved infantile conflicts.
4. Prior to the onset of clinical illness, the intrapsychic conflicts are handled through the idiosyncratic patterning of impulse-defense configurations, character traits, and perhaps more or less ego-syntonic symptoms, which together make up the personality structure of the individual.
5. Through varying combinations of inner and outer stresses (sometimes clearly discernible as "precipitating events"), the previously utilized methods of maintaining homeostatic equilibrium fail and symptoms, or ego-dystonic character traits, or both, appear.
6. The patterning of the symptoms and associated ego-dystonic character traits reveals important elements of the inner conflicts, the ways the ego tries to cope with them, and important aspects of the fundamental character organizations of the individual (Robbins & Wallerstein, 1956).

Three sets of variables, patient (Wallerstein & Robbins, 1956), treatment (Luborsky, Fabian, Hall, Ticho, & Ticho, 1958), and situational (Sargent, Modlin, Faris, & Voth, 1958), were selected and defined and were studied before treatment began, when it terminated, and two years after termination. A naturalistic design was chosen with treatment being determined by the clinical staff and uninfluenced by the research. The initial study was based on the evaluations of the clinical staff with additional data obtained by the research staff only at termination and followup.

On the basis of the assessment of the patient variables a series of specific predictions regarding the treatment course and outcome were made. The assumption underlying each prediction and the evidence needed at termination and followup to confirm or refute it were explicitly stated in advance. Thus it was hoped to learn "to what extent and in what areas both the underlying assumptions and the specific variables chosen do or do not permit accurate prediction . . . and to avoid *post hoc* reconstruction [p. 40]" (Robbins & Wallerstein, 1959).

Over two thousand predictive statements were cast in a formal if- then- because- fashion. For example, "in regard to a patient who sought treatment because of guilt-engendering hostile feelings toward an adopted child which were so intense that she had to return the child to the adoption agency, a prediction statement as follows was made: *if* this patient is treated by psychoanalysis, and *if* she resolves her conflicts with regard to femininity and motherhood, *then* she will behave differently and be able to handle a child of her own (whether adopted or natural) *because* to the extent that a resolution of unconscious conflicts occurs via the expressive interpretive aspects of psychoanalysis, there is an at least proportional change in symptoms, character traits and life style [p. 472]" (White, 1971).

Forty-two cases originally were chosen, equally divided between those being treated by psychoanalysis and those treated by other forms of psychotherapy, with an equal number of late adolescent or adult males and females, without overt psychosis, neurological disease, or mental deficiency. Like so many patients being seen today (Robbins, 1974) most suffered from severe narcissistic character disorders; some were phobic or depressed, and several had addictions or perversions. For reasons of confidentiality, 30 percent of the patients available, many of whom were "good" analytic cases, had to be excluded. Of the 42 patients, 65 percent of whom were analytic patients, 17 (40 percent) were hospitalized before or during treatment.

Six patients were in analysis as a "last resort" (Glover, 1954). The assumption that the support of hospitalization might permit some patients to tolerate an expressive type of therapy despite low anxiety tolerance was not confirmed; in fact several, whose prognoses were poor, regressed.

It was correctly predicted that patients with high ego strength could tolerate increases in anxiety with uncovering treatment. Those whose conflicts were mainly at the phallic level were successfully analyzed. Of the 6 successfully analyzed patients 4 maintained their improvement despite increased responsibilities, whereas 2 had a slight reappearance of symptoms under stress.

Of the analytic cases 9 were suitable, 3 were questionable, and 10 were unsuitable. A major discriminating factor was the ability to tolerate anxiety without disruptive alloplastic or autoplastic defenses. Low anxiety tolerance and alloplastic symptoms were predictive of treatment failure, and the proposition that alloplastic defenses might be replaced by autoplastic defenses was rarely confirmed. This finding supported the prediction that as unconscious unacceptable impulses emerge toward consciousness anxiety increases and characteristic defenses are mobilized.

The concept that proportionate changes in character, symptoms, and life style can occur through "the production by a neutral analyst of a regressive transference neurosis and the ultimate resolution of this neurosis by techniques of interpretation alone [p. 775]" (Gill 1954) was confirmed. However, in approximately 50 percent of the cases significant changes occurred without conflict resolution despite predictions to the contrary.

There was general confirmation of the major transference assumption that in psychoanalysis and expressive psychotherapy, "to the extent that treatment aims consistently to uncover unconscious conflict, transference distortions override the realities of the treatment situation, i.e., the patient's reactions to the therapist are more consistent with genetically determined intrapsychic needs that are active at a given time than with the actual behavior and attitudes of the therapist" (Horwitz, 1974). With supportive therapy the transference tended to conform to the actual personality attributes of the therapist and, particularly if negative, was less intense.

Although the value of a positive transference had been recognized, the concept of the therapeutic alliance later developed by Zetzel (1956) and Greenson (1965) was found to be a *sine qua non* for all types of therapy: "Ideally, both patient and therapist consistently know, believe, or feel—at some level of consciousness—that their primary goal in working together is to help the patient" (Horwitz, 1974). In analysis this was necessary but not sufficient for working through the regressive transference neurosis, but in supportive therapy it often served as the major therapeutic factor.

As predicted, ego-syntonic, passive-dependent traits facilitated the alliance, and for young patients lacking a sense of identity it was further abetted if the therapist offered an active supportive relationship in which their own values were reinforced. The consequent more solid identity apparently fostered further maturation.

The therapeutic alliance requires an optimal amount of need gratification related to specific conflicts. For patients with severe ego defects and disturbed living patterns, the therapist may need to encourage adaptive behavior and controls, assist with reality testing, and, at times, counsel and advise. In some instances needed support and control require hospitalization (Robbins, 1968). Six self-destructive but not addicted patients were predicted to need hospitalization with psychotherapy. Four had successful outcomes; one of the two who did not was not hospitalized and the other was hospitalized only briefly. Hospitalization was also found to be necessary for psychotherapy to be helpful to patients who were addicted to drugs or alcohol. In nine cases it was predicted that a long period would be required to establish a therapeutic relationship. Of the six who had poor impulse control, limited ego strength, low anxiety tolerance, and little psychological mindedness, three established a therapeutic relationship more quickly than predicted, apparently because their therapists in supportive therapy skillfully maintained optimal psychological distance and avoided confrontation of negative transference.

Although supportive therapy was predicted to be less effective and its results less lasting than expressive therapy or analysis, its techniques call for a greater variety of technical operations (Bibring, 1954; Gill, 1951). In four instances of supportive therapy the outcomes significantly exceeded the predictions, which was also true of four other patients who had to be switched from expressive therapy and two from analysis. Nine of these maintained their gains or were further improved at followup with little or no further contact with their therapists. Two who were not improved at termination did show gains at followup two years later.

Oral traits and conflicts could be only partially resolved by analysis. If accompanied by alloplastic features, extreme passivity, or intense narcissism, analysis was contraindicated. All the borderline patients had marked oral fixations and, in analysis, tended to develop delusional thinking.

Poor motivation proved a good contraindicator; in four cases "good" motivation was actually based on the oral anticipation that analysis would be permanently protective and nurturing.

Of the 49 predictions for 21 patients that termination would be accomplished by a recrudescence of symptoms, depression, and desire to continue treatment, 68 percent were confirmed and 37 percent were definitely disconfirmed. Case reviews suggested in many instances that treatment had not been as gratifying as predicted or that termination served as a defense against deeper transference conflicts.

The unanticipated improvements with supportive therapy may have been due to increase of self-esteem, reflecting the therapist's interest, concern, and valuing of the patient; a corrective emotional experience in which the patient's usually evoked responses were reacted to differently by the therapist, leading to a changed perception of himself and others;

transference cures to please the therapist; and identification with the values and the attitudes of the therapist as experienced in treatment.

Improved behavior patterns may have been stabilized through the positive reinforcement and feedback which adaptive change induces. Positive rewards can also be obtained through more adaptive means of relieving tension and receiving gratification.

Of the 36 patients who received the expected treatment, 20 achieved the predicted outcomes and 16 had outcomes which differed from the predictions. The predictions were rather optimistic, tending to overestimate ego strength; this, along with other possible errors in the initial assessment of patient variables, was felt to have been due to inaccuracies in the original clinical evaluations. When reviewed and the 16 best workups compared with the 12 worst, the outcome predictions from the better workups scored 3.3 (on a 4-point scale), where those from the poorer workups scored 1.6 (A. Appelbaum, personal communication).

The assumptions and predictions were generally supported by the findings, but, as anticipated, some additions to and modifications of the original hypotheses are needed. Many of these are reflected in the postdictive assumptions given in Horwitz's (1974) appendix III. Well-motivated patients with strong egos capable of tolerating anxiety can improve with all types of therapy, but they can accomplish most, particularly characterologically, with psychoanalysis. For patients lacking these qualities psychoanalysis does not appear to be indicated, and for those more severely ill, particularly with borderline conditions, it is contraindicated. Many of these, however, were helped with mildly expressive and/or supportive approaches.

Supportive therapy proved to be more effective and the changes it brought about were often more stable than predicted. This broad therapeutic approach requires considerable skill on the part of the therapist: his choice of techniques and handling of the transference reflect his understanding of the patient's conflicts and defenses. This is more than a friendship offering acceptance, support, and concern: "Through his training, understanding and commitment to his patient, the therapist works with the patient's hostility, unreasonable demands and narcissism which would ordinarily alienate the other party to a relationship" (Horwitz, 1974). In a similar vein, Truax and Mitchell (1971) conclude that "the personality of the therapist is more important than his techniques. Conversely, however, techniques that are specific to certain kinds of patients and psychotherapy goals can be quite potent in the hands of a therapist who is inherently helpful, and who offers high levels of empathic understanding, warmth and genuineness, potency, immediacy and who can confront his clients in a constructive manner [p. 341]." Bergin and Strupp (1972) reverse this order, seeing the relationship as a "prerequisite for therapeutic intervention [providing] the matrix within which planful interventions can occur [p. 128]." This interplay of patient-therapist-therapy variables has always been a central psychoanalytic consideration.

The writings of Giovacchini (1972), Kohut (1971), and Kernberg (1968) are consistent with many of these research findings regarding special considerations in the management of transference and the role of conflict resolution. Some psychopathological behaviors must be viewed as the result of faulty ego development as a consequence of constitutional factors (Luborsky & Schimek, 1964) or very early conflicts, rather than only the direct expression of intrapsychic conflicts. Horwitz (1974) concludes that "since one of the well accepted axioms of developmental psychology is that a libidinal tie between parent and child forms the matrix within which major developmental tasks are accomplished, psychotherapy of all types provides a second chance to make up for past developmental failures."

Psychoanalytic theory is a necessary but not a sufficient theory of human behavior, be it normal or abnormal. Both its theory and related therapeutic techniques have been evolving slowly with little assistance from formal research. In the current psychoanalytically based study many predictions were confirmed, but the question remains as to whether the basic assumptions were thereby strengthened or whether some other theory would explain the results as well or better. When predictions were disconfirmed, was this due to methodological errors or theoretical factors? The questions of whether other forms of therapy can achieve similar or better results, and, if so, whether psychoanalysis can enable us to understand how those therapies effect change, are among the many which remain.

REFERENCES

Bergin, A. E., & Strupp, H. H., *Changing frontiers in the science of psychotherapy.* Chicago: Aldine-Atherton, 1972.

Bibring, E. Psychoanalysis and the dynamic psychotherapies. *Journal of the American Psychoanalytic Association,* 1954, 2, 745–770.

Gill, M. M. Ego psychology and psychotherapy. *Psychoanalytic Quarterly,* 1951, 20, 62–71.

Gill, M. M. Psychoanalysis and exploratory psychotherapy. *Journal of the American Psychoanalytic Association,* 1954, 2, 771–797.

Giovacchini, P. L. *Tactics and techniques in psychoanalytic therapy.* New York: Science House, 1972.

Glover, E. The indications for psychoanalysis. *Journal of Mental Science,* 1954, 100, 393–401.

Greenson, R. R. The working alliance and the transference neurosis. *Psychoanalytic Quarterly,* 1965, 34, 155–181.

Horwitz, L. Clinical prediction in psychotherapy. New York: J. Aronson, 1974.

Kernberg, O. F. The treatment of patients with borderline personality organization. *International Journal of Psychoanalysis,* 1968, 49, 600–619.

Kernberg, O. F., Burstein, E. D., Coyne, L., Appelbaum, A., Horwitz, L., & Voth, H. Psychotherapy and psychoanalysis: final report of the Menninger Foundation's psychotherapy research project. *Bulletin of the Menninger Clinic*, 1972, **36**, 1–275.

Kohut, H. *The analysis of the self*. New York: International Universities Press, 1971.

Luborsky, L., Fabian, M., Hall, B. N., Ticho, E., & Ticho, G. R. The psychotherapy research project of the Menninger Foundation, second report: II. Treatment variables. *Bulletin of the Menninger Clinic*, 1958, **22**, 126–147.

Luborsky, L., & Schimek, J. Psychoanalytic theories of therapeutic and developmental changes: implications for assessment. In P. Worchel and D. Byrne (Eds.), *Personality change*. New York: Wiley, 1964, pp. 73–99.

Oberndorf, C. P. Unsatisfactory results of psychoanalytic therapy. *Psychoanalytic Quarterly*, 1950, **19**, 393–407.

Robbins, L. L., Ego psychology and the milieu at the mental hospital. In I. H. Eldred and M. Vanderpol (Eds.), *Psychotherapy in the designed therapeutic milieu*. Boston: Little, Brown, 1968, pp. 65–88.

Robbins, L. L. Implications of a changing hospital population. *Journal of the National Association of Private Psychiatric Hospitals*. 1974, in press.

Robbins, L. L., & Wallerstein, R. S. The psychotherapy research project of the Menninger Foundation: I, orientation. *Bulletin of the Menninger Clinic*, 1956, **20**, 223–225.

Robbins, L. L., & Wallerstein, R. S. The research strategy and tactics of the psychotherapy research project of the Menninger Foundation and the problem of controls. In E. A. Rubinstein and M. B. Parloff (Eds.), *Research in psychotherapy*. Washington, D.C.: American Psychological Association, 1959, pp. 27–43.

Sargent, H. D., Modlin, H. C., Faris, M. T., & Voth, H. M. The psychotherapy research project of the Menninger Foundation: second report, III, situational variables. *Bulletin of the Menninger Clinic*, 1958, **22**, 148–166.

Truax, C. B., & Mitchell, K. M. Research on certain therapist interpersonal skills in relation to process and outcome. In A. E. Bergin & S. L. Garfield (Eds.), *Handbook of psychotherapy and behavior change*. New York: Wiley, 1971, pp. 299–344.

Wallerstein, R. S. The goals of psychoanalysis: a survey of analytic viewpoints. *Journal of the American Psychoanalytic Association*, 1965, **13**, 748–770.

Wallerstein, R. S., & Robbins, L. L. The psychotherapy research project of the Menninger Foundation: IV, concepts. *Bulletin of the Menninger Foundation*, 1956, **20**, 239–262.

Wallerstein, R. S., & Sampson, H. Issues in research in the psychoanalytic process. *International Journal of Psychoanalysis*, 1971, **52**, 11–50.

White, R. B. Psychoanalysis: an evaluation. In J. G. Howells (Ed.), *Modern perspectives in psychiatry*. New York: Brunner-Mazel, 1971, pp. 448–487.

Zetzel, E. R. Current concepts of transference. *International Journal of Psychoanalysis*, 1956, **37**, 369–376.

4 PSYCHOTHERAPY AND THE SENSE OF MASTERY

JEROME D. FRANK

Every person's feelings of security and satisfaction depend to a considerable degree on a sense of being able to exert some control over the reactions of others toward him as well as his own inner states. Inability to control feelings, thoughts, and impulses not only shakes the person's confidence in himself but impedes his ability to control others by preempting too much of his attention and distorting his perceptions and behavior. The feeling of loss of control gives rise to emotions which aggravate and are aggravated by the specific symptoms or problems for which the person ostensibly seeks psychotherapy. In view of this, it is not surprising that all schools of psychotherapy implicitly or explicitly include the aim of enabling the patient to gain increased mastery over himself and his social environment and that their procedures are related to these goals (Strupp, 1970; Frank, 1974).

Interview therapies based on the psychoanalytic model hold that increased control over interpersonal relationships follows from better insight into unconscious sources of subjective disturbances, as implied by Freud's dictum, "Where Id was, there shall Ego be." Insight into the sources of emotional reactions to the therapist typically receives particular emphasis. Sifneos (1972), for example, defines the goal of short-term psychotherapy as that of enabling the patient to find new ways of dealing with the emotional conflicts of the transference, resulting first in a reduction of tension in the interview and later in less stressful relationships with others.

For other forms of insight therapy, the goal of achieving mastery over behavior through changing one's attitudes is more explicit: in particular, reality therapy stresses the importance of assuming responsibility for one's behavior (Glasser, 1965); rational-emotive therapy seeks to help the patient to become aware of and to combat the erroneous "internalized sentences" which cause his problems (Ellis, 1962); and logotherapy has the goal of enabling the patient to gain an increased sense of mastery through the realization that he has the power to determine his attitudes

Jerome D. Frank, M.D., Professor Emeritus of Psychiatry, The Johns Hopkins University School of Medicine.

toward external circumstances, however adverse they may be (Frankl, 1965).

Behavior therapies, such as systematic desensitization or emotional flooding, are based on the view that the route to mastery of fears and similar threatening emotions is not primarily through gaining insight into their origins but through the realization that one can endure such feelings. As a result, the patient becomes able to face and approach the fantasied or real situations rather than avoiding or escaping from them (Watson, 1973).

Those behavior therapists who deny altogether the importance of subjective experiences define the goal of therapy as that of widening the patient's options and placing them under his control (Hunt & Dyrud, 1968). Instead of increased mastery of subjective states leading to more effective behavior, they view the process as running in the reverse direction. They maintain that if the patient learns to control his behavior so as to gain more rewarding reciprocal behavior from others, control over his own feelings will follow automatically. These therapies often stress assertiveness training, through which the patient is encouraged to tackle and master social situations he had previously been unable to handle.

A brief historical digression will demonstrate again that there is nothing new under the sun. Emil Kraepelin recommended an approach similar to that of some behavior therapies for "dread neurosis"—"a more or less constant feeling of anxious suspense which dominates the entire life" (Diefendorf, 1915, p. 400). He writes:

> First one seeks to explain to the patient the basis for his suffering and to convince him that it is not a question of a serious physical illness, as he assumes, but merely the consequences of anxiety. . . .
> After a brief preparatory period of harmless regimes, baths, and bed rest, which serve merely to win the patient's trust and to allow one to get to know him, cautious but planful progressive exercises are begun, as the nature of the symptoms permits. . . . Through calm, friendly, and factual statements that repeatedly bring to the patient's attention the true grounds for his disability, with patience it is usually possible to . . . improve performance step by step, especially if one first supervises the exercises oneself, thereby encouraging the patient and suppressing emerging fears as they arise. . . .
> Once patients are convinced of the true nature of the problem, they usually make rapid progress. They also soon learn to guard themselves against relapses by effectively combating occasional periods of discouragement themselves [p. 1426f.; translated by the author] (Kraepelin, 1913).

As the last sentence implies, a very effective way of increasing the patient's sense of mastery is to convince him that his gains are due to his own efforts. This is implicit in nondirective therapies, in which the therapist disclaims all credit for the patient's progress. It is also high-lighted in those procedures in which the patient, after being taught the method, thereafter conducts his treatment himself. Thus patients have been taught to desensitize themselves through the use of tape recordings of anxiety hierarchies or similar devices (Migler & Wolpe, 1967).

A recent development along the same lines is the use of biofeedback to teach the patient to relax his muscles (Budzynski, Stoyva, & Adler, 1970) or increase his alpha waves on the EEG (Nowlis & Kamiya, 1970). These procedures are closely allied to meditation exercises, which are selfcon-ducted methods of producing tranquility and other desired subjective states.

Space does not permit examining the ways in which group therapies also seek to enhance patients' sense of control. It may suffice to mention one form which focuses exclusively on this goal—the popular self-help movement known as Recovery Incorporated. Its founder, Dr. Abraham Low (who, incidentally, acknowledges indebtedness to Kraepelin), de-scribes the goal of therapy as "to convince [patients] that the sensation can be endured, the impulse controlled, the obsession checked [p. 19] [Low, 1968]. . . . two inner experiences only are subject to control, thoughts and impulses . . . one factor only is capable of controlling them, the Will [p. 132]."

Two features of all forms of psychotherapy which enhance the patient's sense of mastery over himself and his environment are a coherent conceptual framework and the provision of success experiences. Every therapy is based on a set of concepts that explain the patient's distress and how to overcome it. In the course of therapy, the patient is implicitly or explicitly indoctrinated with these concepts, which, by enabling him to organize and label his inchoate feelings and experiences, enhance his sense of control over them. Writers who wish to make something terrifying characterize it as "nameless." To name something is to gain power over it, a truth exemplified by myths as diverse as the story of Rumpelstiltskin and Adam's naming of the animals in Genesis.

Experimental evidence that conceptualization, or "meaning attribu-tion," as the authors term it, is an important component of therapeutic gain is supplied by Lieberman, Yalom, and Miles (1973) in their study of encounter groups. They found that mere emotional release, however gratifying it might be, was unrelated to improvement, which required that the binge be followed by reflections on what had occurred and its implications for changes in behavior.

A second mastery-enhancing component of psychotherapy—provision of success experiences—requires some elaboration. A person has a success experience when his performance exceeds his aspirations (Frank, 1935); that is, it is a fraction of which the numerator is the level of performance and the denominator the level of aspiration. This means that subjective experiences of success can be achieved by lowering one's aspirations as well as raising one's performance. To this end, one object of psychotherapy with some patients is to induce them to lower unrealistic expectations of themselves. As a result, performances which they had felt to be failures now become emotionally neutral. In this presentation, however, I shall be concerned only with the numerator of the fraction, the person's performance.

The first point to note is that level of performance does not produce feelings of success or failure unless the person has formed aspirations in regard to the task. This happens only when he regards his performance as reflecting on his image of himself. The strength of the link between any particular task and self-esteem depends on at least four factors which are relevant to psychotherapy: the patient's personality and past experience, the difficulty of the task, the extent to which he perceives his performance as resulting from his own efforts, and the attitudes of other persons important to him.

For a task to engage a person's aspirations, he must see it as related to personal qualities he regards as important. A nonathletic bookworm may be unmoved by how much time it takes him to run a mile while experiencing a thrill out of being able to identify an obscure passage from Shakespeare, while the reverse might hold true for an unscholarly athlete. In this connection, insight therapies seem especially suited to verbally adept, psychologically minded persons whose self-esteem is tied to their ability to gain new knowledge and formulate it skillfully, while the action-oriented are attracted to therapies stressing performance.

Furthermore, a person forms no aspirations with respect to a task that he regards as much too easy or much too hard, so performance on such tasks yields feelings neither of success nor of failure. A person whose piano-playing skill extends to picking out popular tunes does not feel crushed at his inability to play the "Moonlight Sonata" or elated because he can play the scale of C major. The best way to assure that a task lies within the range that will produce success or failure experiences is to let the person choose the level of difficulty himself. This principle is implicit in all therapies that use structured hierarchies, which enable the patient to experience a series of successes as he masters one level after another.

In this connection, performances which the patient regards as due to his own efforts would be expected to reflect more strongly on his self-esteem than those which he attributes to factors beyond his control, whether they be mere chance, a medication, or the help of someone else. In recognition of this, as already mentioned, psychotherapists of all persuasions convey to the patient that his progress is the result of his own efforts. Nondirective therapists disclaim any credit for the patient's acquisition of new insights, and directive ones stress that the patient's gains depend on his ability to carry out the prescribed procedures.

The most important determinant of whether performance in a task is linked to self-esteem, however, is probably the attitude of those whose opinion is important to the person's self-image. For our patients the psychotherapist is such a person, so performance in any task he sets becomes a potential source of experiences of success or failure. Furthermore, he can heighten the effect of successes by praise and ameliorate the effects of failures by indicating that poor performance has not diminished his respect for the patient. In this connection, one reason young therapists come to grief with schizophrenics is that, by demanding that the patient work on his problems, they set him a task he cannot do, leading to failure experiences which aggravate his condition.

If this analysis of the role of mastery in psychotherapy is valid, then enhanced sense of mastery should be related to clinical improvement. Only in recent years have scales directly related to this concept been introduced, so information is still scanty. What is available, however, supports the hypothesis. These I-E (Internal-External) scales (Rotter, 1966) and powerlessness scales (Seeman & Evans, 1962) measure the relative extent to which the patient feels that the locus of control over his own life lies within himself or feels that it lies in external events.

One researcher, using such a scale, tested hospitalized patients on admission and again on discharge, after they had received primarily milieu treatment. He found a highly significant increase in reported feelings of control over both internal and external events. In his words: "The more control one experiences *over* internal and external forces as compared to the control one experiences *from* internal and external forces, the more likely is one to display a higher level of adjustment [p. 314] [Tiffany, 1967]". This finding is supported by four studies of psychotherapy of outpatients (Gillis & Jessor, 1970; Smith, 1970), two of them our own. All found a shift in locus of control toward the internal side to be correlated with improvement.

Many features of psychotherapy can lead to temporary relief of distress, among them arousal of the patient's favorable expectations, the mere sense of relief from the discovery that his apprehensions about going crazy were unfounded, and the discovery of someone to listen to his troubles. It seems reasonable to assume, however, that continued improvement will depend on the patient's willingness to come to grips with problems which he previously avoided and to handle them more successfully that he had before treatment. One important component of his ability to do this should be an enhanced sense of mastery. Clinical support for this hypothesis is implied by Kraepelin's finding that his patients learned to guard themselves against relapses, thus implicitly attributing maintenance of improvement to the patients' increased ability to master their symptoms by their own efforts. He added that those whom he had been able to follow remained well, many for more than twenty years. In a recent study Lieberman et al. (1973) compared a group of participants in encounter groups who had maintained their gains one year after the conclusion of treatment with those who had not. They found that those who maintained their gains stressed the importance of thinking about what one is doing, and of pausing to analyze problem situations. They "stressed an active internal process rather than one in which the person is simply the passive recipient of influence." Those who did not maintain their gains, by contrast, expressed the attitude that a person "could be squelched or supported by a broad, undifferentiated force . . . which he does not direct or could not counteract [p. 403]."

Such observations imply that patients who attribute relief of distress to their own efforts will be able to achieve it for longer periods after treatment is ended than those who attribute it to a medication. The latter would be expected to relapse when the medication is withdrawn. An ingenious experiment offers support for this assumption. Persons who complained of trouble falling asleep were all given the same dose of chloral hydrate and instructed in relaxation exercises for seven days, after which the drug was discontinued. Half were then told that they had received an optimal dose; the rest were told that the dose was really too weak to shorten the time of falling asleep, so that their improvement must have resulted primarily from the exercises. Those who were led to attribute their improvement to their own efforts maintained their gains over a four-day period better than those who attributed greater speed in falling asleep to the medication (Davison, Tsujimoto, & Glaros, 1973).

To investigate the role of a sense of mastery in maintaining therapeutic change following psychotherapy, we devised an experiment to compare the immediate and long-term effects of two therapies: one in which we tried to lead patients to attribute therapeutic gains to their own efforts and one in which improvement was attributed to a placebo.[1] We hypothesized that, because of the many nonspecific factors in both treatments, both would be equally effective in producing immediate benefit, but that patients who attributed improvement to their own efforts would maintain it better after the treatment ceased. We further hypothesized that at followup these patients would show greater shift in locus of control toward the internal side than those who had received a placebo.

The sample consisted of 32 psychiatric outpatients diagnosed as suffering from neuroses or personality disorders which might respond to psychotherapy. All received an initial evaluation followed by eight sessions at weekly intervals in which they carried out three tasks: one measuring reaction time, one requiring them to describe a scene on a tachistoscopically presented picture, and a third which ostensibly measured their galvanic skin response to various disturbing, pleasant, and neutral visual and auditory stimuli. Efforts were made to link performance in the tasks to aspects of the patients' personal problems as determined at the initial interview. At the end of each session the patient was shown a graph of his performance on each task which accentuated his actual progress.

In addition, at the start of each session, each patient had an opportunity to talk into a tape recorder uninterruptedly for half an hour and, at the start of the next session, received a written comment on it from a therapist whom he never met. The purpose was to give patients an opportunity to talk about their problems while discouraging the formation of a therapeutic relationship which might overshadow the experimental manipulation.

Half the patients received a placebo throughout the period of the study, to which their improvement in the tasks was attributed (the "placebo" condition). At the final session the placebo was discontinued with the explanation that the treatment program had been completed and that the gains it produced would be expected to continue. The other half received no medication and were led to believe that improvement on the tasks was due solely to their own efforts (the "mastery" condition).

To measure locus of control, we devised three scales, partly based on Seeman's powerlessness scale (Seeman & Evans, 1962), which were combined to yield a single index. Clinical improvement was evaluated by patients' and therapists' global improvement scores and the Discomfort Scale derived from the Hopkins Symptom Checklist (Derogatis, Lipman, Rickels, Uhlenhuth, & Covi, 1974).

All patients were evaluated immediately at the close of treatment and again three months later. On the average, all patients showed significant improvement at the end of therapy, and there was no difference in improvement between the mastery and placebo groups. Three months after the close of therapy, however, patients in the mastery condition had maintained their improvement better than those in the placebo condition, confirming our first hypothesis.

With respect to clinical improvement and locus of control, the population as a whole showed a significant shift toward the "internal" side, concomitant with improvement, although degree of improvement at three months did not correlate significantly with the extent of the shift.

Comparison of patients who scored in the top and bottom thirds of the locus of control scales (the most internally controlled and the most externally controlled, respectively) revealed an interesting, statistically significant interaction with type of therapy. At the three-month followup point, the more internally controlled showed more improvement in the mastery condition than a similar group in the placebo condition, while the more externally controlled showed the reverse, as shown in Figure 1. This finding has implications for the use of a locus of control measure as

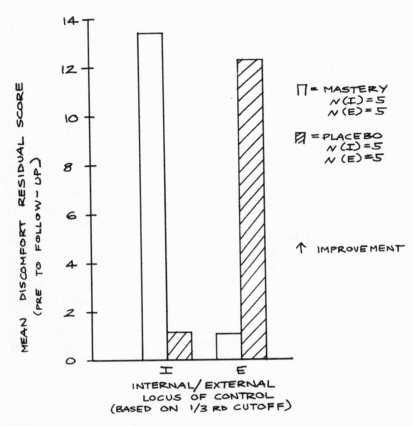

FIG. 1. Pre- to followup Discomfort Scale residual scores for mastery and placebo conditions with reference to internal and external locus of control.

a criterion for selection of patients for different types of therapy which warrant further exploration.

To summarize the findings of this rather complex experiment, both placebo and mastery groups improved to the same degree during the period of therapy itself. Three months after its completion, however, those who had been led to attribute progress to their own efforts maintained their clinical improvement significantly better than those who attributed their progress to a pill.

The similarity in improvement of the two groups during therapy may perhaps be attributable to a feature common to both—communication with an unseen therapist by means of a tape[2]—as well as to the probability that both the placebo and mastery conditions stimulated the patients' favorable expectations.

A probable explanation of the discrepancy in the improvement of the two groups after three months is this: persons who attribute improvement in a course of therapy to an outside agent are more apt to relapse when the course is completed and the therapist assures them that they no longer need the medication than are those persons who attribute improvement to themselves and thereby gain a heightened sense of mastery which encourages them to approach and deal with their problems more effectively.

To sum up, this paper has reviewed clinical and experimental data suggesting that the feeling of being able to control internal and external events is related to clinical improvement in therapy, and that whether the patient feels able to control, or feels controlled by, external events may affect his responsiveness to therapies which attribute progress to his own efforts or to an external agent.

NOTES

1. This study was supported in part by U.S. Public Health Service Research Grant MH-04618. The other members of the research staff were Rudolf Hoehn-Saric, M.D., Stanley D. Imber, Ph.D., Bernard Liberman, Ph.D., and Anthony R. Stone, Ph.D., who acted as therapists and trainers, and Mr. Fred Ribich, Research Assistant.

2. Of the 31 patients on whom the information is available, 25 found the taping sessions helpful and 16 found them more helpful than either the tasks or the placebo. Clearly, the opportunity to unburden oneself, even to an unseen listener, can be therapeutic.

REFERENCES

Budzynski, T., Stoyva, J., & Adler, C. Feedback-induced muscle relaxation: application to tension headache. *Journal of Behavior Therapy and Experimental Psychiatry*, 1970, **1**, 205-211.

Davison, G. C., Tsujimoto, R. N., & Glaros, A. G. Attribution and the maintenance of behavior change in falling asleep. *Journal of Abnormal Psychology*, 1973, **82**, 124-133.

Derogatis, L. R., Lipman, R., Rickels, K., Uhlenhuth, E. H., & Covi, L. The Hopkins Symptom Checklist (HSCL): a self-report symptom inventory. *Behavioral Science*, 1974, **19**, 1-15.

Diefendorf, A. R. *Clinical psychiatry: a text-book for students and physicians abstracted and adapted from the 7th. German edition of Kraepelin's "Lehrbuch der Psychiatrie."* New York: Macmillan, 1915.

Ellis, A. *Reason and emotion in psychotherapy.* New York: Lyle Stuart, 1962.

Frank, J. D. Individual differences in certain aspects of the level of aspiration. *American Journal of Psychology*, 1935, **48**, 119-128.

Frank, J. D. Psychotherapy: the restoration of morale. *American Journal of Psychiatry*, 1974, **131**, 271-274.

Frankl, V. E. *The doctor and the soul: from psychotherapy to logotherapy.* New York: Knopf, 1965.

Gillis, J. S., & Jessor, R. Effects of brief psychotherapy on belief in internal control: an exploratory study. *Psychotherapy: Theory, Research and Practice*, 1970, **7**, 135-137.

Glasser, W. *Reality therapy: a new approach to psychiatry.* New York: Harper, 1965.

Hunt, H., & Dyrud, J. Commentary: perspective in behavior therapy. In J. M. Shlien (Ed.), *Research in psychotherapy*, Vol. 3. Washington, D.C.: American Psychological Association, 1968, pp. 140-152.

Kraepelin, E. *Psychiatrie, achte Auflage, III Band.* Leipzig: Johann Ambrosius Barth, 1913.

Lieberman, M. A., Yalom, I. D., & Miles, M. B. *Encounter groups: first facts.* New York: Basic Books, 1973.

Low, A. A. *Mental health through will-training.* 16th ed. Boston: Christopher, 1968.

Migler, B., & Wolpe, J. Automated self-desensitization: a case report. *Behavior Research and Therapy*, 1967, **5**, 133–135.

Nowlis, D. P., & Kamiya, J. The control of electro-encephalographic alpha rhythm through auditory feedback and the associated mental activity. In T. Barber, L. V. DiCara, J. Kamiya, N. E. Miller, D. Shapiro, and J. Stovya (Eds.), *Biofeedback and self-control.* Chicago: Aldine-Atherton, 1971, pp. 283–291.

Rotter, J. B. Generalized expectancies for internal vs. external control of reinforcement. *Psychological Monographs*, 1966, **80**(1), 1–28.

Seeman, M., & Evans, J. W. Alienation and learning in a hospital setting. *American Sociological Review*, 1962, **27**, 772–782.

Sifneos, P. E. *Short-term psychotherapy and emotional crisis.* Cambridge: Harvard University Press, 1972.

Smith, R. E. Change in locus of control as a function of life crisis resolution. *Journal of Abnormal Psychology*, 1970, **75**, 329–332.

Strupp, H. H. Specific vs. non-specific factors in psychotherapy and the problem of control. *Archives of General Psychiatry*, 1970, **23**, 393–401.

Tiffany, D. W. Mental health: a function of experienced control. *Journal of Clinical Psychology*, 1967, **23**, 311–315.

Watson, J. P. Prolonged exposure in the therapy of phobias. In J. Masserman (Ed.), *Current psychiatric therapies.* New York: Grune & Stratton, 1973, pp. 83–90.

5

DISCUSSION:
Comments on the Menninger Project

DOUGLAS M. McNAIR

I first learned of the Menninger Project when I was helping out on the sidelines at the first American Psychological Association Psychotherapy Conference in 1958. The Project has taken about twenty years from inception to the so-called final report.[1] (I understand more reports and books are to come.) The sample was made up of 42 patients, 21 in psychoanalysis and 21 in several other therapies, or about two cases per year. According to the credits in the report, 36 researchers at the Ph.D. or M.D. level were involved in the Project at one time or another. There were nine additional expert research consultants. The design was "naturalistic," with all that implies. Extrapolating from the time involved, the small number of patients per treatment method, and the vast professional and financial resources required for the study, my guess is that it will be about the year 3000 before clinical trials will provide satisfactory evidence of the true role of psychoanalysis among our treatment regimens. At the earliest, everyone now living and their children's children will be dead. Actually, I doubt that such evidence ever will be presented. One reason, probably not the major one, is the very real difficulties involved in any psychotherapy research. A more important reason is that the people in positions to do the studies and provide the research data do not appear really interested. The main reason is that psychoanalysis may be simply bypassed in favor of other treatments. There are briefer treatments such as psychopharmacology, the many variants of short-term and time-limited psychotherapy, and behavior therapy; there are the family and group approaches, at least some of which involve radically different concepts of disorder, of patienthood, of therapist-patient relationships, and of treatment.

Some points in the Menninger Report interested me. Others bothered me. Some did both. One troublesome issue concerns the measurement of patient variables. As most of you probably know, the scaling of patient variables involved a very complex paired comparison procedure in which two independent raters used clinical notes and summaries as the data base

Douglas M. McNair, Ph.D., Professor of Psychiatry and Psychology, Boston University School of Medicine.

from which to derive comparisons of every patient with every other patient on 12 dimensions. Most of the rated dimensions were derived from psychodynamic concepts. Factor analyses of these ratings at the initiation of treatment, at termination, and at followup consistently yielded one major factor defined by 10 of the 12 rated characteristics. *Severity of Symptomatology* turned out to be an excellent marker of the principal factor, correlating about .85–.90 with the factor. Symptom Severity was at least as good a marker as any of the other measured characteristics, most of which were defined in more psychodynamic terms (Patterning of Defenses, Ego Strength, Level of Psychosexual Development, etc.). The other two factors represented among the patient scales hardly qualify as major. They accounted for only a small proportion of the variance, and they were each defined by only a single scale.

Many of us in our research rely rather heavily on the measurement of manifest symptomatology and psychopathology as criteria of outcome. Sometimes we have been charged with emphasizing the superficial at the expense of what is really relevant and meaningful, or of even worse errors. I secretly find it delightful to learn that what we have been measuring all along overlaps so much with what is psychodynamically real and relevant. But I also find it disappointing that this vast effort did not identify some important, reliably measurable patient dimensions that were relatively independent of symptom severity. I wish the Project had correlated its method of rating severity of disorder with similar measures based on patient self-ratings and observer's assessments via clinical rating scales. My hunch is that the correlations would be very high, but we will never know.

To quantify the treatments, the Project started with 19 scales, and 14 survived various reliability and discriminability tests. A factor analysis yielded two large and two small treatment factors. The major factors were Use of Psychoanalytic Techniques (Interpretation, Dream and Fantasy Analysis, Focus on Childhood, Transference, and Avoidance of Attention to Current Life Situations) and what appeared to be an interesting Competence Factor (Skill with the Specific Case, Absence of Therapist Tension, Achievement of Therapist's Goals, Keeping the Therapist's Personality in the Background, and Liking for the Patient). It would have been helpful to know whether, and, if so, how, the four treatment methods differed in terms of these factors, but these data were not given.

The six major criteria of change all appeared to tap a single factor. You have to ignore the usual criterion for number of factors (latent roots > 1.00) to extract more than one dimension of change. It was again disappointing to learn that such an extensive, expert, analytic effort identified only the unidimension of global improvement.

There were many features of the Project that I found extremely troublesome. Some of these may be dealt with in earlier reports which I have not read or have forgotten. A central issue is that the basic data base was not the same from patient to patient. The clinical summaries and the progress notes which were the basis for the tedious scaling procedures varied widely in comprehensiveness and completeness. Nowhere did I find simple descriptive statistics on the patients and the treatments. Basic demographic statistics such as age, sex, race, and marital status are not presented, nor are their relations to outcome considered in the final report. The same is true for prior clinical histories. Nowhere could I find the numbers of patients assigned to Expressive Psychotherapy, to Supportive Psychotherapy, or to Expressive-Supportive Psychotherapy. Presumably these were subsets of the 21 patients not assigned to psychoanalysis. Nowhere did I find any mention of psychotropic drugs. Were they not used? Nowhere are there comparisons at the beginning of treatment of the kinds of patients who were *not* randomly assigned to the four treatment methods. Again, nowhere did I find a description of the length of the various treatments in hours, months, or years. I could go on, but this gives you an idea of my reservations about the study.

The application of the Guttman-Lingoes Multidimensional Scalogram Analysis (MSA) will be of great interest to many researchers. As far as I know, it's the first application of MSA to treatment research. I have neither the expertise nor the time to go into the mathematics of MSA. It is a nonmetric method of profile similarity analysis. The data comprising the profiles are categorical rather than continuous variables. The method determines, for example, whether Profile A is more similar to Profile B or to Profile C, but it does not retain information on the actual distance between profiles. It assigns similar profiles to the same spatial region and dissimilar profiles to different regions but does not preserve information on distances within or between regions. MSA tends to represent relationships in a smaller space than does factor analysis. The usual output is a two-dimensional plot representing projections from a larger space.

As I understand the Project report, the MSA clustered the profiles into sub-regions, and the clusters of profiles differed in degree of Global Change, in the treatment methods applied, and in several highly correlated initial patient characteristics. One way to interpret the results is to say that the different treatments produced different degrees of improvement and that the effectiveness of the particular treatments depended on the presenting characteristics of the patients. Psychoanalysis, for example, looked most effective, but effectiveness differed depending on patient characteristics such as Ego Strength, Motivation, and Anxiety Tolerance (i.e., in Severity of Symptomatology).

However, I am concerned about possible confounding in the MSA results. As there was no random assignment to treatments, the patients in the different treatments probably differed markedly at admission. I think it is very likely that the MSA results reflect the confounding of treatments and initial severity plus the well-known fact that pretreatment status nearly always has a strong relationship to outcome.

Turning from the MSA results to the more conventional analyses of relationships among the sets of variables, in the final report approximately 100 hypotheses were stated and tested concerning expected relationships among the patient, treatment, situational, and outcome variables. Nearly half the hypotheses predicted that treatment characteristics would affect outcome. Further, nearly all of these treatment hypotheses were variations on the theme of how therapist competence and the extent of use of psychoanalytic techniques should influence improvement. About half these hypotheses were confirmed. Most of those confirmed indicated positive relationships between therapist skill and outcome. I found these results on competence impossible to interpret. The researchers tried unsuccessfully to obtain a global measure of each therapist's competence that was independent of any specific treatment case. They were forced to rely instead on an assessment of the skill which each therapist demonstrated during his treatment of each patient in the study. This may well simply amount to another way of measuring outcome.

Another 30 of the hypotheses predicted relationships between patient characteristics and improvement. Most of these were variants of the general theme that improvement would depend upon the degree of psychopathology present at admission or that improvement in one dimension would correlate positively with improvement in another. About half of these hypotheses also were confirmed. I found it possible to restrain my excitement over these findings.

Only about 20 hypotheses dealt with social and environmental influences on improvement. Apparently the researchers' attention to the patients' surroundings reflects the influence of a pre-ecological era. Only about 10 percent of these hypotheses were supported. The Project appeared to be plagued throughout with difficulties in evaluating and assessing situational variables.

As a final comment, I cannot help raising a "what might have been" fantasy. Suppose that, twenty years ago, a psychoanalytic institute had adopted a simple, brief, standardized assessment program that provided a uniform, quantitative data base on all cases. The assessment battery would have included demographic, history, and clinical variables, brief patient self-rating devices, and clinician rating scales. It would have been administered at three points in time: admission, end of treatment, and followup. Large numbers of cases would have been accumulated. Analyses of relationships would have been conducted easily and inexpensively. After, say, five to ten years prediction studies might have revealed that identifiable kinds of patients improved markedly while others did not.

Someone might then have planned, conducted, and reported controlled studies on whether it was the treatment method that produced the improvement; someone else might have experimented with and reported the results of alternative treatments for the non-improver types; and so on. Would the yield of such a program have been more, less, or about the same? My Manifest Bias Scale score must be obvious.

One way of ending might be to say that the time is long overdue for psychoanalysts to produce some treatment evaluations and research worthy of serious attention. This is hardly original. I have been hearing it for twenty-five years. I once thought it was an important issue. I am no longer convinced that it is. The analysts and their patients can decide for themselves.

NOTE

1. My comments represent my opinions about a specific research project and the current status of research on the effects of psychoanalysis. They are not opinions about psychoanalysis as a treatment method.

6

DISCUSSION:
How Long the Tower of Babel?

LESTON L. HAVENS

I want to underline a problem suggested by several of these papers and add what seems to me the means for its solution.

The paper of Luborsky, Singer, and Luborsky strengthens the impression, given so strongly and consistently by their work, that they are sophisticated and critical, on the one hand, and sympathetic to the great difficulties of this research, on the other. We are all the more motivated to seek a solution to the problem with which they close the paper: what are "the components of a helping relationship"?

I suggest that attempts to deal with this problem have been hindered by the state of the art; that is, we are poorly placed to define components of a helping relationship. It seems to me that the other papers in the group illustrate this, too.

The first authors write: "The most potent explanatory factor is that the different forms of psychotherapeutic treatment have a major common element—a helping relationship with a therapist is present in all of them, along with the other related nonspecific effects such as suggestion and abreaction." This sentence makes my point nicely. What is "a helping relationship"? Does it mean principally an intention to help plus the presence of someone to be helped? Is that any more "specific" than the various "nonspecific" components, such as suggestion and abreaction, or the provision of the patient "with a plausible explanatory system," to which the authors and Dr. Frank allude favorably? We cannot even assume there is a *single* "major common element." Many components may help; not all of them are shared by all the methods. Penicillin and surgery both sometimes help; both generally require a "helping relationship." In the case of penicillin, however, the helping relationship can be with oneself; not every patient who treats himself has a fool for a doctor. (At least, no one has felt like stating that about Freud's self-analysis!) The point is that we cannot assume that a single factor is at work or that a helping relationship is present or that any component is nonspecific.

Let me illustrate this further by three sentences from Dr. Kernberg's paper. "Our general conclusion was that while high initial *Ego Strength*

Leston L. Havens, M.D., Professor of Psychiatry, Massachusetts Mental Health Center, Harvard University Medical School.

62

implies a good prognosis for all modalities of treatment within a psychoanalytic frame of reference, psychoanalysis may bring about the highest degree of improvement in such patients." On the other hand, patients "with low initial *Ego Strength* treated by therapists with high skill improved to a significantly greater extent when the focus on the transference . . . was high. Therefore, we concluded that the lower the initial *Ego Strength* of the patient, the more important is the work with the transference in determining the outcome of the treatment."

The accepted teaching is that transference interpretation is the *sine qua non* of psychoanalysis. Work with the transference is regarded as the essential element in determining the outcome of the treatment. On the other hand, Dr. Kernberg finds that those patients who do least well in psychoanalysis most require work with the transference. Here there is either a paradox or the much sought "major common element." Both the high and low ego strength patients require work with the transference!

The paradox is resolved and the major common element preserved by specifying *how* one works with the transference. Presumably this was done by interpretation in the psychoanalyses. In the case of the low initial ego strength patients the technical methods are not so clear. Such patients required "a special modality of treatment which could be described as a modified expressive or supportive-expressive approach." My point again is that the description of the psychotherapeutic components is unsatisfactory. How, for example, does one work with the transference non-analytically? Some hints are available in the Sullivanian literature (Havens, 1973). The work takes a quite different shape in existential psychiatry (Havens, 1974). No more than a start has been made in describing these new methods with a degree of precision comparable to that of psychoanalysis and some of the objective-descriptive techniques.

In Dr. Frank's paper we encounter still a third "major common element." "Two features of all forms of psychotherapy which enhance the patient's sense of mastery over himself and his environment are a coherent conceptual framework and the provision of success experiences." Many different means lie at hand for producing these results. Their effectiveness depends upon the extent to which they do. That, Dr. Frank might argue, would explain the results of the first paper. The various means, group or individual therapy, this school's method or that, matter less than the "two features." Therefore everyone can win a prize.

Dr. Frank's idea could also explain a good part of Dr. Kernberg's presentation. Surely the patient's "sense of mastery over himself and his environment," his having "a coherent conceptual framework," even the occurrence of "success experiences" must be highly correlated with what Dr. Kernberg calls high ego strength. Indeed, Dr. Frank's two features can be directly translated into a cognitively and experientially strong ego.

(No one to my knowledge, since Ives Hendrick, has attempted to locate the sense of mastery outside the ego, in the id.) In short, psychotherapy should be ego-strengthening.

Difficulties, it seems to me, enter from two directions. Dr. Frank explains both too little and too much. He explains too little in that he overlooks other ways to help, for example, by changes in restrictive consciences or revisions of our grasp of the past. It is true that the endpoint of these efforts, too, may be increased cognitive and experiential mastery, but that is to fall into the second error of explaining too much. Dr. Frank would not then be describing a major component of psychotherapeutic work; he would be describing a major endpoint or ideal. Few would question that increased mastery is a major endpoint or even that such a phrase may perhaps be used to subsume all other goals without stretching its meaning too outrageously. The problem, however, is a technical one. Our goals provoke far less disagreement than do the means we have to reach them.

Insofar as clinical methods produce mastery they are effective: most, as I say, would agree to that. But what are the best technical means to achieve mastery in this particular case or that? There the schools part company. We do not even have the conceptual framework within which to describe and compare methods.

REFERENCES

Havens, L. L. *Approaches to the mind: movement of the psychiatric schools from sects toward science.* Boston: Little, Brown, 1973, pp. 182–203, 305–312.

Havens, L. L. The existential use of the self. *American Journal of Psychiatry*, 1974, **131**, 1–10.

GENERAL DISCUSSION

DR. JOSEPH ZUBIN:* I can't help but feel that there is perhaps a middle ground between Dr. McNair's pessimism and Dr. Haven's optimism. Let me point out from my own experience how the picture of psychoanalysis has altered over the last forty years. When I entered the field forty years ago at the Psychiatric Institute I came fresh with my psychometric tools and experimental designs ready to apply them to the assessment of the mentally ill. To my great chagrin I discovered that the reigning spirit was psychoanalysis, which had no use for measurement, and, as a matter of fact, I was told that to measure these patients interferes with their therapeutic progress. This did not deter me from entering the field, and despite my colleagues' objections I made several attempts at evaluation.

The next development that comes to mind is the last meeting of this Association devoted to evaluation of psychotherapy some ten years ago. There for the first time I noticed that evaluation had been laid aside in favor of an escape into process. Since therapy could not be evaluated, it was decided to look at the process itself and forget about evaluation.

Now I am delighted to see that at this meeting we have turned matters around and come back to the possibility of evaluation, even with all the convolutions evident in the preceding papers. Furthermore, it is possible that studying the process itself may reveal the components necessary for evaluation.

DR. ISAAC MARKS:† Well, a few thousand years ago somebody said "To them that hath it shall be given even more," and a pervasive finding we get from many studies seems to be that people who already have a lot of assets gain more from a wide variety of treatments.

I don't think we can use this generalized finding to explain everything about psychotherapy or psychoanalysis. I think we will get a more fruitful idea about the many different facets of psychotherapy which might be potent if we divide variables into at least two kinds, those that transcend techniques and problems and those which are specific to particular techniques or to patients with particular kinds of clinical difficulties. The example of mastery which Professor Frank gave us may be one instance

---

*Biometrics Research Unit, New York State Department of Mental Hygiene.
†Institute of Psychiatry, University of London.

of a transcendental variable, although it is not yet clear under what conditions mastery may be important and under what conditions not.

Another question to which we need to pay attention is just how large a difference is significant. In Professor Frank's figures it was clear that the difference between mastery and non-mastery was relatively small. In other words, the concept is useful but it does not produce a massive effect. We must use it and build it in as part of our therapeutic armamentarium. But what about all the rest of the variables that can lead to improvement? The paper contained very interesting asides about the way patients valued a chat with a tape recorder, with subsequent feedback on tape from a psychiatrist. Maybe in this area we will get an even bigger payoff.

So we should not think only in terms of single dominant variables but also of many factors acting together. Furthermore, what is therapeutic in one set of mental disorders may not be in another. Influences governing the relief of depression may have little relevance to the reduction of compulsive rituals. We need to be more specific in our thinking—specific with respect to techniques and to different clinical problems—while recognizing that there are also variables which transcend methods and diagnoses.

DR. FRITZ A. FREYHAN:* Just a note: we have heard multiple references to "strong and weak egos." To lend some measure of specificity to such terms we need a psychopathological frame of reference. While ego strength is hardly measurable, it should at least relate to such dimensions as mood disorders, obsessive neuroses, etc.

DR. KERNBERG: I would like to address myself first to Dr. McNair's comments. I am sorry that Dr. McNair could address himself only to the report "Psychotherapy and psychoanalysis: final report of the Menninger Foundation's Psychotherapy Research Project," and not to the paper I presented here today. I think that some of his questions may have been answered in my presentation here, particularly the analysis of the relevance of our findings for future psychotherapy research and our own thinking regarding strengths and weaknesses of the methodology applied. A number of Dr. McNair's questions and criticisms have been focused upon in earlier reports and discussions, for example, the one recently published in the *International Journal of Psychiatry* (Discussion of psychotherapy and psychoanalysis: final report of the Menninger Foundation's Psychotherapy Research Project, 1973, **11**, 95-103). I will limit myself here to some salient observations by Dr. McNair.

Regarding the Paired Comparisons procedure—in which two independent raters used clinical notes and summaries as the data base—this procedure is really not complex at all from the viewpoint of the raters; in

*Editor-in-Chief, *Comprehensive Psychiatry*.

fact, it corresponds to the natural tendency of clinicians to compare two patients from a certain angle or viewpoint. Our main retrospective criticism of this procedure was the inordinate length of time needed to carry it out for all the variables at all points of time; however, the Paired Comparisons permitted us—for the first time, we believe—to quantify clinically significant and conceptually complex variables within psychoanalytic psychotherapy and psychoanalytic theory at large.

Dr. McNair finds it disappointing that our Project did not identify some other important, reliably measurable patient dimensions that were relatively independent of symptom severity, and wishes that we had utilized patient self-ratings and observer assessments via clinical rating scales. One of the major objectives in our efforts to evaluate patient variables was to determine whether overall quantitative measures of change—including various qualitative dimensions—were feasible, in contrast to evaluating change along several relatively independent dimensions. The Health-Sickness Rating Scale reflected such an integrated, quantitative instrument, and its high correlation with the Paired Comparisons of Change provided, it seems to me, crucial support for the use of simplified integrative quantitative scales for evaluating improvement. At the same time, our small sample of 42 cases may very well have precluded the differentiation of other patient variables which were merged in the overall factor of *Ego Strength*. Although it is true that *Severity of Symptoms* turned out to be an excellent marker of *Ego Strength*, I do not think that we know whether future statistical analyses of larger patient populations will reveal the importance of other variables and point to other *Ego Strength* factors. Clinically speaking, there are patients who have definite manifestations of ego weakness and yet a remarkable absence of manifest symptoms, such as patients with severe narcissistic character features and antisocial trends. For the sophisticated clinician, a simple measure of improvement along a symptom list does not, it seems to me, convincingly cover the field.

I also wish to stress—in referring to Dr. McNair's wish that patient self-ratings and observers' assessment had been included—that the design, in order to be a truly naturalistic one, attempted to leave the natural treatment setting undisturbed, and that neither patients nor therapists were aware at the initial time or during the entire duration of the treatment that their patients were part of our research population.

Dr. McNair mentions that the data base was not the same from patient to patient and that he did not find simple descriptive statistics on the patient and the treatments, such as basic demographic statistics and their relations to outcome. Some of these data have been referred to in earlier publications, and others will be included in the case histories which Dr. Robert Wallerstein is preparing at this time for publication. The general demographic data were largely unrelated to outcome, as was the number of treatment hours and the total duration of treatment as such. As mentioned in the final report on the quantitative studies, such relationships as did emerge involved the nature of the therapeutic techniques, ego strength, the therapists' skill, etc.; I referred to this more extensively in my paper.

In discussing the MSA results, Dr. McNair states that, as there was no random assignment to treatment, the patients in the different treatment groups probably differed markedly at admission and that MSA results may reflect the confounding of treatment and initial severity. I disagree; both quantitative studies reveal that patients assigned to psychoanalysis and psychotherapy did not differ in their initial *Ego Strength* and severity of psychopathology in general.

Regarding our selection criteria, we explicitly assigned patients on a non-random basis to what was believed to be best for each patient, and, therefore, to some extent at least, the results of the study are produced by the treatment selection criteria of the therapist. Under these circumstances our findings, which were opposite to what we expected from the viewpoint prevalent at the time of the initiation of the study, are I think particularly meaningful. In retrospect, some of the treatment indications were done erroneously on the basis of traditionally accepted recommendations of certain treatment modalities for certain types of patients; this, we believe, strengthens our findings which go against "researcher bias."

Dr. McNair mentioned repeatedly the fact that about half of the treatment hypotheses were confirmed, perhaps to imply that these may have been chance correlations. One reason for carrying out the two independent quantitative studies was to evaluate all our hypotheses within a comprehensive, overall predictive statement, and our combined analyses of both quantitative findings differentiate overriding consistencies from correlations affecting only subgroups or partial issues.

Dr. McNair questions the assessment of the therapist's skill with individual cases, suggesting that this may well have amounted to just another way of measuring outcome. We found that the skill demonstrated in each particular case was highly correlated with the therapist's general level of skill.

As I have mentioned in my presentation, we fully agree with Dr. McNair's comment that the Project was plagued throughout with difficulties in evaluating and assessing situational variables.

Now, regarding Dr. McNair's final comment about "what might have been," I want to stress that when this project started, about twenty years ago, there was no agreement as to the major variables which influence treatment outcome, no agreement as to whether these variables could be quantified, and no agreement as to whether outcome itself—or sophisticated conceptions of it—could be quantified at all. This Project was able to define crucial variables in psychoanalysis and psychoanalytic psychotherapy and to quantify some of these variables in ways which did justice to their clinical complexity and yet were relatively simple for research evaluation. The testing of the relationships among such relatively sophisticated, clinically valid, and reliable variables represents, it seems to me, an important contribution to the field of psychotherapy research and practice. The overall findings of the Project indicate that patients with ego weakness need treatment techniques different from those used with patients with better ego functioning and suggest the possibility of specifying the kind of treatments that are needed for such patients. These findings are, it seems to me, exciting, and have already influenced the clinical field of psychoanalytic psychotherapy.

After the battle, everybody is a general. Probably, if we had to start all over again now, knowing all that we have learned, we would do things differently. However, the findings derived from the Project, it seems to me, not only warrant the lengthy effort but also explain the fact that this has been one of the very few psychotherapy research projects which have effectively influenced treatment practices (beyond the narrow range of the researchers directly involved). This is important, particularly because psychotherapy researchers frequently complain that clinicians pay little attention to them or that research findings have not made much impact on daily practice.

In response to Dr. Freyhan's question, I think that it is possible now to define patients along a dimension of *Ego Strength* which would clinically be independent from the dimension of *Severity of Symptoms*. I think that we can now, in part because of the findings of the Project, establish a better selection of patients along the dimensions of what I call "high level," "intermediate level," and "low level" of ego organization or *Ego Strength*, having characteristics independent of the dimension of severity of symptoms such as depression, anxiety, etc. And, therefore, I think that we can now carry out a better selection of patient populations for outcome studies.

DR. McNAIR: One of the hazards of being a "wise critical discussant" is that people hear and react to you as "critic," but never as "wise." First, the simple reason why I did not read Dr. Kernberg's paper in advance is that he did not submit it in advance. Second, in my view, almost none of my questions and reservations about the Menninger Project were answered satisfactorily by the presentation today.

The data for the Paired Comparisons procedure consisted of a one-paragraph summary for each of the 42 cases derived from clinical notes. A batch of 12 of these paragraphs were selected, and these 12 patients were compared, two at a time, with each other. The procedure was repeated for each characteristic measured. Then six patients from the first batch were included in the next batch of 12, etc., so that seven batches were required to rate the 42 cases. The end result was presumed to represent a comparison of every patient with every other patient. Dr. Kernberg clearly recognizes the complexity of this procedure. Also the quality of the original clinical notes and the selectivity that goes into generating the condensed summaries raise enormous methodological and substantive issues. Dr. Robbins presented data this morning (see p. 44) suggesting that the improvement ratings were positively related to the quality of the clinical workups.

The *Severity of Symptoms* Paired Comparisons scaling consistently (at three points in time) had the highest correlations with the other 12 measures. *Severity of Symptoms* also loaded very highly on the major factor identified, *Ego Strength*, and it was as good an indicator as any of the meaning of this factor. Also, as I recall, the *Ego Strength* and *Severity of Symptoms* correlations ranged from about .80 to .95. This means to me that these measures are largely redundant. Obviously, whenever there is a correlation of less than 1.00 between two measures, some cases may score high on one and low on the other. Such examples would be extremely rare, however, in a sample of only 42.

I want to make three other points quickly. First, if you do not randomly assign patients to treatments, you simply cannot attribute different outcomes to the different treatments as opposed to such confounding factors as, for example, pretreatment patient differences. It is the investigator's job to show, at least, that such alternative explanations are implausible. Dr. Kernberg's comments further indicate that alternative explanations are not only plausible but likely. Second, how does he determine that a general measure and a specific measure of therapist competence are "highly correlated" when he clearly states in the final report that it was not possible to obtain a satisfactory measure of general competence? Finally, it is asserted that the findings of the Project have influenced psychoanalytic practice. I would like to see the evidence that these findings, in fact, have stimulated changes in techniques, and I would caution that any such changes may prove to be ill-founded.

DR. ROBBINS: I want to reiterate that originally we made a commitment to a naturalistic design. This precluded the random assignment of patients to different types of treatment, the type of treatment having been determined by the clinical staff using their clinical criteria and judgments. Had we, for example, assigned patients with low ego strength to each type of psychotherapy in order to have an equal number in each cell, this would have been a totally different project. The use of a naturalistic design also limited the use of certain statistical approaches and the employment of others such as the method of Paired Comparisons and the Multidimensional Scalogram Analysis.

During the time prior to 1954 when this project was being originally conceptualized by Drs. Paul Bergman, Helen Sargent, and others, no one had anticipated the length of time it would take, the problems that would be encountered, and the inconclusiveness of the findings. In retrospect, I feel that if I had to do this all over again, I wouldn't do it, although I cannot think of a better way to have done what we tried to do.

It should be kept in mind that this was, basically, neither a hypothesis testing nor an outcome study, but rather a hypothesis finding and hypothesis refining project. In addition it was an effort to develop and test new methodologies such as using clinical judgments as primary data, employing the method of Paired Comparisons, etc.

This project began over twenty years ago, covering over half the period of time to which Dr. Zubin referred. Since then psychoanalytic concepts have evolved and changed to some extent, and new forms of therapy such as behavior modification have developed. When this project began, the two principal psychotherapy schools were the nondirective, client-centered approach and psychoanalysis.

In response to Dr. Freyhan's question about our having chosen such variables as *Ego Strength* without attaching them to well-established clinical syndromes, I must first state that it was our feeling and experience that diagnostic categories, in themselves, are not sufficiently precise nor predictive. For example, during World War II 90 percent of the conditions seen were character disorders not described in our diagnostic manuals. The classifying of clinical syndromes is constantly changing, as evidenced, for example, by the current discussion regarding homosexuality. Feeling that formal diagnostic categories were too limited, Dr. Wallerstein and I attempted to determine what patient variables were used by clinicians in deciding the type of psychotherapy to recommend. We then attempted in each case to make the implicit clinical judgments and predictions based upon them as explicit as possible. We hoped thereby to reach greater accuracy than we felt could be achieved by employing the usual diagnostic categories.

DR. DONALD F. KLEIN:* I think it is a real headache, as Dr. McNair pointed out, that the patients received different treatment depending on their naturalistic state. Therefore I don't see how it can be claimed that the borderline patients responded to one specific type of treatment when the type of treatment they got was determined by their initial state.

Another thing that disturbs me somewhat is that I don't have any real feel for the amount of improvement that we are talking about. What we have been discussing is the comparison of differential effectiveness between "different treatment methods and different levels of ego strength," but I don't know whether these did wonders, worked medium

*Long Island Jewish-Hillside Medical Center.

okay, worked just barely okay, or worked very badly. If I am going to decide whether to use one treatment method or another, it is because I want to make a real impact on the situation. I would appreciate if Dr. Kernberg could speak to that point.

It certainly has been my limited personal psychotherapy experience, augmented by observing a fair amount of psychotherapy, that people treating borderlines do get involved in complex emotional interactions and that often these interactions are ignored in a passive way until the whole situation blows up.

So it strikes a responsive chord with me to hear Dr. Kernberg say the treatment relationship of borderline patients is a primary concern. Dr. Havens was also saying that you must deal with this not in a passive interpretive framework but in an active participant framework.

DR. KERNBERG: The initial philosophy of the Project was geared toward the study of change. We assumed that change would proceed in various directions, which had to be predicted individually in terms of the specific problems of each patient. There was a general theoretical reluctance to think of one overall dimension of improvement in contrast to multiple dimensions of change. The statistical analysis, however, indicated that the dimensions of change were highly related and that evaluation of an overall dimension of change in the direction of improvement was, indeed, feasible. The high correlation of the Paired Comparisons of Change with the Health-Sickness Rating Scale was one important piece of evidence in this regard.

Thus our attitude changed, and we started to talk about improvement rather than about change. Our main dimensions were the Paired Comparisons of Change and the Health-Sickness Rating Scale. We have been impressed by the research potentials of the Health-Sickness Rating Scale, and I have referred to this in detail in my paper.

Regarding the question by Dr. Klein about the treatment of borderline patients, it is true that the techniques of supportive psychotherapy were less precisely defined than those of standard psychoanalysis. On the basis of our instruments, and from the viewpoint of the quantitative analyses, we were not able to define supportive techniques except along the two dimensions referred to in my paper: these dimensions were the degree to which interpretive techniques were used, and the extent to which there was provision of supportive techniques. Supportive techniques included active suggestion, advice, and manipulative techniques. All of these were in contrast to expressive techniques such as clarification and interpretation.

One new and I think important finding was that if the therapist remained in a relatively neutral position from a technical viewpoint and provided relatively little support—while the patient obtained important structuralization of his life outside of therapy—the treatment results with borderline patients were better than in the contrary case, that is, when external support was lacking, and the psychotherapy proper was purely supportive. You may be aware that in other studies that I have carried out in recent years regarding the diagnosis and treatment of borderline patients I have reached similar conclusions.

DR. GEORGE MURPHY:* I would like to come back to the fact that basic to the evaluation of therapy in medicine is a knowledge of the natural history of the disease being treated. Now it has been shown today and elsewhere that it is possible in some ways to evaluate changes in patients who are exposed to various therapies. But we can't tell whether the treatment, as opposed to the natural history of the disorder treated, is relevant to change. The poor state of our knowledge of the natural history of some psychiatric illnesses, as alluded to by Dr. Robbins, is not an excuse. We have to recognize where we are and do what we can to improve that situation.

Psychotherapy seems to deal with a more heterogeneous population, whereas in pharmacotherapy target populations are more clearly defined, and exciting results are forthcoming. Not until we know more clearly the natural history of the diseases being treated is much to be expected from studies of the results of psychoanalysis. Untreated undescribed patients will not serve as a control. This is not offered as a put-down of psychotherapy, in which I have a considerable professional investment, but simply as a comment.

*Washington University School of Medicine.

7 PRESIDENTIAL ADDRESS: Brain Function, Verbal Behavior, and Psychotherapy

MAX FINK

In the proceedings of a recent symposium of the American Psychopathological Association, Freyhan (1972) noted that the founders were physicians, mostly neurologists, who actively treated the severe mentally ill. They were not satisfied to approach their patients from a neurologic framework alone, to view the mind and behavior as reflex expressions; nor did they view "mind" as a byproduct of the history of the subject, removed from the functions of the brain. In their discussions, they attempted to integrate the mechanistic views of the structural neurologists and neuropathologists with the dynamic views of the individual psychologists. This session of the Association is dedicated to an evaluation of psychological therapies, particularly the joint use of psychological and pharmacologic interventions. It seems timely to review studies of the interaction of changes in brain function and changes in language, attitude, and perception for their contributions to the problems of this conference.

In relating somatic and psychotherapies, psychotherapy is usually defined as "supportive," focused on present-day interpersonal relations in work, family, and social situations. Outcome criteria are rarely defined in psychologic terms but usually as changes in social or family adjustments or in symptoms measured by self-rating scales. Lacking in studies of combined therapies (i.e., psychotherapy and pharmacotherapy in schizophrenia, depression, and neuroses) is a theoretical framework with predictors and outcome measures, derived from psychological constructs.

More than twenty years ago, David M. Rioch and Edwin A. Weinstein, influenced by the psychological views of Harry Stack Sullivan, W. Alanson White, and Clara Thompson and the neurophysiologic observations of Kurt Goldstein and Karl Lashley, described systematic changes in

Max Fink, M.D., Department of Psychiatry, Health Sciences Center, State University of New York at Stony Brook; President, American Psychopathological Association, 1973-1974.

The work was supported in part by National Institute of Mental Health Research Grants MH-15561, MH-20872, and MH-24020.

language following acute brain injury and suggested that the altered syntax, form, and rate of speech served defensive and adaptational purposes. In an extraordinary volume, *Denial of Illness*, Weinstein and Kahn (1955) described changes in language in patients with brain damage before and after the administration of amobarbital. While patients with brain damage may exhibit disorientation and denial of illness before amobarbital, these adaptations were so characteristic after amobarbital as to be recommended as a diagnostic test for diffuse organic brain dysfunction. The concepts of adaptive responses to altered brain function, particularly in language, mood, and attitude, provided interesting and testable hypotheses relevant to the interaction of somatic and psychological therapies, to the evaluation of outcome, and to the definition of predictors.

LANGUAGE AS ADAPTIVE RESPONSE

One application of this view was in the question of whether defensive operations could be defined during experimentally induced brain dysfunction, as in convulsive therapy. In 1958 we described the effects of amobarbital on the language of patients in whom seizures were induced three times a week under standard conditions (Kahn & Fink, 1958). Interviews were held prior to the first treatment, after four to six, and again after seven to nine convulsions. Amobarbital was given at a fixed rate of 0.05 grams/minute until nystagmus, slurred speech, drowsiness, and errors in counting backward were noted. A standardized series of questions was used.

Patients' speech changed progressively during treatment. They used third-person references rather than first person; answered questions by another question or evasion; used many more qualifiers, such as "kind of," "sort of," and "possibly"; used the past tense rather than the present, even for present-related statements; and displaced or minimized symptoms. They frequently used cliches and stereotyped expressions. After amobarbital, these changes became more prominent and developed earlier in the course of treatment, and two new adaptations were observed—cryptic responses, and withdrawal or failure to respond to questions (Kahn, Fink, & Weinstein, 1955, 1956). We interpreted these language changes as manifestations of denial and distance—as adaptations which served a therapeutic aim.

These syntactic language changes during treatment were related to the outcome evaluations: patients rated as much improved exhibited more syntactic language changes and did so earlier in their treatment course than patients evaluated as unimproved. In the two-thirds of the patients who responded best to convulsive therapy, these denial language patterns were prominent in amobarbital interviews before treatment was started, suggesting that their presence was a predictor of response. The language changes were also positively related to independent measures of brain change—increases in EEG slow-wave (2–6 Hz) activities. When we examined other relations of pre-treatment denial language patterns, we found not only a relation to outcome evaluations but also a relation to the degree of measured neurophysiologic change—the higher the pre-treatment denial language score, the greater the percent time slow-wave activity induced during treatment (Kahn & Fink, 1958).

This investigation, based on a highly structured interview, focused on the syntactic aspects of the subject's responses. To describe language changes in an unstructured interview, and their effects on the observer, Jaffe (1957) applied an analysis of speech diversity, the Type-Token Ratio (TTR). This is a measure of the redundancy of words of both patient and therapist: the lower the ratio, the greater the repetitiveness. In a population similar to that in the amobarbital study, we determined the TTR for 25-word units in the first 500 words of clinical interviews in 25 ECT-treated and 10 control patients (Jaffe, Fink, & Kahn, 1960). With repeated seizures, the mean TTR decreased and the standard deviation increased, reflecting an increased repetition of words. This increase was accompanied by a qualitative stereotypy, as in the increased use of cliches. As in the denial language analyses, the decrease in TTR was related to an increase in EEG slow-wave activity.

We next examined the effects of diethazine, a phenothiazine derivative said to increase EEG slow waves, on the language of schizophrenic patients. Diethazine not only failed to increase EEG slow-wave activity but sharply reduced it (Fink, 1958). We used diethazine in a fashion similar to amobarbital in examining convulsive therapy patients at various stages of their treatment. Prior to treatment, diethazine increased the diversity of speech and the number of self-references and reduced the syntactic changes we had learned to associate with increased EEG slow-wave activity. These effects were even more marked during treatment, when diethazine sharply reduced EEG slow-wave activity. Surprisingly, this change in cerebral measures was accompanied by a reduction in syntactic changes, a decrease in redundance of speech, and an increase in symptoms reported by the patients. The reversal in language and symptoms was so marked that we curtailed these studies as too uncomfortable for the patients.

The association of a reduction in post-convulsive EEG slow waves with increased variability of speech, increased use of present tense, and lesser use of cliches and evasive responses was further examined by testing other compounds known to inhibit post-seizure EEG slow-wave activity: anticholinergics like benactyzine and ditran; the antihistamine diphenhydramine; and the stimulants amphetamine and lysergide (LSD-25). With each substance, when cerebral slow-wave activity decreased, patients exhibited a greater diversity of speech and a reduction in the syntactic measures of denial which we had identified as "improvement" in the convulsive therapy process (Fink, Jaffe, & Kahn, 1960; Fink, 1960).

Similar studies were undertaken in schizophrenic patients receiving repeated administrations of lysergide (LSD-25). Don, Stevens, and Fink (1965) examined the effect of 1 mcg/kg LSD on the TTR during a five-hour observation period. They observed an increase in the diversity of speech associated with the reduction in EEG slow waves and an increase in fast (beta) frequencies.

ATTITUDE AS ADAPTIVE RESPONSE

Attitudinal measures also change as brain function is altered by repeated convulsions. The modified California F-Scale consists of ten statements of the type "No sane, normal, decent person could ever think of hurting a close friend or relative," and "If people would talk less and work more, everybody would be better off" (Kahn, Pollack, & Fink, 1960a). The subject is asked to indicate the degree of his agreement or disagreement with these statements on a seven-point scale, with high scores indicating maximal agreement. The scale is said to measure stereotypy in thinking and authoritarianism and was derived from studies of political attitudes.

As with the linguistic measures, we observed a systematic increase in F-Scale scores with increasing numbers of treatments. We also found a positive correlation between the increase in the F-Scale score and the amount of EEG slow-wave activity. Indeed, there was an unusual predictive quality for the F-Scale score: patients with the higher initial scores developed greater degrees of physiologic change and greater increases in the F-Scale scores with equivalent numbers of treatments.

Further, the greater the increase in F-Scale score with treatment, the greater the degree of behavioral change and the better the improvement ratings. High-scoring patients are considered to be stereotyped in their thinking, to have difficulty in introspection, and to use language with a limited variability in words—attributes that we believe contributed to their selection for a non-verbal therapy and to the increase in repetitiveness, use of cliches, and denial which characterized their improvement process (Fink & Kahn, 1961).

PERCEPTUAL CHANGE IN ADAPTATION

The perceptual changes associated with brain change also contribute to the adaptive process. In perceptual studies in the same population, we observed the decreases in performance on recent and remote memory tasks, in measures of recall, in the perception of tachistoscopic figures, and in the critical flicker fusion rate (Fink, Kahn, & Pollack, 1959; Karp, Pollack, & Fink, 1962; Korin, Fink, & Kwalwasser, 1956; Pollack, Kahn, Karp, & Fink, 1962). We also found an impairment in performance in the Gottschaldt Hidden Figures Test (Kahn & Fink, 1957; Kahn, Pollack, & Fink, 1960b). This test measures the discrimination of visual geometric figures from a complex background. It is a timed, twenty-five-item task with progressively more difficult figures as earlier figures are completed. With increasing numbers of seizures, errors increase, and this increase is related to the increase in EEG slow-wave activity. As was found in the case of the California F-Scale scores, patients with the poorest pre-treatment performance showed the greatest increase in the degree of EEG slow-wave activity.

We interpreted the decrease in ability to discriminate figure from background and the increase in stereotypy and conformity on the attitude scale as processes supporting the adaptive changes of denial, minimization, cliches, and repetitive speech which characterized earlier studies. We found some confirmation of this belief in studies of Rorschach criteria as predictors of outcome (Kahn & Fink, 1960); in characterizing the behavioral responses to convulsive therapy (Fink & Kahn, 1961); in defining the characteristics of patients who are selected for convulsive therapy (Kahn & Fink, 1959; Kahn & Pollack, 1959; Kahn, Pollack, & Fink, 1957, 1959); and in defining the characteristics of patients who refuse convulsive therapy (Pollack & Fink, 1961). From these diverse studies, we were encouraged to view the relation between changes in brain function and changes in behavior as part of a general theory of the association of brain change and interpersonal behavior in man.

CASE REPORT

Before approaching a more general view as a theory, I would like to relate one set of observations in which the interpersonal and physiologic data were studied in a therapeutic situation. At the time of these studies, my coworkers R. L. Kahn and J. Jaffe suggested that we observe directly the therapeutic interactions of resident therapists with their patients, particularly those referred for convulsive therapy. We established a supervisory seminar about the case load of a resident therapist, Dr. Harold Esecover (Jaffe, Esecover, Kahn, & Fink, 1961).

One patient, a forty-four-year-old widow and mother, had been hospitalized for three months for depression, anxiety, anorexia, physical complaints, and feelings of unreality and isolation. After three months' observation and psychotherapy, she was referred for convulsive therapy, and her case was included in the supervisory seminar. The supervisory sessions were informal, the therapist presenting his cases as he wished. Some observations during the three months of supervision are shown in Figure 1.

In this patient's treatment, two forms of somatic therapy were utilized, a 27-day period of subconvulsive treatments (three applications a week for twelve treatments) followed by twelve convulsive treatments (days 29 to 59) and a followup period of 35 days. The therapist, the patient, and the members of the supervisory group were not aware that the initial treatments were subconvulsive, nor did they know that the mode of treatment changed at day 29. Although patient and therapist expected a therapeutic benefit from convulsive therapy, no changes in their interaction or symptoms occurred throughout the period of subconvulsive administrations. The first changes were noted on the 38th day—the day after the fifth *convulsive* treatment—when the therapist reported some slight changes in the interaction. These were clearly identified by the therapist and by the patient on the 45th day—after the seventh convulsive treatment—at a time when the physiologic measures showed an increase to 13 percent slow-wave activity. During the twenty days of measurable physiologic changes, the patient exhibited reductions in symptoms and increased euphoria, denial, and language changes; the therapist showed increasing interest, recording a greater number of pages of notes; and the variety and intensity of their interactions increased. Even with the regression in physiologic changes following the end of the induced seizures (after day 60), the language and communication patterns maintained their changed mode, leading eventually to a satisfactory therapeutic evaluation.

The change in therapeutic interactions was occasioned not only by referral for somatic therapy, with its symbolic interpretations, but by the neurophysiologic consequences and the accompanying perceptual, linguistic, and mood changes following repeated seizures.

A THEORETIC CONSTRUCT

In 1968, in reviewing the effects of different psychoactive compounds on the EEG, we and others were able to identify at least four, and probably seven, classes of EEG effects (Fink, 1968, 1969) (see Table 1). Using these classes, it was possible to pigeonhole the known psychoactive compounds according to their EEG patterns, and it was thereby found that compounds with similar clinical uses exhibited similar EEG effects. This classification has since been used to predict the therapeutic range and applications for numbered psychoactive drugs in Phase-I clinical studies (Fink, 1974). I believe these observations lend themselves to a calculus of the interaction of verbal behavior in the psychotherapeutic relationship with the brain changes induced by the administration of psychoactive

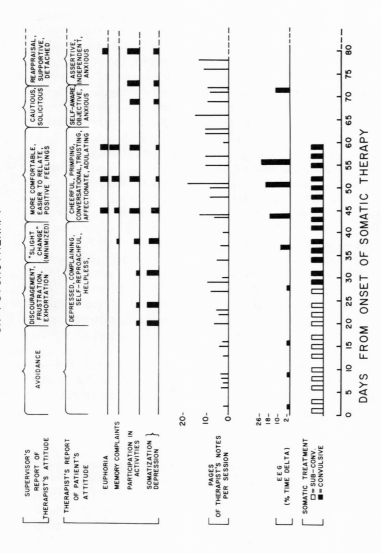

EFFECT OF CHANGING BRAIN FUNCTION
ON PSYCHOTHERAPY

FIG. 1. Course of observations in supervised therapy of forty-four-year-old woman who received subconvulsive and convulsive therapy concurrently. (Source: Jaffe, Esecover, Kahn, & Fink, 1961, p. 48.)

Table 1. EEG Effects of Psychoactive Drugs

	Frequency (Hz)								Amplitude		Pattern	Example
	Mean	Varia-bility of Mean	Delta (0.1–3.5)	Theta (3.5–7.5)	Alpha (7.5–13.0)	Slow Beta (13.0–18.0)	Beta (18–26)	Fast Beta (26–35)	Total Energy	Varia-bility		
Ia	-	-	+	++	±	-	--	--	++	+	bursts	ECT, chlorpromazine
Ib	-	-	+	++	++	-	--	--	+	-		butaperazine
IIa	+	+	±	+	-	+	++	+	+	-	spindles	amobarbital
IIb	+	+	-	-	++	+	±	0	-	+	"desynchronized"	LSD, d-amphetamine
IIIa	-	+	+	++	--	+	++	+	±	+		imipramine
IIIb	-	+	++	+	-	++	++	+	++	+		atropine
IV	+	-	±	±	++	+	0	0	++	-		cannabis

Source: Adapted from Fink, 1968, p. 499.

++, marked increase
+, some increase
0, no change
±, variable response
-, some decrease
--, marked decrease

substances (or, as in these studies, by other "somatic" therapies designed to change brain functions).

Referring to the EEG classification in Table 1, we find that available compounds may either increase or decrease the amount of slow-wave activity; decrease alpha amplitudes and increase the amounts of irregular fast frequencies; increase the amount of alpha activity; increase rhythmic beta activities with an increase of theta frequencies at higher dosages; and produce additional combinations of these frequency and pattern changes. I suggest that by using combined pharmacologic and psychological therapies it is possible to predict the types of linguistic, mood, perceptual, and attitudinal changes occasioned by specified changes in brain function, and to select appropriate psychoactive substances to enhance the adaptations regarded most useful by the therapist.

Thus, barbiturates have been used by many authors for abreaction and unblocking of catatonic states. They have utilized the decreased perceptual acuity and the increase in speech redundancy, denial, and euphoria which accompanied the synchronization, beta spindling, and slowing of EEG patterns as means through which anxious thoughts and ideas can gradually be expressed, can be verbalized, and can be presented to the conscious self.

Others have used lysergide (LSD), mescaline, desoxyn, and methamphetamine to elicit EEG desynchronization and increased fast frequencies with an attendant increase in awareness and imagery and a decrease in denial. These compounds serve to diversify speech and to increase the range of therapist-patient interactions, particularly in subjects in whom speech patterns are redundant, limited, or blocked.

The phenothiazines, butyrophenones, and thioxanthenes elicit an increase in slow waves and a decrease in fast frequencies similar to those found during induced convulsions, with resulting decreases in perceptual acuity, increased repetitiveness of speech, decreased discrimination of figure from background, decreased imagery, and increased syntactic use of the displacement, denial, and minimization characteristic of ECT. In successful pharmacotherapy, these changes can be measured; where the physiologic changes fail to occur, these adaptive changes are frequently lacking and the therapeutic results are considered poor.

The thymoleptic substances have different neurophysiologic effects, characterized by an increase in slow frequencies (similar to those caused by the antipsychotic drugs), with an increase in the fast frequencies as well. At higher doses, these substances elicit delirium with obtunded consciousness, increased imagery, increased motor restlessness, decreased perceptual acuity, and repetitive speech. At the usual clinical doses of thymoleptics, these effects are less: speech is repetitive, cliches increase, denial is prominent, and motor activity is increased, as is revery, imagery, denial, and euphoria.

Recently, transcendental meditation and the inhalation of cannabis have been recommended to reduce anxiety and tension and to increase imagery, revery, and language diversity. Seen from a neurophysiologic framework, these maneuvers may be most successful in short-term situations, since enhanced alpha activities are rarely sustained by these means.

It is possible today to directly examine the neurophysiologic effects of compounds. Just as one is accustomed to use blood levels of substances such as lithium as a guide to dosage and treatment goals in that therapy, the neurophysiologic consequences of psychoactive drugs or somatic therapies may also be selected so that the adaptive changes and altered interpersonal transactions that are best suited to the disordered individual will be elicited. The goal may be to increase or decrease perceptual acuity, to diversify or increase repetitiveness of speech, to enhance imagery, to increase or decrease the use of denial, or to stimulate or reduce recall and memory. In these cases the present somatic methods are sufficient to allow less reliance on the clinical stereotypes of antipsychotic drugs for the psychotic, anti-anxiety drugs for the neurotic, and thymoleptics or convulsive therapy for the depressed. The information at hand is sufficient for an integration of the neurophysiologic effects of diverse compounds with personality typologies to produce an endless range of changes in interpersonal behaviors.

Such a calculus requires, in addition to the available neurophysiologic specificities, greater attention to psychological characterization of patients in order to define their habitual modes of adaptation and to predict the consequences of neurophysiologic change. Rather than defining populations by clinical nosology, which is so sensitive to changing social and political values, we must seek ways to define habitual adaptations by measures of language, attitude, and perception. The application of these views to studies of repeated seizures has been most useful in our understanding of the convulsive therapy process (Fink, 1972; Fink, Kety, McGaugh, & Williams, 1974). It has provided predictors in attitudinal, perceptual, and neurophysiologic measures and defined testable outcome measures with relevance to the clinical condition. In the present investigations of combined pharmacotherapy and psychotherapy, attention seems to be focused on issues which have limited long-term and theoretic value, such as clinical phenomenology based on phenotypic characteristics; fixed doses of drugs without attention to the individual differences in metabolism and the measurement of individual physiologic indices; and outcome criteria that are global and social, so responsive to the vagaries of the observer and the setting as to have limited generalizability to other populations. The experiences cited here suggest that with more attention to neurophysiologic variables, to tests of attitude, perception, language, and cognition as predictors and process variables, and to adaptive models as outcome criteria we may yet elucidate a useful theory of combined psychiatric therapies based on brain function and individual psychology.

Many years ago while viewing a performance of the Rockettes at the Radio City Music Hall, I was impressed by the changes in imagery resulting from changes in lighting. At one moment, the line consisted of a hundred dancing girls; at the next, I saw only the rhythmic movements of heels and hands suspended in a black space, to be followed by waving headdresses undulating slowly, yielding an image of grass moving in the wind. We see our patients and they see us in the light of the changing patterns of brain functions which we occasionally alter, thereby changing the imagery with which they respond to us and to their environment.. Changes induced in their neurophysiology affect their speech and perception and, both subtly and directly, affect our own speech and perception. Given the wealth of our present alchemy, we may yet learn to use the chemistry at our disposal to help the individual patient by viewing the therapeutic process as the interaction of cerebral physiology and perception, mood, and language operating in a dyadic relationship.

SUMMARY

Studies of combined psychotherapy and somatic therapy generally use clinical diagnostic criteria for the selection of the somatic therapy and evaluate results by changes in symptoms and global social ratings. In studies of induced convulsions (ECT), a physiologic-adaptive view led to studies of language, perception, and attitude as predictors and outcome criteria of adaptive response to altered brain function.

Using these experiences as a model, a theoretic construct for combined therapies is developed: a specific somatic therapy may be selected because of its defined neurophysiologic effects, which are monitored to account for individual differences in metabolism; predictors of adaptive response are defined by attitudinal, linguistic, and perceptual tests; and outcome is defined by changes in adaptation in the dyadic relationship. The theoretic model is an integration of the individual psychologic characteristics of the subject with the induced neurophysiologic effects of the various somatic therapies now available.

REFERENCES

Don, A., Stevens, J., & Fink, M. *Changes in language, EEG, and behavior induced by LSD in schizophrenic subjects.* St. Louis: Psychiatric Research Foundation, 1965.

Fink, M. Effects of anticholinergic agent, diethazine, on EEG and behavior: significance for theory of convulsive therapy. *Archives of Neurology and Psychiatry*, 1958, **80**, 380–387.

Fink, M. Effect of anticholinergic compounds on post-convulsive EEG and behavior of psychiatric patients. *Electroencephalography and Clinical Neurophysiology*, 1960, **12**, 359–369.

Fink, M. EEG classification of psychoactive compounds in man: review and theory of behavioral associations. In D. Efron, J. Cole, J. Levine, and J. R. Wittenborn (Eds.), *Psychopharmacology—a review of progress, 1957–1967.* Washington, D.C.: U.S. Government Printing Office, 1968, pp. 497–507.

Fink, M. EEG and human psychopharmacology. *Annual Review of Pharmacology,* 1969, **9,** 241–258.

Fink, M. CNS effects of convulsive therapy. In J. Zubin and F. Freyhan (Eds.), *Disorders of mood.* Baltimore: Johns Hopkins University Press, 1972, pp. 93–112.

Fink, M. EEG applications in psychopharmacology. In M. Gordon (Ed.), *Psychopharmacological agents,* Vol. 3. New York: Academic Press, 1974.

Fink, M., Jaffe, J., & Kahn, R. L. Drug-induced changes in interview patterns: linguistic and neurophysiologic indices. In G. J. Sarwer-Foner (Ed.), *The dynamics of psychiatric drug therapy.* Springfield, Ill.: C. C. Thomas, 1960, pp. 29–44.

Fink, M., & Kahn, R. L. Behavioral patterns in convulsive therapy. *Archives of General Psychiatry,* 1961, **5,** 30–36.

Fink, M., Kahn, R. L. & Pollack, M. Psychological factors affecting individual differences in behavioral response to convulsive therapy. *Journal of Nervous and Mental Disease,* 1959, **128,** 243–248.

Fink, M., Kety, S., McGaugh, J., & Williams, T. (Eds.), *Psychobiology of convulsive therapy.* Washington, D.C.: V. H. Winston and Sons, 1974.

Freyhan, F. The psychopathologist—what man of science? In J. Zubin and F. Freyhan (Eds.), *Disorders of mood.* Baltimore: Johns Hopkins University Press, 1972, pp. 1–16.

Jaffe, J. An objective study of communication in psychiatric interviews. *Journal of Hillside Hospital,* 1957, **6,** 207–215.

Jaffe, J., Esecover, H., Kahn, R. L., & Fink, M. Modification of psychotherapeutic transactions by altered brain function. *American Journal of Psychotherapy,* 1961, **15,** 46–55.

Jaffe, J., Fink, M., & Kahn, R. L. Changes in verbal transactions with induced altered brain function. *Journal of Nervous and Mental Disease,* 1960, **130,** 235–239.

Kahn, R. L., & Fink, M. Perception of embedded figures after induced altered brain function. *American Psychologist,* 1957, **12,** 361.

Kahn, R. L., & Fink, M. Changes in language during electroshock therapy. In P. Hoch and J. Zubin (Eds.), *Psychopathology of communication.* New York: Grune and Stratton, 1958, pp. 126–139.

Kahn, R. L., & Fink, M. Personality factors in behavioral response to electroshock therapy. *Journal of Neuropsychiatry,* 1959, **1,** 45–49.

Kahn, R. L., & Fink, M. Prognostic value of Rorschach criteria in clinical response to convulsive therapy. *Joural of Neuropsychiatry,* 1960, **1,** 242–245.

Kahn, R. L., Fink, M., & Weinstein, E. A. The amytal test in patients with mental illness. *Journal of Hillside Hospital,* 1955, **4,** 3–13.

Kahn, R. L., Fink, M., & Weinstein, E. A. Relation of amobarbital test to clinical improvement in electroshock. *Archives of Neurology and Psychiatry* (Chicago), 1956, **76,** 23–29.

Kahn, R. L., & Pollack, M. Prognostic application of psychological techniques in convulsive therapy. *Diseases of the Nervous System,* 1959, **20,** 180–184.

Kahn, R. L., Pollack, M., & Fink, M. Social factors in selection of therapy in a voluntary mental hospital. *Journal of Hillside Hospital,* 1957, **6,** 216–228.

Kahn, R. L., Pollack, M., & Fink, M. Sociopsychologic aspects of psychiatric treatment in a voluntary mental hospital: duration of hospitalization, discharge ratings and diagnosis. *Archives of General Psychiatry,* 1959, **1,** 565–574.

Kahn, R. L., Pollack, M., & Fink, M. Social attitude (California F-Scale) and convulsive therapy. *Journal of Nervous and Mental Disease,* 1960, **130,** 187–192. (a)

Kahn, R. L., Pollack, M., & Fink, M. Figure-ground discrimination after induced altered brain function. *Archives of Neurology and Psychiatry* (Chicago), 1960, **2,** 547–551.(b)

Karp, E., Pollack, M., & Fink, M. Critical flicker frequency and EEG alpha: a reliability study. *Electroencephalography and Clinical Neurophysiology,* 1962, **14,** 60–63.

Korin, H., Fink, M., Kwalwasser, S. Relation of changes in memory and learning to improvement in electroshock. *Confinia Neurologica,* 1956, **16,** 88–96.

Pollack, M., & Fink, M. Sociopsychological characteristics of patients who refuse convulsive therapy. *Journal of Nervous and Mental Disease*, 1961, **132**, 153–157.

Pollack, M., Kahn, R. L., Karp, E., & Fink, M. Tachistoscopic perception after induced altered brain function: influence of mental set. *Journal of Nervous and Mental Disease*, 1962, **134**, 422–430.

Weinstein, E. A., & Kahn, R. L. *Denial of illness*. Springfield, Ill.: C. C Thomas, 1955.

PART II:
ASPECTS OF
BEHAVIOR THERAPY

8

A BEHAVIORAL CONSULTATION PROGRAM FOR PARENTS AND TEACHERS OF CHILDREN WITH CONDUCT PROBLEMS

K. DANIEL O'LEARY and RONALD N. KENT

A few years ago we conducted an outcome survey of the Child Psychological Clinic at Stony Brook. Basically, we were interested in the extent to which all parents who received service at our clinic felt they had been helped to deal with the behavioral problems of their children. Second, we wanted to know how parents viewed their therapists. While recent reviews have documented the efficacy of behavioral procedures with children in the home (Patterson, 1969) and classroom (O'Leary & O'Leary, 1972; O'Leary & O'Leary, in press), the utility of behavioral modification procedures in child outpatient clinics remains unsubstantiated. Many behavioral interventions have been conducted under circumstances which probably were more conducive to success than if those interventions had occurred in a strictly clinical environment. Clinicians in an outpatient facility do not have incentives at their disposal to help ensure that the requests they make of teachers and parents are implemented (e.g., course credit, grades contingent upon successful behavioral intervention, payment for participation, and completing forms or recording data). Thus, it

K. Daniel O'Leary, Ph.D., Professor of Psychology, State University of New York, Stony Brook.

Ronald N. Kent, Ph.D., Research Associate and Visiting Assistant Professor of Psychology, State University of New York, Stony Brook.

The work was sponsored by National Institute of Mental Health Grant MH-21813.

The authors are particularly indebted to the therapists, Drs. Kenneth Kaufman, Susan O'Leary, Lisa Serbin, and Mary Starke, who contributed significantly to the development of the therapy program as well as to the positive outcomes. We are also especially indebted to research assistants Sandra Armel and Joan Fisher. Mr. Ray Barber, Director, Pupil Personnel Services, and school psychologists John Greer, Peter Lombardo, and Robert Schur, of Middle County School District, Centereach, N.Y., were helpful throughout the program.

seemed desirable to assess the efficacy of behavioral treatment procedures in an environment closely resembling that of the outpatient practitioner in private practice or in a community clinic.

In this case, the facility was a university Child Psychological Clinic where the service was implemented by graduate students in clinical psychology. As in the case of most outpatient clinics, the presenting complaints varied greatly. Problems included social withdrawal, temper tantrums, delinquent acts, immaturity and lack of independence, academic retardation, self-destructive behavior, and conflicts in family relationships. Treatment ranged from approximately one month to one year, and the average number of consultations per case was 14.

The details of this evaluation have been published by O'Leary, Turkewitz, and Taffel (1973), but basically the findings were as follows: ratings obtained from therapists at termination and parents six months following termination indicated overall improvement in 87 percent and 90 percent of the cases, respectively; 96 percent of the parents (70 families) liked their therapist; and the personal characteristics most frequently noted by the parents were warmth, understanding, and sincere interest in the client.

The rates of improvement we found were quite striking when compared to those recorded in the existing literature. In fact, in the 17 followup studies reported by Levitt (1957), the average improvement rate was 78 percent. However, as in all clinic surveys, the spontaneous improvement rate was unknown, and improvement with specific populations (e.g., enuretics, delinquents, and hyperactives) was unclear. Thus, we decided to evaluate in a controlled study, the effects of a behavioral intervention program for second- to fourth-grade elementary school children with both academic and social difficulties.

Referrals were made by teachers after a meeting with the coinvestigators, who described the type of treatment offered. Treatment and control children were selected on the basis of observed levels of disruptive classroom behavior (O'Leary, Kaufman, Kass, & Drabman, 1970), aggression scores on the Louisville School Behavior Checklist (Miller, 1972), and reading level as measured on the California Achievement Test. Families to be offered treatment were notified of our consultation services by the school psychologists. It was necessary to contact 20 families to obtain the necessary 16 treatment cases; 16 other children in 16 other classrooms were included in a no-treatment control group. Thus, in all, 32 classrooms, 16 with treated target children and 16 with untreated target children, were involved.

A preliminary comparison of subjects selected for treatment and control groups is presented below:

	Treatment	Control	F test
Total disruptive behaviors per 20 sec intervals	1.32	1.45	n.s.
CAT reading	29th percentile	31st percentile	n.s.
Louisville School Behavior Checklist aggression z scores	2.52	2.45	n.s.

Our behavioral consultation program emphasized four factors whose individual effectiveness had already been documented:

1. Instructions and feedback to parents and teachers concerning praise for appropriate behavior and ignoring of disruptive behavior (Becker, Madsen, Arnold, & Thomas, 1967).

2. A report card from the teacher to the parent which provided daily evaluations of the child's progress on individual target behaviors, such as completing math assignments, bringing in homework, not fighting in class. When the daily report indicated improvement, parents were asked to give the child special privileges (e.g. a specific dessert, reading a story to the child, and extra TV). On occasion, hourly teacher evaluations were used as a supplement to the daily report where it was judged by the child's therapist that the child would not respond to daily reports. On two occasions, children were taught to evaluate their own behavior (Bailey, Wolf, & Phillips, 1970; Hawkins, Sluyter, & Smith, 1972).

3. Soft reprimands (reprimands audible only to the child being reprimanded) rather than loud reprimands (O'Leary et al., 1970).

4. Having the child spend ten to fifteen minutes per day four times per week on a programmed reading series (in this case, Sullivan Readers) with his parents (Ryback & Staats, 1970).

The four therapists spent approximately 20 hours per case, dividing the consultation almost equally between parents and teachers. All 16 families who contacted us for service remained throughout the treatment. Fifteen of the 16 teachers participated throughout the program: one teacher-therapist relationship was strained by scheduling difficulties and, in addition, a personality clash. Fortunately, in the latter instance, parent cooperation was very high and teacher consultation was maintained by sporadic phone contact. A typical assessment and treatment case sequence is depicted in Table 1. Marital problems, impending divorces, and individual problems of parents, such as depression, prevented therapists from following this schedule in any rigid fashion. However, even in cases where personal and family problems were evident, the therapists tried to spend some portion of each session on the implementation of the intervention program.

Table 1. Typical Case Sequence

Assessment: Sessions 1–4

Parent: collect demographic data and discuss school and home problems
Child: discuss school with child; give verbal section of WISC
Teacher: discuss past involvement with child and specific current problems
Teacher: establish base rate measures of academic and social problems

Treatment: Sessions 5–20

Parent: build natural incentive system for daily report implementation
Teacher: start praise, soft reprimands, and daily report
Parent and child: discuss daily report
Teacher: observe and give feedback regarding praise, soft reprimands, and daily report
Parent: model proper tutoring techniques
Parent and child: observe and give feedback on tutoring techniques of parents
Teacher: change targets on daily report if progress is evident; give feedback to teacher
          regarding rates of praise
Parent and child: discuss school problems;* if progressing well, expand general reinforce-
          ment techniques to home problems
Parent: discuss general conceptual framework and learning principles and how parent
          would apply them to new problems of child
Sessions 19–20: emphasize changing targets, withdrawing frequency of daily report,
          maintenance of change, need for novel reinforcers, crucial nature of
          teacher and parent attention, and recommendations for following year

---

*Several of these discussions were by phone.

The results of our consultation program revealed that the treated children improved significantly more ($p < .05$) than control children on three major types of dependent measures: classroom observations of disruptive behavior, factorially derived measures of aggression based on a teacher checklist, and teacher ratings of specific academic and social target behavior. I will now briefly elaborate on the findings regarding these types of measures.

1. *Classroom Observations at Therapy Termination.* There were ten categories of behavior in our code. They included items such as interference with others, clowning, vocalization, noncompliance, and physical and verbal aggression. A composite measure of undesired behavior was computed by summing the frequencies on the ten categories. In addition, to account for great variability in classroom levels of disruptiveness, difference scores were used in our analysis which compared target children with randomly selected classmates. Two twenty-minute observations in June revealed that treated children improved significantly more than control children on the composite measure of disruptive behavior.

2. *School Behavior Checklist Scores.* First, treated children improved significantly more than control children on the aggression factor of the Louisville Checklist. Second, we excluded socially desirable items from

the extraversion factor (e.g., he is friendly) so that it contained largely undesirable items (e.g., he tries to be the center of attention). On the basis of the undesirable extraversion items, treated children showed greater improvement than untreated children. Third, there was a tendency ($p < .13$) for treated children to show greater improvement on a Low Need Achievement Factor reflecting academic motivation.

3. *Teacher Ratings of Improvement in Specific Academic and Behavioral Targets.* Ratings by treatment and control teachers of specific academic and behavioral areas of difficulty were obtained. These ratings indicated that treated children improved more than control children in specific problem areas in both academic and behavioral realms.

Questionnaire data from both teachers and parents of treated children were quite positive. We employed a 7-point rating scale on which 4 was defined as neutral, 1 as very negative, and 7 as very positive. On this basis it may be concluded that parents liked their therapists ($\bar{X} = 6.9$) and felt they were concerned with their problems ($\bar{X} = 6.2$). Using a 7-point rating scale (4 was neutral, 1 very negative, and 7 very positive), teachers described their therapists as likeable ($\bar{X} = 6.5$), committed ($\bar{X} = 6.4$), competent ($\bar{X} = 6.5$), and concerned with their problems ($\bar{X} = 6.3$).

We are quite enthusiastic about our ability to demonstrate both rating and observational changes in children usually labeled "conduct problems" (Quay & Peterson, 1967; Quay, 1972) and by parent and teacher evaluation of our therapists. The absence of differences between therapists —either in terms of demonstrable effect on classroom behavior or in terms of parent and teacher perception—was important, indicating that all therapists were evaluated as being very competent, likeable, and concerned with their problems.

In contrast, rather discouraging results were obtained on the reading section of the CAT. Both treatment and control subjects gained only 3.5 months in a 6-month period. The teachers' ratings, however, indicated that treated children improved more than control children on specific academic target behaviors. Such improvement ratings may indicate that children receiving therapy have improved in work or study habits. Post-CAT scores were obtained in June. Since some children were accepted for treatment as late as March 1, it is possible that our intervention was simply not of sufficient duration to exact academic change on standardized achievement tests. Alternatively, it may be that parents who are not selected for their ability to supervise tutoring may be unable to exact change regardless of the number of weeks of intervention. In fact, we found two parents who were so punitive that we decided not to suggest that they implement the tutorial program.

This year we have made two very substantial changes in our consultation program. First, we are using a Macmillan tutorial program for children whom the teachers feel need remedial aid. Tutoring is implemented by undergraduates who see the child 30 times for 30 minutes. Second, we are comparing the effects of our consultation program as implemented by clinical psychologists with the effects as implemented by clinical psychologists and a co-therapist with a B.A. who implements two-thirds of the program. Three of our four B.A. therapists are former teachers. The fourth has experience in a social work setting with children, though she does not have a social work degree. All four B.A. therapists participated in forty hours of training in behavioral procedures, assessment, and interview strategies. Basically, we are interested in developing a treatment program which is empirically effective and applicable for psychologists or psychiatrists working with a co-therapist trained in behavior therapy who travels from school to school consulting with teachers. We feel that if a child has school problems, it is imperative that some intervention occur in the school. Unfortunately, because of scheduling and monetary considerations, many clinical psychologists and psychiatrists are not prone to contact schools (Berkowitz, 1968). Our hope is that our co-therapist team approach will represent not only an effective intervention but an economic and practical one.

REFERENCES

Bailey, J. S., Wolf, M. M., & Phillips, E. L. Home-based reinforcement and the modification of the predelinquents' classroom behavior. *Journal of Applied Behavior Analysis*, 1970, 3, 223–233.

Becker, W. C., Madsen, C. H., Arnold, C. R., & Thomas, D. R. The contingent use of teacher attention and praise in reducing classroom behavior problems. *Journal of Special Education*, 1967, 1, 287–307.

Berkowitz, H. A preliminary assessment of the extent of interaction between child psychiatric clinics and public schools. *Psychology in the Schools*, 1968, 5, 291–295.

Hawkins, R. P., Sluyter, D. J., & Smith, C. D. Modification of achievement by a simple technique involving parents and teacher. In M. Harris (Ed.), *Classroom uses of behavior modification*. Columbus, O.: Charles Merrill, 1972, pp. 101–120.

Levitt, E. E. The results of psychotherapy with children: an evaluation. *Journal of Consulting Psychology*, 1957, 21, 189–196.

Miller, L. C. School behavior checklist: an inventory of deviant behavior for elementary school children. *Journal of Consulting and Clinical Psychology*, 1972, 38, 134–144.

O'Leary, K. D., Kaufman, K. F., Kass, R. E., & Drabman, R. S. The effects of loud and soft reprimands on the behavior of disruptive students. *Exceptional Children*, 1970, 37, 145–155.

O'Leary, K. D., & O'Leary, S. G. *Classroom management: the successful use of behavior modification*. New York: Pergamon Press, 1972.

O'Leary, S. G., & O'Leary, K. D. Behavior modification in the school. In H. Leitenberg (Ed.), *Handbook of behavior modification*. Englewood Cliffs, N.J.: Prentice Hall, in press.

O'Leary, K. D., Turkewitz, H., & Taffel, S. J. Parent and therapist evaluation of behavior therapy in a child psychological clinic. *Journal of Consulting and Clinical Psychology*, 1973, 41, 279–283.

Patterson, G. R. A community mental health program for children. In L. A. Hamerlynck, P. O. Davidson, & L. E. Acker (Eds.), *Behavior modification and ideal mental health services*. Alberta, Canada: University of Calgary, 1969, pp. 130–179.

Quay, H. C. Patterns of aggression, withdrawal and immaturity. In H. C. Quay and J. S. Werry (Eds.), *Psychopathological disorders of children.* New York: Wiley, 1972, pp. 1–29.

Quay, H. C., & Peterson, D. R. *Manual for the behavior problem checklist.* Urbana: University of Illinois, 1967.

Ryback, D., & Staats, A. W. Parents as behavior therapy-technicians in treating reading deficits (dyslexia). *Journal of Behavior Therapy and Experimental Psychiatry,* 1970, **1,** 109–119.

9

OUTCOME RESEARCH STRATEGIES IN BEHAVIOR THERAPY: Issues and Evidence from the Treatment of Alcoholics

G. TERENCE WILSON

Of fundamental importance to any discussion of psychiatric outcome research strategies is Bandura's (1969) distinction between *physical* and *psychological* methods of treatment. The familiar concepts of "cure," "spontaneous remission," and "relapse" which describe physical disease processes are less appropriate in conceptualizing changes in behavior which are under the control of social-psychological variables. Unlike physical disease, deviant or disturbed behavior is, for the most part, a function of antecedent and consequent environmental events and internal cognitive mediating processes which may vary in different situations, in different people, and at different times even in the same person. As Bandura (1969) notes, this "would be analogous to having malignancies appear in a given person under one set of social circumstances and disappear under others [p. 57]." In evaluating the relative efficacy of psychological therapies the focus is on the initial *induction* of behavioral change, its *generalization* beyond the hospital or consulting office to the patient's natural environment, and the *maintenance* of the treatment-produced gains over time. It is often important to distinguish between these processes since they may be governed by somewhat different factors. Failure to do so clouds the interpretation of the results of therapeutic outcome studies.

This problem, and the wider issues involved in assessing outcome research with complex psychiatric disorders, can be illustrated with reference to the behavioral treatment of alcoholics using aversion therapy, which perhaps still remains the most common and the preferred behavior therapy technique in the treatment of alcoholics. Evaluation of

G. Terence Wilson, Ph.D., The Psychological Clinic, Rutgers University.

The work was supported by National Institute of Alcohol Abuse and Alcoholism Grant AA00259-04.

previous outcome studies has been based upon subjective judgments of whether the patient is abstinent (success) or not (relapse) at various followup periods ranging anywhere from three to about fifteen months in duration. The data from studies of this sort provide little unequivocal support for the efficacy of electrical aversion therapy in producing lasting improvements (e.g., Hallam, Rachman, & Falkowski, 1971; MacCulloch, Feldman, Orford, & MacCulloch, 1966; Regester, 1972; Vogler, Lunde, Johnson, & Martin, 1970). However, the absence of any clear-cut treatment effect several months after therapy has been discontinued does not necessarily mean that aversive conditioning techniques are ineffective. It might be that these methods induce initial therapeutic gains which are short-lived because of the failure to ensure the appropriate conditions for generalization and maintenance, which as Baer, Wolf, and Risley (1968) remind us, must be "programmed rather than expected or lamented [p. 97]."

Since the use of aversion therapy is predicated on the assumption that it suppresses drinking directly by endowing the alcohol with negative properties, the logical first step in conducting outcome research on these methods would be to demonstrate this hypothesized suppressant effect in the laboratory setting before testing its efficacy in a complex clinical outcome study. Should aversion therapy prove to suppress drinking effectively, then it might be profitably included in a more encompassing treatment program designed to produce generalization and maintenance of therapeutic improvement. If no immediate treatment effects are induced, then the technique would be better discarded. This initial laboratory-centered approach would also permit rigorous, objective measurement which is necessary in order to specify the theoretical mechanisms responsible for behavior change. Aside from these conceptual issues, the methodological problems involved in accurately measuring whether individuals are drinking excessively or not at followup evaluations make it difficult to interpret findings. Evaluation procedures which rely on patients' self-report, even in those instances where attempts are made to corroborate these reports by interviewing significant others in the patients' environment or by checking arrest or rehospitalization records, are of questionable reliability and validity (Summers, 1970).

The present series of investigations assessed the effects of different aversive control procedures using a free operant drinking baseline in the semi-naturalistic situation of the Rutgers University Alcohol Behavior Research Laboratory (ABRL). This four-bed inpatient research facility, which has been described in detail elsewhere (Nathan, Goldman, Lisman, & Taylor, 1972), allows continuous observation and measurement of free operant drinking behavior. All subjects were gamma-type male alcoholics who were therapeutic failures from New York and New Jersey state institutions, were medically and psychiatrically screened, were treatment-motivated, and had voluntarily consented to undergo a course of aversion therapy from which they understood they were free to withdraw at any point.

In Study 1, four subjects were allowed ad libitum access to a maximum of 30 ounces of 86-proof whiskey over each of three consecutive twenty-four hour periods with the single limitation that their blood alcohol level (BAL)[1] never exceed 250 mg/100cc. A crossover design was used which allows both between- and within-subject comparisons of the effects of different treatments. Two subjects received 120 trials of aversive escape conditioning over a four-day period while the other two received an equal number of backward conditioning trials as a control form of treatment. Following a second ad lib drinking baseline period the treatment procedures were reversed for a further four-day treatment phase. A final post-treatment baseline drinking period evaluated the effects of the second treatment regimen.

The escape conditioning paradigm was modeled on the clinical procedure employed by Blake (1965) and Vogler et al. (1970) and recently recommended by Eysenck and Beech (1971) as the "optimal" treatment of choice with alcoholics. Subjects were seated in a simulated bar setting with Beckman electrodes attached to the index and middle fingers of the non-dominant hand. They were instructed to look at, smell, and then sip some whiskey without swallowing. A shock, administered contiguously with the sip, was terminated by subjects' spitting the alcohol into a small bucket. Shock levels in this and subsequent studies were individually determined according to subjects' subjective report of what was painful and a clear flexion of the arm. The intensities used ranged 4 to 8 milliamps, which are comparable to those reported in the clinical treatment literature. As in all the studies reported here, efforts were made to foster high expectations of therapeutic success in both the subjects and the nursing and research staff in the ABRL, such that the demand characteristics of the situation called for little or no alcohol consumption.

The results of Study 1 are summarized in Table 1. It is clear that the treatment procedures had little impact on drinking except in the case of subject 3, who showed a substantial reduction in ounces of alcohol consumed following the escape conditioning treatment. However, this subject returned to drinking within a week of being released from the ABRL and was rehospitalized. The strikingly negative results obtained with subjects 1, 2, and 4 have been replicated using similar procedures in four additional subjects (Wilson, Leaf, & Nathan, 1975). Subjects' attitudes toward alcohol as measured by daily administrations of evaluative scales of the Semantic Differential did not differ during escape and backward conditioning phases, although attitudes during both treatment

Table 1. Mean Number of Ounces of Alcohol Consumed, Study 1

	Baseline 1	Treatment 1	Baseline 2	Treatment 2	Baseline 3
Subject 1	21.3	escape conditioning	21.5	backward conditioning	23.0
Subject 2	13.7	escape conditioning	15.0	backward conditioning	15.5
Subject 3	28.0	backward conditioning	25.5	escape conditioning	1.5
Subject 4	24.3	backward conditioning	25.5	escape conditioning	26.5

phases were significantly less favorable than during baseline periods 1 and 2 (see Fig. 1). These attitudinal responses indicate transient placebo effects as opposed to any aversive conditioning process, and together with the drinking data provide scant support for the efficacy of this form of aversion therapy with alcoholics. In an analogue outcome study, Miller, Hersen, Eisler, and Hemphill (1973) similarly showed that the escape conditioning procedure fared no better than an attention-placebo control treatment.

Another widely used aversion therapy technique is known as covert sensitization (Cautela, 1967). In this technique, imaginal representation of the thoughts, feelings, and behavior which lead to drinking is repeatedly associated with noxious images of nausea and vomiting as aversive stimuli. Several potential advantages recommend the use of this method. First, as an aversive stimulus, nausea appears to be more biologically appropriate for establishing conditioned aversive responses to alcohol per se than such an artificial event as electric shock (cf. Wilson & Davison, 1969). Second, covert sensitization is a self-control technique which enhances generalization since the client can readily re-create the aversive image to control the desire to imbibe in the natural environment (Mahoney, 1972). Finally, there are both practical and ethical considerations which favor its use over painful electric shock. Enthusiastic reports of the successful application of aversive imagery methods to the treatment of alcoholism have, unfortunately, been limited to uncontrolled clinical studies and case reports (e.g., Ashem & Donner, 1968), and controlled outcome studies have been conspicuously lacking.

Studies 2a and b compared the effects of associating alcohol-related stimuli with symbolically induced aversion to an electric shock procedure similar to that described in Study 1. An important difference between Studies 1 and 2 was that in the latter the aversive stimulus was paired with the imaginal representation of various components of the entire complex

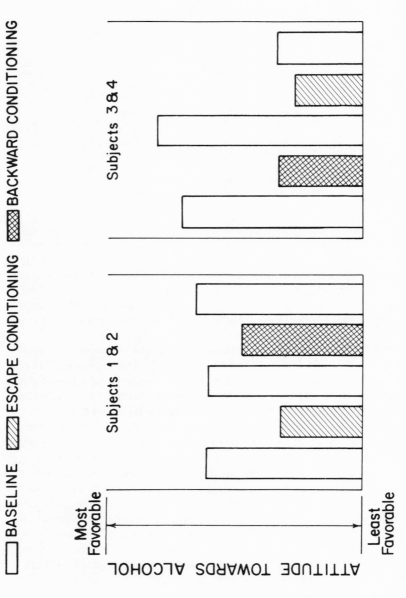

FIG. 1. Ratings of subjects' attitudes toward alcohol on scales of the Semantic Differential.

pattern of internal and external stimuli leading to drinking. Using the same crossover design, subjects received twice-daily sessions of ten trials each for four days of either type of aversion therapy procedure following a two-day baseline drinking phase. The two subjects assigned to the shock condition decided against continuing the treatment program after one and two days, respectively, stating that they found the procedure too anxiety-evoking. The other two subjects completed the scheduled treatment reversal phase together with the second and third post-treatment baseline drinking assessment periods of four days, respectively.

The results are presented in Table 2, Group 1. Subjects 1 and 2 showed sizeable percentage reductions in alcohol consumption of approximately 49 and 71 percent, respectively, following the aversive imagery treatment. Subject 1 showed a slight increase in drinking following the second treatment phase, whereas subject 2 ceased drinking. These findings cannot be unequivocally interpreted because the loss of data from subjects 3 and 4 precluded any between-treatments comparison and because the single-subject reversal design is inevitably confounded should the pre-treatment baseline frequency of the target behavior not recover following the first treatment intervention (Leitenberg, 1973). Accordingly, a replication of this experiment was conducted with four other subjects (Group 2 in Table 2). In addition to directly recording drinking behavior, psychophysiological measures of subjects' response to directed imagery of alcohol and actually viewing a bottle of alcohol were taken before, during, and after each treatment phase, using GSR and EMG recordings.

Both covert sensitization and faradic shock conditioning produced substantial decrements in drinking from pre-treatment baseline levels of 36 and 41 percent, respectively, but did not differ significantly from one another. Although not superior in outcome efficacy, covert sensitization

Table 2. Mean Number of Ounces of Alcohol Consumed, Study 2

	Baseline 1	Treatment 1	Baseline 2	Treatment 2	Baseline 3
Group 1					
Subject 1	27.5	aversive imagery	14.0	electric shock	18.0
Subject 2	14.5	aversive imagery	3.75	electric shock	0.0
Subject 3	26.0	electric shock	—	aversive imagery	—
Subject 4	12.0	electric shock	—	aversive imagery	—
Group 2					
Subject 1	27.25	electric shock	18.25	aversive imagery	21.50
Subject 2	25.25	electric shock	12.25	aversive imagery	10.00
Subject 3	21.50	aversive imagery	14.75	electric shock	10.75
Subject 4	24.00	aversive imagery	14.00	electric shock	16.50

was clearly less stressful than the electric shock procedure, as shown by subject attrition in Study 2a and confirmed by anecdotal reports in Study 2b. Callahan and Leitenberg (1973) make similar observations on the use of these two methods in the modification of deviant sexual behaviors. The reduction in drinking which was obtained in Study 2 cannot be unambiguously attributed to the effects of the specific treatment techniques employed. The relative improvement of these subjects' drinking behavior, when contrasted to that of the same type of subject in Study 1, could plausibly be due to the inclusion of more representative and important antecedent controlling stimuli during the conditioning sessions (cf. Berecz, 1972). However, the role of placebo factors cannot be discounted even though they have been shown to have little impact when specifically controlled for, as in Study 1 and Study 4 (see below). It is noteworthy that Miller et al. (1973) achieved a 36 to 37 percent reduction in drinking in both their aversive conditioning and attention-placebo groups (a decrease remarkably similar to that obtained in Study 2b), which led them to conclude that "the effects of electrical aversion therapy may be more related to such factors as therapeutic instructions, expectancy, specificity of the procedure or experimental demand characteristics than the conditioning factors [p. 491]." A preliminary scan of the psychophysiological measures indicates no clear evidence of the development of conditioned anxiety responses to the image or sight of alcohol following either form of treatment. Hallam et al. (1971) previously reported little change in either cardiac or skin resistance measures in alcoholics treated by electrical aversion therapy.

These results are far from impressive, even if we assume that they were attributable to the treatment procedures themselves and not to the effects of uncontrolled placebo influences. The failure to suppress drinking more completely within the confines of a protective milieu, free from the stress and conflict which so typically characterizes the alcoholic's life in the natural environment, augurs poorly for the therapeutic efficacy of these classical conditioning techniques. In contrast to the classical conditioning paradigm, which attempts to control drinking by devaluing the positively valenced properties of alcohol, the treatment might more productively emphasize operant conditioning principles and attempt to modify alcohol consumption directly by manipulating the response-contingent consequences of which it is a function.

Study 3 investigated the effects of a punishment procedure, i.e., response-contingent aversive stimulation, on drinking behavior. A crude ABAB single-subject reversal design was used in which the treatment variables were consecutively introduced and then withdrawn while subjects' drinking was continuously recorded. Following an initial two-day baseline assessment phase, subjects received a two-second shock ranging

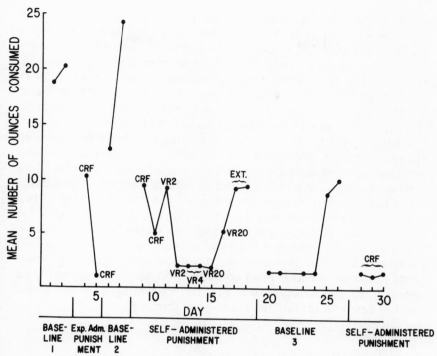

FIG. 2. Mean number of ounces of alcohol consumed across baseline drinking and experimenter- and self-administered shock conditions.

from 3 to 10 milliamps in intensity whenever they consumed a one-ounce shot of alcohol. As shown in Figure 2, all four subjects showed a rapid reduction of drinking under these conditions. However, alcohol consumption returned to its initial baseline level immediately coincident with the removal of the punishment contingency (days 6 and 7). Suppressed intake again followed the reintroduction of the aversive contingency despite the fact that shock was self- rather than experimenter-administered and despite the fading out of shock on an increasingly intermittent punishment schedule (days 9 to 18). Returning the subjects to baseline conditions during days 20 to 26 resulted in a maintenance of reduced alcohol intake, although the trend indicated a gradual recovery towards pretreatment levels.

The findings from Study 3 suggest that drinking by alcoholics is, at least in part, a function of its consequences. Unfortunately, the design of this study does not make it possible to conclude that the punishment contingency per se was responsible for the changes in amount of alcohol consumed. Study 4 employed a more sophisticated crossover design in demonstrating that the systematic application of the aversive contingency is critical in regulating drinking. Following baseline, subjects 2 and 3 were yoked to subjects 1 and 4, respectively, who were placed on a 100 percent punishment schedule. Thereafter treatment conditions were reversed, with subjects 2 and 3 determining the number and sequencing of shocks for themselves and their yoked partners. The yoked or noncontingent treatment condition effectively controls for the role of nonspecific social influence processes such as expectancy and demand characteristics.

Figure 3 clearly shows that the contingent relationship between drinking behavior and aversive stimulation was both necessary and sufficient for most effective suppression of alcohol consumption. Noncontingent aversive stimulation failed to influence drinking significantly. The efficacy of this punishment procedure has been replicated in two subsequent studies (Wilson & Tracey, 1974). This demonstration of the operant control of drinking is consistent with Cohen, Liebson, Faillace, and Allen's (1971) findings that alcoholics could voluntarily restrict their drinking to less than five ounces per day if this moderation was contingently rewarded by access to an enriched environment as opposed to an impoverished laboratory setting. Free or noncontingent access to the enriched environment resulted in excessive drinking.

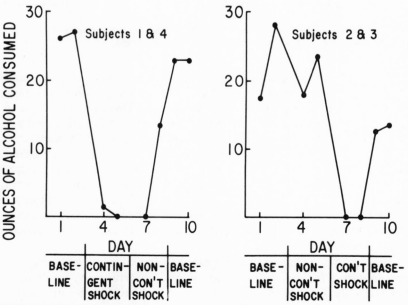

FIG. 3. Mean number of ounces of alcohol consumed during baseline drinking and under conditions of contingent and noncontingent shock.

These findings establish that dramatic, clinically relevant changes in alcohol intake can be induced by altering the reinforcing consequences of drinking behavior. They suggest that alcoholism can be fruitfully conceptualized within a social learning framework, and they challenge the disease theory of alcoholism with its emphasis on loss of control in which any drinking is presumed to trigger off the addictive process and the subsequent inability to regulate intake (Jellinek, 1960), a notion which has been widely contradicted of late (e.g., Marlatt, Demming, & Reid, 1973; Sobell & Sobell, 1973). The real problem lies in implementing this social learning analysis of drinking so as to produce generalization and long-term maintenance of either abstinence or appropriately controlled drinking.

One strategy is to use *contingency contracting* in the natural environment. Wilson and Rosen (1976), for example, had an alcoholic agree to a contract which limited his drinking to controlled, social situations. Any violation was "punished" by having the patient forfeit some portion of a money deposit to be spent in a manner extremely aversive to the patient, i.e., a contribution to an organization he most despised. Adherence to the contract was explicitly reinforced by his wife's affection and support. Followup evaluations revealed a maintenance of treatment-produced moderate drinking. In a similar manner, Hunt and Azrin (1973) employed a massive community-reinforcement treatment program for chronic alcoholics in which vocational, social, and familial reinforcers which had been previously lacking were developed and then made contingent on continued sobriety. Excessive drinking resulted in temporarily withdrawing a reinforcer, i.e., time out from positive reinforcement. Compared to a control group which received a conventional hospital program for alcoholics, patients from the reinforcement program showed considerable improvement. Throughout an independently conducted six months following evaluation they spent significantly less time drinking, showed less unemployment, earned more money, and left their families less.

The impressive nature of these data is attributable to the joint or separate action of several factors. Generalization of treatment-produced change was directly accomplished by rearranging the reinforcing consequences of drinking in the patients' work and home environments. Maintenance of treatment gains after patients were released from hospital was deliberately fostered by programmed home visits which were gradually phased out over time. These visits ensured that the program procedures were being followed and attempted to solve any additional problems which patients encountered. Finally, the solution to producing durable therapeutic effects is more a function of the scope of the treatment program than of the technical niceties of the conditioning paradigm employed (Bandura, 1969; Lazarus & Wilson, in press). Hunt and Azrin

(1973) used a multifaceted behavioral treatment program which effected generalization across different times, situations, and behaviors by teaching the patients broad problem-solving competencies and social skills. Sobell and Sobell (1973) have also conceptualized abusive alcoholic drinking as a discriminated operant response and have treated hospitalized alcoholics with an individualized, broad-spectrum behavioral approach. Although not free from methodological problems (O'Leary & Wilson, 1975), Sobell and Sobell's findings at both one- and two-year followups showed success rates (defined as either abstinence or controlled drinking) of close to 90 percent. Complex psychiatric disorders such as alcoholism are usually controlled by several factors which must all be dealt with if lasting therapeutic benefit is to result.

Future research must address itself to sorting out the diverse effects and critical ingredients of different generalization and maintenance strategies and to determining how they interact with various treatment-induced changes in producing long-term therapeutic gains. Improvements in methodology for assessing behavioral change in the natural environment are particularly important. The approach described here satisfies both the logical and the empirical requirements for meaningful outcome research on psychological forms of treatment.

NOTE

1. Breathalyzer readings of each subject's BAL were taken three times a day. A computer program which summed the number of drinks consumed in conjunction with a "real time" clock and each subject's alcohol metabolism constant provided continuous estimates of BALs.

REFERENCES

Ashem, B., & Donner, L. Covert sensitization with alcoholics: a controlled replication. *Behaviour Research and Therapy*, 1968, 6, 7–12.
Baer, D. M., Wolf, M. M., & Risley, T. R. Some current dimensions of applied behavior analysis. *Journal of Applied Behavior Analysis*, 1968, 1, 91–97.
Bandura, A. *Principles of behavior modification.* New York: Holt, 1969.
Berecz, J. Modification of smoking behavior through self-administered punishment of imagined behavior. *Journal of Consulting and Clinical Psychology*, 1972, 38, 244–250.
Blake, B. G. The application of behaviour therapy to the treatment of alcoholism. *Behaviour Research and Therapy*, 1965, 3, 75–85.
Callahan, E. J., & Leitenberg, H. Aversion therapy for sexual deviation: contingent shock and covert sensitization. *Journal of Abnormal Psychology*, 1973, 81, 60–73.
Cautela, J. R. Covert sensitization. *Psychological Reports*, 1967, 20, 459–468.
Cohen, M., Liebson, I. A., Faillace, L. A., & Allen, R. P. Moderate drinking by chronic alcoholics. *Journal of Nervous and Mental Disease*, 1971, 53, 434–444.
Eysenck, H. J., & Beech, H. R. Counter conditioning and related methods. In A. E. Bergin & S. L. Garfield (Eds.), *Handbook of psychotherapy and behavior change.* New York: Wiley, 1971, pp. 543–611.
Hallam, R., Rachman, S., & Falkowski, W. Subjective, attitudinal, and physiological effects of electrical aversion therapy. *Behaviour Research and Therapy*, 1971, 10, 1–13.

Hunt, G. M., & Azrin, N. H. A community-reinforcement approach to alcoholism. *Behaviour Research and Therapy*, 1973, **11**, 91–104.

Jellinek, E. M. *The disease concept of alcoholism*. New Haven, Conn.: College and University Press, 1960.

Lazarus, A. A., & Wilson, G. T. Behavior modification: clinical and experimental perspectives. In B. B. Wolman (Ed.), *Treatment methods of mental disorders: a handbook for practitioners*. New York: Van Nostrand Reinhold, in press.

Leitenberg, H. The use of single-case methodology. *Journal of Abnormal Psychology*. 1973, **82**, 87–101.

MacCulloch, M. J., Feldman, M. P., Orford, J. F., & MacCulloch, M. L. Anticipatory avoidance learning in the treatment of alcoholism: a record of therapeutic failure. *Behaviour Research and Therapy*, 1966, **4**, 187–196.

Mahoney, M. J. Research issues in self-management. *Behavior Therapy*, 1972, **3**, 45–63.

Marlatt, G. A., Demming, B., & Reid, J. B. Loss of control drinking in alcoholics: an experimental analogue. *Journal of Abnormal Psychology*, 1973, **81**, 233–241.

Miller, P. M., Hersen, M., Eisler, R. M. & Hemphill, D. P. Electrical aversion therapy with alcoholics: an analogue study. *Behaviour Research and Therapy*, 1973, **11**, 491–497.

Nathan, P. E., Goldman, M. S., Lisman, S. A., & Taylor, H. A. Alcohol and alcoholics: a behavioral approach. *Transactions of the New York Academy of Sciences*, 1972, **34**, 602–627.

O'Leary, K. D., & Wilson, G. T. *Behavior therapy*. Englewood Cliffs, N.J.: Prentice-Hall, 1975.

Regester, D. C. Change in autonomic responsivity and drinking behavior of alcoholics as a function of aversion therapy. Paper presented at the American Psychological Association Annual Convention, Hawaii, 1972.

Sobell, M. B., & Sobell, L. C. Evidence of controlled drinking by former alcoholics: a second year evaluation of individualized behavior therapy. Paper presented at the American Psychological Association Annual Convention, Montreal, Canada, 1973.

Summers, T. Validity of alcoholics' self-reported drinking history. *Quarterly Journal of Studies on Alcohol*, 1970, **31**, 972–974.

Vogler, R. E., Lunde, S. E., Johnson, G. R., & Martin, P. L. Electrical aversion conditioning with chronic alcoholics. *Journal of Consulting and Clinical Psychology*, 1970, **34**, 302–307.

Wilson, G. T. & Davison, G. C. Aversion techniques in behavior therapy: some theoretical and metatheoretical considerations. *Journal of Consulting and Clinical Psychology*, 1969, **33**, 327–329.

Wilson, G. T., Leaf, R., & Nathan, P. E. The aversive control of excessive drinking by chronic alcoholics in the laboratory setting. *Journal of Applied Behavior Analysis*, 1975, **8**, 13–26.

Wilson, G. T., & Rosen, R. C. Training controlled drinking in an alcoholic through a multifaceted behavioral treatment program: a case study. In J. D. Krumblotz & C. E. Thoresen (Eds.), *Counseling methods*. New York: Holt, Rinehart & Winston, 1976, in press.

Wilson, G. T., & Tracey, D. A. An experimental investigation of the effects of covert sensitization on excessive drinking by chronic alcoholics. Unpublished manuscript, Rutgers University, 1974.

10 "PSYCHOLOPHARMACOLOGY": The Use of Drugs Combined with Psychological Treatment

ISAAC M. MARKS

The use of pharmacological agents in psychiatric disorder is of memorable vintage. Less old is their combination with psychological treatments, and only recently has there been systematic study of the interaction between psychotropic drugs and psychotherapeutic techniques. The main principles of interaction are still unknown. This new area is of such potential importance that it could be called "psycholopharmacology" if we did not already have sufficient long words in psychiatry.

The joint use of psychotherapy and drugs has mainly been in syndromes in which anxiety or depression are prominent. This report dwells largely on phobic disorders. The commonest psychological techniques employed have been of the exposure genre like desensitization or flooding in fantasy and in vivo, sometimes used systematically and at other times only indirectly, by suggestion. Although most reports in this area are uncontrolled, an increasing number have adopted double-blind procedures and require more attention.

ABREACTION

Abreaction is one of the oldest procedures to deliberately combine drugs and psychotherapy. The drugs concerned include those which are inhaled (chloroform, ether, or nitrous oxide) or given intravenously (barbiturates such as hexobarbitone, pentobarbitone or amylobarbitone, methamphetamine or diazepam). There is no evidence that drugs are essential for abreaction. Abreaction or catharsis can occur spontaneously or be triggered by sudden noises, alcohol, discussion about combat, or in psychotherapy. It can be induced by hypnosis, psychodrama, films, or simple suggestion. The clinical features and consequences of abreaction

Isaac M. Marks, M.D., Reader in Experimental Psychopathology, Institute of Psychiatry, University of London.
This work was supported in part by a grant from the Bethlem-Maudsley Research Fund.

appear similar regardless of the way in which the emotion has been induced. As yet we do not know which events decide whether abreaction is desensitizing, habituating, or simply ineffective.

INTRAVENOUS AGENTS

There is little doubt that several classes of oral drugs can reduce anxiety or depression at least temporarily (reviewed by Lader & Marks, 1972). From time to time it becomes fashionable to administer these classes of drugs intravenously, though there is little evidence that intravenous is any better than oral administration beyond instilling a sense of potency in the doctor. Intravenous drugs carry two disadvantages. They can be dangerous and usually require the presence of a doctor at the patient's side during treatment. Oral drugs do not require a medical presence beyond the act of prescribing and a minimum of monitoring thereafter. This is an important consideration at a time when therapy is being given increasingly by non-medical personnel. Convincing controlled data are mandatory to justify the routine use of intravenous agents. Such data are sadly lacking.

In 1959, King and Little (1959) contrasted intravenous thiopental with placebo injections and with psychotherapy. Although the thiopental group showed more improvement than controls during a followup of up to three months, the controls included patients who had not had an injection and the report gave too few details to allow adequate assessment.

Intravenous thiopental was also studied by Husain (1971), who contrasted its effects with that of a saline infusion in patients with agoraphobia or social phobias. Patients had either flooding or desensitization in fantasy assisted either by thiopental or saline intravenously. Thiopental facilitated flooding but made no difference to desensitization in fantasy. The design involved crossover of treatments, which precludes conclusions about persistence of effects during followup.

Another intravenous barbiturate, methohexitone, is often recommended as an adjuvant to desensitization in fantasy. Three studies have examined this with some kind of control, but none have yet included the crucial control for the effect of an injection alone. Yorkston, Sergeant, and Rachman (1968) found discouraging results in severe agoraphobics. In less severe phobics, Mawson (1970) noted that intravenous methohexitone significantly enhanced the value of desensitization compared to that of muscular relaxation without an injection. This was a crossover design which did not allow assessment of followup beyond a few days. In another study of severe agoraphobia, Lipsedge et al. (1973) reported that methohexitone desensitization in fantasy reduced phobias more than did desensitization with simple muscular relaxation, but again there was no saline injection control.

Another sedative, propanidid, has been used intravenously during exposure in vivo of agoraphobics (Hudson, Tobin, & Gaind, 1972), and the tricyclic clomipramine has been used intravenously in obsessives (Capstick, 1971; Rack, 1971). All these were uncontrolled.

In brief, the value of intravenous drugs used in combination with psychological treatment has yet to be substantiated from experimental evidence; this combination carries distinct disadvantages compared to oral drugs of the same class.

Inhalations of carbon dioxide have occasionally been tried for the reduction of anxiety in neurotic patients. Slater and Leavy (1966) administered these to 12 anxious inpatients who served as their own controls for three treatments: (1) a carbon dioxide-oxygen mixture, (2) hyperventilation, and (3) full inhalation of air. Ten minutes after treatment a carbon dioxide mixture resulted in a significantly greater reduction in anxiety on self-ratings, but this change was not significant after twenty-four hours. Haslam (1971) gave lactate infusions to 16 patients with anxiety states. Of the 10 who developed anxiety with this procedure, 9 were said to be calmed by subsequent carbon dioxide inhalation. Of the 6 who showed no anxiety with lactate infusion, only 1 improved with carbon dioxide inhalation. Ratings were obtained immediately after the inhalations. Evidence for the persistent value of carbon dioxide inhalation is thus still negligible, and longer-term studies are desirable.

Evidence in anxiety syndromes for the value of *oral* drugs with psychological treatment is of a firmer kind. Table 1 summarizes controlled work in the field.

"ANTIDEPRESSANTS"

Imipramine has been the subject of two double-blind controlled studies. In agoraphobics Klein (1964) found that imipramine reduced panic more than did a placebo and suggested that this helped patients to enter their phobic situations. In school phobics (Gittelman-Klein & Klein, 1971), more imipramine children, compared to a placebo group, returned to school and improved on ratings of global help, depression, physical complaints, and school phobias. These differences were not present at three weeks, and only developed after six weeks. This might have been related to dose rather than time, as the mean medication at three weeks was 107 mgs. a day, compared to 152 mgs. at six weeks. Patients and families had been seen weekly; case workers instructed the families to maintain a firm attitude towards school attendance and acted as a liaison with the school. The authors suggested that this played an essential part in producing the greater improvement seen in children treated with imipramine. They thought that imipramine alone, without insistence on return to school, would have led to children being happier while staying at home, without returning to school. Feeling better did not automatically lead to school return. Of the children on imipramine who felt better, not all went back to school. Imipramine was seen as instrumental in reducing general anxiety, which then facilitated the effect of parental pressure on the child to expose himself to the feared school situation.

MONOAMINE OXIDASE INHIBITORS

These drugs are frequently prescribed outside the U.S.A. There have been two controlled studies, one in England and one in Canada. At the Maudsley, phenelzine was studied by Tyrer, Candy, and Kelly (1973) in chronic agoraphobics and social phobics. Patients entered a double-blind trial of phenelzine vs. placebo in a flexible dosage for two months. Throughout the trial all patients were advised to expose themselves gradually to phobic situations so that the effect of the tablets could be evaluated. Of the 40 patients who entered the trial, 32 completed it, among whom there were 14 matched pairs. Phenelzine patients improved significantly more on overall assessment, secondary phobias, and work. There was no correlation between dose and response in the phenelzine group. The average dose was 45 mgs. daily. As in the study by Gittelman-Klein and Klein (1971) with imipramine, the superiority of phenelzine took time to emerge; though it began at the four-week rating, it was only significant by the eight-week rating. Despite this, initial depression did not correlate with outcome.

In this study, improvement of phobias was measured on the scale described by Gelder and Marks (1966). The degree of improvement was very similar to that obtained (Gelder, Marks, & Wolff, 1967) with desensitization in fantasy in a comparable population. Desensitization in fantasy is a weak form of exposure compared to exposure in vivo. Thus the effect of phenelzine, though significant, was not large. An interesting future study would be a comparison of phenelzine plus exposure in vivo rather than in fantasy.

An independent study in Canada (Solyom, Heseltine, McClure, Solyom, Ledwidge, & Steinberg, 1973) also investigated phenelzine in 10 comparable phobic patients using similar scales. Patients treated with phenelzine showed equivalent degrees of improvement to those in the preceding studies. Again, improvement was significant but small, and of the same magnitude as that of a comparison group which had desensitization in fantasy without drugs. The phenelzine group received no systematic instructions regarding exposure. As with Tyrer et al. (1973), the

Table 1. Controlled Studies of Drugs and Exposure Treatments in Phobic Patients

Drug	Population IP = inpatients OP = outpatients	Author	Type of exposure	Comments
Sedatives				
Inhalation of CO_2	anxious IP	Slater and Leavy, 1966	–	outcome measured immediately post-treatment
	anxious IP	Haslam, 1971	–	outcome measured immediately post-treatment
Intravenous barbiturates				
thiopental	anxious phobics	King and Little, 1959	–	50 percent of control subjects had no injection, scanty detail
thiopental	anxious phobics	Husain, 1971	df + ff	no injection control
methohexitone	agoraphobic IP	Yorkston et al., 1968	df	no injection control
methohexitone	agoraphobic OP	Lipsedge et al., 1973	hp, df	no injection control
methohexitone	mixed phobic OP	Mawson, 1970	df	
Benzodiazepines				
diazepam	specific phobic OP	Marks et al., 1972	P	crossover design; outcome measured two days post-treatment
	agoraphobic IP	Johnston and Gath, 1973	ff + P	crossover design; outcome measured one day post-treatment (N = 4 only)
	agoraphobic OP	Hafner and Marks, 1976	P + hp	group exposure; parallel design
Beta blockers				
alprenelol	agoraphobic OP	Ullrich et al., 1972	P + hp	alprenelol helped anxiety, not avoidance
Antidepressants				
tricyclics–imipramine	agoraphobics	Klein, 1964	hp	
imipramine	school phobic OP	Gittelman-Klein and Klein, 1971	hp	delay before improvement

Table 1. (Continued)

monoamine oxidase inhibitors				
phenelzine	agora- and social phobic OP	Tyrer et al., 1973	hp	delay before improvement, relapse when drug stopped
phenelzine	agora- and social phobic OP	Solyom et al., 1973	–	delay before improvement, relapse when drug stopped
iproniazid	agora- and social phobic OP	Lipsedge et al., 1973	–	delay before improvement, relapse when drug stopped iproniazid helped anxiety, not avoidance

Drugs given orally unless otherwise stated.

- = not systematic
df = desensitization in fantasy
ff = flooding in fantasy
P = exposure in practice (vivo)
hp = home program of P

average dose of phenelzine was 45 mgs. daily. Tyrer et al. had noted that patients who stopped the drug had minor relapses. Solyom et al., too, found that 6 of the 10 phenelzine subjects who stopped taking the drug relapsed.

The same tendency to relapse on stopping monoamine oxidase inhibitors was noted by Lipsedge et al. (1973) with iproniazid in severe agoraphobics. Sixty outpatients were assigned at random to one of six groups in a 2 × 3 factorial design. The main comparison relevant here is that of iproniazid versus placebo. During treatment all patients were encouraged to carry out a daily home program of graded exposure and to keep a daily diary of these activities, and were praised for improvement. Dosage of iproniazid was up to 150 mgs. daily over eight weeks. While still on medication at the end of treatment, iproniazid patients showed significantly more improvement than placebo patients on anxiety but not on avoidance. Withdrawal of iproniazid was followed by frequent relapse. Interestingly, on the Gelder-Marks phobia scales the effect of iproniazid plus home exposure in vivo was greater than that of placebo with the same program, but was not improved by the addition of desensitization in fantasy.

In brief, the three controlled studies of monoamine oxidase inhibitors agree that this class of drug has a significant if limited effect and that there is a high relapse rate following drug withdrawal. The way in which these drugs interact with systematic exposure treatment is still obscure.

BETA-BLOCKERS

A systematic combination of alprenelol with exposure in vivo of agoraphobics was made by Ullrich, Ullrich, Crombach, and Peikert (1972) in a double-blind trial. Patients received two hours of exposure in vivo daily for fourteen days after they signed a contract not to escape from the situation. During exposure they received either alprenelol or placebo. Two other groups either had exposure in vivo without placebo or were put on a waiting list. Exposure with alprenelol produced a superior reduction in autonomic anxiety which became apparent by the second week. Alprenelol did not enhance decrease in avoidance. This greater reduction in anxiety than in avoidance parallels the findings of Lipsedge et al. (1973) with phenelzine.

BENZODIAZEPINES

Three controlled studies have examined the combination of diazepam with exposure in vivo in phobics. In 4 agoraphobic inpatients, Johnson and Gath (1973) contrasted the effect of 20 mgs. of oral diazepam with placebo and with the presence of a dummy syrup to which patients attributed drug effects. Treatment was on three consecutive days a week for four weeks, for a total of twelve sessions in an incomplete Latin square design. Exposure consisted of 45 minutes of flooding in imagination followed by 60 minutes of in vivo practice of hierarchy items. Exposure treatment was more effective when given together with diazepam. Improvement was unaffected by the patient's attribution of effects to a dummy syrup. Outcome was measured the day after each treatment block, and the crossover design did not allow assessment of followup effects.

This result was in accord with that of an earlier similar study done at the Maudsley on twelve specific phobics. This and a subsequent larger study will be discussed in some detail to highlight a few of the problems which beset the researcher in this area. The designs tried to get over the hypothesized presence of drug dissociation and aimed to make exposure treatment more pleasant. In clinical practice phobics often become able to enter their phobic situation under the influence of sedatives, but as the drug effect wears off they begin to escape from the situation once more. This might be a form of state-dependence or drug dissociative behavior. In animal experiments, behavior learned in a sedative-drug state often fails to transfer to the undrugged state (Miller, 1964). It seems probable that this effect might be more pronounced during the phase of peak drug effect and less when the drug effect is wearing off. In rats, exposure to the phobic situation during slow withdrawal of sedative drugs has been effective in extinguishing conditioned avoidance responses (Sherman, 1967). Whether this was true for humans was tested in this study. A "waning" experimental condition involved exposure in vivo during the transitional phase from a drug to a non-drug state while drug effects were presumed to be declining. A "peak" group was exposed while psychotropic effects were presumed to be at their highest. A third group was exposed with placebo.

In the first study, a crossover design, Marks, Viswanathan, and Lipsedge (1972) treated 18 outpatients with chronic specific phobias. Patients were allocated at random to exposure for two hours to the real phobic situation in one or two out of three possible treatment conditions; i.e., exposure starting (1) four hours after oral diazepam 0.1 mgs. per kgm. ("waning" group); (2) one hour after oral diazepam 0.1 mgs. per kgm. ("peak" group); or (3) four hours or one hour after oral placebo. Each patient had two treatment sessions in a balanced sequence. Assessment was blind for the patient, therapist, and independent rater. The design of the first study is detailed in Figure 1. The average dose was 7.5 mgs. The dose of diazepam was small enough not to produce obviously visible sleepiness, and patients were not asked about the effect of their elixir so as to avoid clues being given to the therapist about their treatment condition. Outcome was measured two to three days after the end of treatment.

Table 2.   Experimental Design of study by Marks et al. (1972)

Time: 9 A.M.	10	11	12	1 P.M.	2	3	4 P.M.
Session I, day 1: 1st assessment	elixir[a] drunk	IV blood sample		elixir[b] drunk	IV blood sample	continuous exposure to real phobic situation →	IV blood sample / patient rates session unpleasantness
Session II, day 4: 2nd assessment	as for day 1						
day 8: 3rd assessment	no treatment						

[a] Contained diazepam if exposure was during "waning" diazepam; otherwise contained placebo.
[b] Contained diazepam if exposure was during "peak" diazepam; otherwise contained placebo.

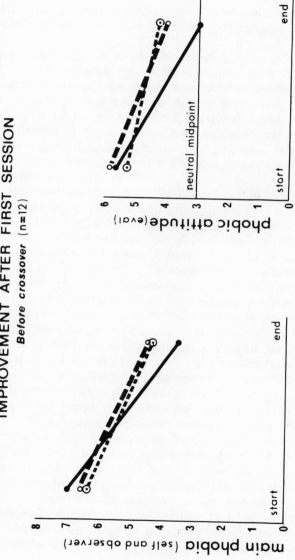

IMPROVEMENT AFTER FIRST SESSION
Before crossover (n=12)

FIG. 1. Improvement after first session: before crossover. (Source: Marks et al., 1972.)

Exposure in vivo under all three conditions produced significant improvement. However, the waning group was significantly superior to placebo and the peak group was in between. The trend of superiority was consistent for clinical, attitudinal, and physiological ratings. The trend was already present significantly after the first treatment session, before crossover (Fig. 2).

There was no evidence of drug dissociation at the moderate dosage employed because the peak group, if anything, did slightly better than the placebo group. The absence of drug dissociation was interesting. Perhaps dissociation might have occurred had exposure been for but a few minutes rather than for two hours. A third possibility might be that the psychotropic effect, like the serum level, was waning even between one and three hours after ingestion, so that the so-called peak group was actually a partially waning group, which might account for its slight superiority to placebo. No measure of psychotropic effect was made that was independent of the phobia. Theoretically one might speculate that the rate of degradation or excretion of diazepam is affected by an individual's activity. Perhaps during great anxiety the rate is accelerated, thus obscuring differences in serum level in the two diazepam groups which might otherwise be apparent. Conversely, anxiety might equally well retard the rate of breakdown of diazepam.

One aim of the research had been to make exposure treatment more pleasant without impairing its efficacy. This aim was not achieved, as all three treatment conditions were rated by the patients as equally unpleasant. The degree of unpleasantness was less than expected—only slightly unpleasant on semantic differential and analogue scales. This was surprising in view of the great anxiety which patients showed during confrontation with the phobic object and their physiological arousal during the process. Therapists exposed patients to the phobic situation as rapidly as patients would allow. This pace was unwittingly rather faster under diazepam than under placebo, so that the diazepam groups may have had more intense exposure during a given session, which might account for their superior results. Under diazepam patients touched the phobic object for the first time rather earlier in the first session than they did under placebo. It might be that patients can tolerate only a particular maximum of anxiety during exposure before they escape, and that the same maximum is reached higher up the hierarchy under influence of a sedative than with placebo. In other words, mild sedation may increase the amount of confrontation that is possible. However, this might also increase the amount of anxiety and unpleasantness in the session to the same level as under placebo.

Serum levels of diazepam fluctuated so widely among individuals that it was of little value in studying differences between groups (Fig. 3). Nevertheless, individual patients had reliably similar serum levels when

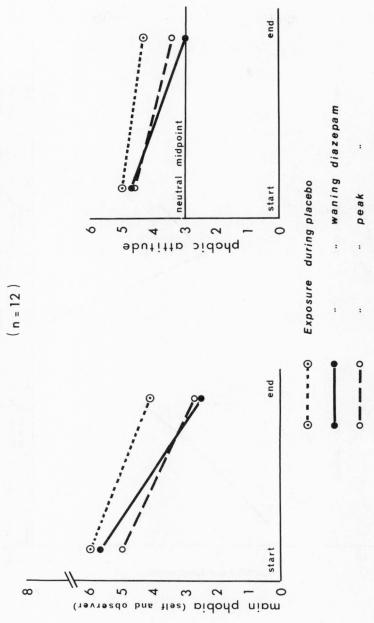

FIG. 2. Improvement after first session: before and after crossover. (Source: Marks et al., 1972.)

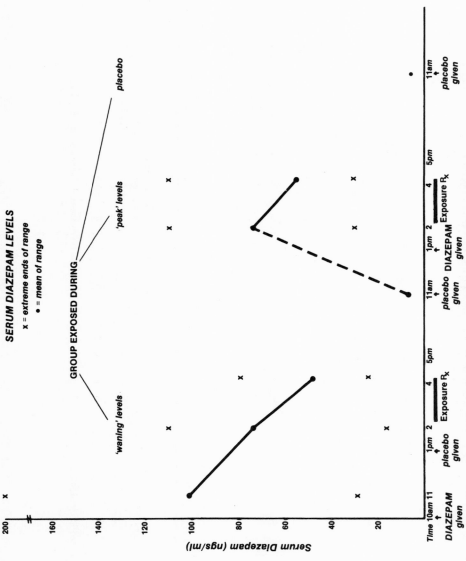

FIG. 3. Serum levels of diazepam between groups. (Source: Marks et al., 1972.)

they took the drug on successive sessions (Fig. 4). Serum levels of diazepam bore no obvious relation to its psychotropic effect as measured by subjective anxiety. Present technology does not allow us to measure levels of drug or active metabolites in those parts of the brain which might reflect psychotropic activity.

The outcome of this study suggested that phobics might be treated better by exposure in vivo which began several hours, not immediately, after oral sedation and continued for several hours while psychotropic effects were declining. A partial replication of this idea was tried by Hafner and Marks (1976), but variations in the experimental design might affect conclusions which can be drawn. They assigned 42 agoraphobic out-patients randomly to treatment in one of three conditions of exposure in vivo given in four sessions over two weeks. Each session of exposure was three-and-one-half hours long and began half an hour after 0.1 mg. per kgm of oral diazepam in the "peak" condition, three-and-one-half hours later, in the "waning" condition, or after similar time intervals following placebo in a third condition. An important difference from the previous study was that exposure in vivo was given in groups of 6 patients at a time, not individually, as in the first experiment. Every group of 6 contained 2 patients in each of the three drug or placebo conditions. A fourth randomly assigned condition (N = 12) consisted of individual exposure in vivo with placebo. Another difference from the previous study was that this was a parallel design without crossover so that followup effects could be studied; each patient was treated in only one exposure condition. A final difference was that patients here were agoraphobics, not specific phobics.

Outcome two days after treatment showed only a slight nonsignificant trend for superiority of phobia reduction in the waning diazepam group, and this difference disappeared totally by one-, three-, and six-month followup. Once more there was little difference in anxiety or unpleasantness of sessions in diazepam and in placebo conditions. An attempt was made to measure psychotropic effects of diazepam by measuring critical flicker fusion thresholds. These did not discriminate in any way between drug and placebo conditions. Serum drug levels were not measured.

The largest most consistent trend was for patients in all three group-exposure conditions to do better than patients who were exposed in vivo individually. This group effect might have washed out any differences due to drugs in at least two ways; first, groups in their own right might be as calming as diazepam. Second, the pace of exposure in vivo was set by groups as a whole and was not tailored to any one person, unlike the situation with individual exposure in the preceding study by Marks et al. (1972). In the present experiment every group of patients contained subjects in waning, in peak, and in placebo conditions. If diazepam works

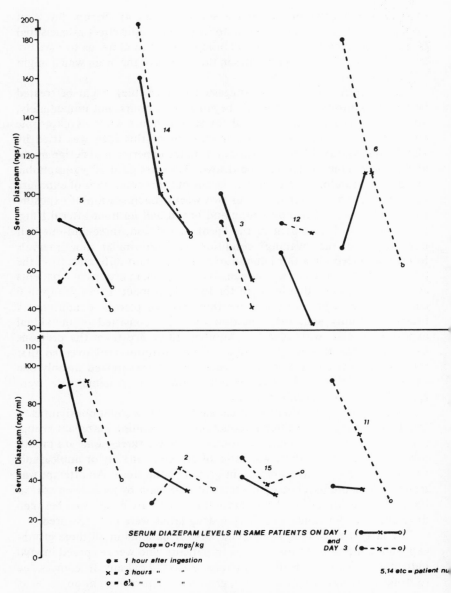

FIG. 4. Serum levels of diazepam: individual reliability. (Source: Marks et al., 1972.)

at all, it might be by allowing a more rapid pace of exposure to the phobic situation. Future studies will need to measure this pace of exposure more carefully. Results from this and the previous study might also have differed because diazepam could conceivably affect specific phobics and agoraphobics differently, but this is speculative. Because of the contrast in designs this investigation cannot be regarded as a total failure to replicate the preceding one.

ISSUES IN RESEARCH

The foregoing studies illustrate some pitfalls which have to be overcome in future research in the area. It goes without saying that designs must provide for ratings which are blind with respect to the drugs and to the psychological treatments which are being manipulated. The designs need to include at least two factors: (1) drug vs. placebo, and (2) the psychological technique in question vs. the control technique appropriate for the hypothesis being tested. The interaction between these two factors is also crucial. So far the only study to manipulate both drug and psychotherapeutic factors is that of Lipsedge et al. (1973).

Badly needed are good measures of psychotropic effects of drugs which are independent of the phobias or obsessions. Most physiological measures are too remote from subjective states to be of value. No good measures of this kind are yet available. Also unavailable at present are techniques to measure levels of drugs or their active metabolites in the cerebrospinal fluid or brain. Serum levels are too far from the operative events to be of great use, though they have some value in indicating drug metabolism. Drug dosage is also obviously important.

Less obvious is the importance of dosage not only of the drug but also of the psychological treatment being given. It makes a difference whether the exposure is in fantasy or in vivo, how soon after drug administration it begins, how long it continues afterwards and the speed with which the patient is brought into contact with the phobic situation in all its frightening aspects. It is also important to know how much anxiety or unpleasantness occurs during exposure treatment. Though benzodiazepine drugs are traditionally regarded as sedatives and anxiolytics, the evidence that they decrease subjective anxiety during exposure is not impressive. Though diazepam does decrease skin conductance activity, subjective discomfort was not greatly altered with the moderate dose (average of 7.5 mg) employed in the Maudsley studies or even with much higher doses used in uncontrolled work by McCormick (1972). It is still an open question how far sedative drugs actually prevent anxiety during exposure. Diazepam and its congeners might be less anxiolytic than has been supposed hitherto.

Another theoretical and practical problem is whether and when drug dissociation exists, i.e., when does learning fail to transfer from drug to non-drug state or vice versa? The evidence in humans is inconclusive. If drug dissociation does exist, it is likely to vary with many circumstances.

We have seen that current labels for drugs can be misleading and that anxiolytic drugs need not be very anxiolytic. "Antidepressant" drugs may have actions beyond the reduction of depression. Where "antidepressants" have been useful in phobic disorders improvement in phobias did not correlate with change in depression. Yet on these drugs improvement relative to placebo usually took several weeks to become manifest, a time interval similar to the lag usually seen in relief of depression by antidepressant drugs. Perhaps this indicates a common mechanism underlying both actions of these drugs. Relapse on cessation of these drugs might perhaps be prevented by more vigorous exposure in vivo.

This paper has been concerned only with the use of drugs and psychological treatments in anxiety syndromes. We have not touched on their potential interplay with other problems and techniques, e.g., the operant training of schizophrenics or subnormals. Most of this area is unexplored, and progress is likely to be slow. Each of the many questions discussed above will take years of effort and thousands of dollars to answer. Nevertheless, the payoff in this field may be sufficiently great to make the effort well worth while. The alternative is to continue spending vast amounts of money on drugs and psychotherapies whose effects are uncertain.

SUMMARY

Until recently the actions of drugs and of psychological treatments have tended to be examined in isolation from one another. However, the possibility of interactional effects requires study of their combined use, e.g., state-dependent learning is well attested in animals and might interfere with treatment in humans. In phobias, tricyclics (imipramine) and monoamine oxidase inhibitors (phenelzine, iproniazid) have been of significant benefit compared to placebo, the effect not being of an antidepressant kind. During exposure in vivo β-adrenergic blockers have reduced autonomic symptoms in phobics more than placebo, though avoidance was not affected.

In specific phobics one double-blind study of oral diazepam during individual exposure in vivo found that fear was reduced significantly more after exposure was given during its waning psychotropic phase than after placebo. Exposure during the peak psychotropic phase of diazepam was intermediate in its effect. There was no evidence of state dependence with diazepam at this moderate dosage (0.1 mgs./kg) and no relationship between outcome of blood level of diazepam, which varied greatly between individuals but was constant for the same individuals over different occasions. It was surprising that subjective anxiety was similar during exposure with or without diazepam, but patients in the waning diazepam phase allowed earlier direct contact with the phobic object during exposure in vivo.

Another double-blind study examined group exposure in vivo of agoraphobics during waning and peak phases of diazepam and placebo. Each group of 6 patients contained 2 in each condition. Preliminary analysis suggests that overall decrease in phobias was similar in each treatment condition, though patients on diazepam entered the phobic situation alone rather earlier than did placebo patients. Diazepam only slightly reduced subjective anxiety during exposure to the phobic situation. Diazepam may be less anxiolytic in its action than has hitherto been supposed.

REFERENCES

Capstick, N. Anafranil in obsessional states—a followup study. Paper presented at the Fifth World Congress of Psychiatry, Mexico, 1971.

Gelder, M. G., & Marks, I. M. Severe agoraphobia: a controlled prospective trial of behaviour therapy. *British Journal of Psychiatry*, 1966, **112**, 309–319.

Gelder, M. G., Marks, I. M., & Wolff, H. Desensitisation and psychotherapy in phobic states: a controlled enquiry. *British Journal of Psychiatry*, 1967, **113**, 53–73.

Gittelman-Klein, R., & Klein, D. F. Controlled imipramine treatment of school phobia. *Archives of General Psychiatry*, 1971, **25**, 204–207.

Hafner, J., & Marks, I. M. Exposure in vivo of agoraphobics: the contributions of diazepam, group exposure, and anxiety evocation. *Journal of Psychological Medicine*, 1976, in press.

Haslam, M. T. The relationship between the effect of lactate infusion on anxiety states, and their amelioration by carbon dioxide inhalation. Paper presented at the Fifth World Congress of Psychiatry, Mexico, 1971.

Hudson, B. L., Tobin, J. C., & Gaind, R. Followup of a group of agoraphobic patients. Paper presented at the Second Annual Conference of Psychiatry, Mexico, 1972.

Husain, M. Z. Desensitization and flooding (implosion) in treatment of phobias. *American Journal of Psychiatry*, 1971, **127**, 1509–1514.

Johnston, D., & Gath, D. Arousal levels and attribution effects in diazepam-assisted flooding. *British Journal of Psychiatry*, 1973, **122**, 463–466.

King, A., & Little, J. C. Thiopentone treatment of the phobic-anxiety-depersonalization syndrome. *Proceedings of the Royal Society of Medicine*, 1959, **52**, 595–596.

Klein, D. F. Delineation of two drug-responsive anxiety syndromes. *Psychopharmacologia*, 1964, **5**, 397–408.

Lader, M., & Marks, I. M. *Clinical Anxiety*. New York: Grune and Stratton, 1972.

Lipsedge, M., Hajioff, J., Huggins, P., Napier, L., Pearce, J., Pike, D. J., & Rich, M. The management of severe agoraphobia: a comparison of iproniazid and systematic desensitisation. *Psychopharmacologia*, 1973, **32**, 67–80.

Marks, I. M., Viswanathan, R., Lipsedge, M. S., & Gardner, R. Enhanced relief of phobias by flooding during waning diazepam effect. *British Journal of Psychiatry*, 1972, **121**, 493–505.

Mawson, A. N. Methohexitone-assisted desensitisation in the treatment of phobias. *Lancet*, 1970, **1**, 1084–1086.

McCormick, W. O. Drug-assisted desensitisation of phobias. Paper presented at the Conference on Behavioural Engineering, Wexford, Ireland, 1972.

Miller, N. E. In H. Steinberg (Ed.), *Animal Behaviour and Drug Action.* London: Churchill, 1964.

Rack, P. H. Intravenous anafranil and obsessional states. Paper presented at the Fifth World Congress of Psychiatry, Mexico, 1971.

Sherman, A. R. Therapy of maladaptive fear-motivated behaviour in the rat by the systematic gradual withdrawal of a fear-reducing drug. *Behaviour Research and Therapy,* 1967, **5**, 121–129.

Slater, S. L., & Leavy, A. The effects of inhaling a 35% CO_2-65% O_2 mixture upon anxiety level in neurotic patients. *Behaviour Research and Therapy,* 1966, **4**, 309–316.

Solyom, L., Heseltine, C. F. O., McClure, D. J. Solyom, C., Ledwidge, B., & Steinberg, G. *Canadian Psychological Association Journal,* 1973, **18**, 25–32.

Tyrer, P. J., Candy, J., & Kelly, D. H. W. Phenelzine in phobic anxiety: a controlled trial. *Psychological Medicine,* 1973, **3**, 120.

Ullrich, R., Ullrich, R., Crombach, G., & Peikert, V. Three flooding procedures in the treatment of agoraphobics. Paper presented at the Second European Conference on Behaviour Modification, Wexford, Ireland, 1972.

Yorkston, N., Sergeant, H., & Rachman, S. Methohexitone relaxation for desensitising agoraphobic patients. *Lancet,* 1968, **2**, 651–653.

11

DISCUSSION:
Behavior Therapy.
Some Critical Comments

MICHAEL J. MAHONEY

The current status of behavior therapy as an enduring field of clinical research and scientific inquiry can scarcely be contested. Claims of "faddism" have not been borne out by the data—behavior therapy has not only survived a turbulent youth but has grown into an impressive body of theory and research which is quickly becoming familiar in a variety of disciplines. I shall not here devote time to some of the formal criticisms of the behavioral approach. Those criticisms and their validity have been taken up elsewhere (Mahoney, Kazdin, & Lesswing, 1974). What I would like to do here is to offer some criticisms of my own.

The time has come, I think, for behavior therapists to engage in some constructive self-criticism. As Lazarus (1971) has pointed out, we are not in danger of extinction. Behavior therapy has come of age and it is time to abandon the energetic (and often myopic) defensiveness of our adolescence. If we aspire to genuine scientific ideals, we must subject our hypotheses—and even our model(s)—to stringent and frequent reevaluation. My comments today stem from a firm conviction in the viability of an empirical approach to human behavior. I feel that behavior therapy has taken a large step in the direction of identifying and therapeutically utilizing significant descriptive principles. While this "first step" is, I think, in the right direction, our journey is a long one. It is my opinion that the pace of our travel could be appreciably increased if behavior therapy researchers would take a long pragmatic look at some of the following methodological issues.

1. *Innovation versus replication.* Unfortunately, most of the professional pellets in contemporary behavioral research fall to the creative theorist and innovative researcher. The arduous task of systematic replication and parametric refinement receive little attention despite their critical role in scientific self-correction. This problem, of course, is not restricted to behavior therapy. However, in a field so young and rudimen-

Michael J. Mahoney, Ph.D., Associate Professor of Psychology, Pennsylvania State University, University Park, Pennsylvania.

tary, the empirical foundations of pioneering research are even more crucial. Directions are more important early in a journey than late. We need to systematically reassess some of our staid landmarks in behavioral research. With our current knowledge of human behavior, we should be well equipped for the task of appropriately redistributing the professional rewards.

2. *Single-subject versus group research.* There seems to be a clandestine feud between behavior therapists who pursue single-subject inquiries and those who view group research as the only avenue for scientific progress. It would be very easy to classify the factions, but that is not my purpose. My point is that both types of research offer powerful paradigms for empirical inquiry. They vary in the types of questions they allow and in the answers they provide, but neither is inherently more legitimate or scientific than the other. I shall belabor this point only enough to provide references to support my position. Single-subject research offers practical utility in (1) demonstrating an effect, (2) generating hypotheses, and (3) providing a clinically relevant paradigm for the individualization of therapy. Excellent defenses of these functions can be found in Lazarus and Davison (1971), Thoresen (1972), and Kazdin (1973). Group research, on the other hand, offers advantages in (1) comparing the effects of independent variables, (2) identifying predictors of inter-subject variability, and (3) making probabilistic generalizations to other populations. These functions are described by Campbell and Stanley (1963) and Paul (1969).

Dichotomous arguments have frequently been aired by both factions in this feud. Proponents of the group paradigm have relegated almost all single-subject research to a pre-scientific purgatory. They have remained ignorant of methodological refinements which transcend the early monotony of ABAB designs and uncontrolled case histories. Data from single cases, according to the nomothetic researcher, are only "suggestive" and can never qualify as good experimental evidence. The often heated interchanges between these methodological factions are well illustrated in the comment of one worker that the only problem with "idiographic" research was that someone left out the "t" between the "o" and the "g."

On the other hand, single-subject researchers have often been remiss in their wholesale rejection of inquiries based on group designs and statistical controls. There is nothing inherent in group research which demands that it ignore "transition states" and behavior change processes. Group averages and probabilistic predictors are far from clinically useless.

I have belabored the point enough. Suffice it to say that the feud is neither functional nor justified. Science progresses according to degrees of confidence, and both single-subject and group research offer their own legitimate and unique contributions.

3. *Maintenance and generalization.* The issues of therapeutic transfer and post-treatment maintenance have become increasingly acknowledged topics in behavior therapy research. During our youth we were frequently content to carry out and publish what Gerald Patterson has called "whoopee" studies. In these early inquiries a specific circumscribed behavior was modified via some monstrously large reinforcer. This effect was quickly written up for publication, and the behavior therapist rushed on ambitiously to further demonstrations of his expertise. More recent self-examination by behavioral researchers, however, has suggested that we need to pay far more attention to the analysis and programming of post-treatment maintenance and transfer. Since these issues have begun to receive their empirical due, my comments are more salutatory than critical.

4. *The cognitive inquisition.* For a variety of historical and methodological reasons, behavior therapy researchers have been reluctant to examine cognitive-symbolic processes in behavior change. Covert events —while readily acknowledged at cocktail parties and *ex cathedra* discussions—have been formally attacked as unscientific, unparsimonious, and illegitimate.

The roots and logical status of this "cognitive inquisition" have been extensively dealt with elsewhere (cf. Mahoney, 1974). I shall only point out here that contemporary behavior therapists continue to adopt a "prime mover" assumption in human behavior which posits that the "first" and most important causes of human actions come from "without" rather than from "within." Humanistic psychologists, of course, have proposed the exact opposite. It is my opinion that both are wrong. There is no first cause.

Cognitive factors undoubtedly play a significant role in human action. The empirical evidence is overwhelming—covert events can function as antecedents, mediators, and consequences of overt responses. Moreover, notwithstanding the arguments of some of my more radical colleagues, I believe that we now have adequately sophisticated technologies for measuring many of these covert processes.

If we, as behavioral researchers, have any pretensions of developing a comprehensive model of human behavior, then we must begin to examine those phenomena which monopolize the life of the adult *homo sapiens* —i.e., private events.

5. *Prohibited variables.* A closely related issue has to do with the currently "approved" elements in behavior therapy research. There are some rather unfortunate prohibitions which limit not only our empirical horizons but also our theoretical breadth. For example, even though the typical behavior therapist views his client as a complex biological organism, biological variables are virtually "taboo" in his research.

Pharmacological effects, nutritional factors, and sleep deprivation are seldom explored.

Likewise, there is a strong aversion to such influences as placebo effects, expectancy, and relationship factors in behavior therapy. These terms have acquired strongly negative connotations. An effect produced by "placebo" is considered illegitimate and discarded, rather than becoming a stimulus for inquiries regarding the processes involved. Expectancy and demand characteristics are similarly stigmatized. Nonspecific variables are occasionally invoked to explain unpredicted results, but are otherwise ignored. I should like to state here my own agreement with Albert Bandura (1969) that the term "nonspecifics" should be dropped from our methodological vocabularies. In a deterministic science, there are no "nonspecific variables," only unspecified ones.

Relationship variables sound too ambiguous and dangerously traditional for most contemporary behavioral researchers. The prospect that other theoretical models and systems of therapy might have something to offer the behavior therapist is a radical (and perhaps blasphemous) suggestion. However, most behaviorists would concede that the behaviors and cues associated with a therapist may affect therapeutic outcome. With very little translation, these and other prohibited variables could be readily explored from the anchor-point of a behavioral model.

6. *The conditioning model.* My final criticism has to do with what might be called a "conceptual chauvinism." Many contemporary behavior therapists adopt a conditioning model of human functioning to the virtual exclusion of any other. Alternative models are seen as competing with, rather than complementing, our knowledge of "basic learning principles." With a patriotic fervor which can scarcely be ignored, many wave the banner of "learning theory" and "conditioning therapies" as if these were the undisputed avenues to Behavioral Truth. Procrustean formulas are not an unfamiliar sight: when data and model conflict, the data are ignored, transformed, or attributed to experimental error.

My own views on the inadequacy of a peripheral conditioning model are not unique. It has become increasingly apparent in the last few years that that model is in dire need of help if it is to claim any degree of conceptual breadth or explanatory adequacy. While basic learning principles do seem to offer a firm empirical foundation upon which to build our understanding of human behavior, their *in*sufficiency can hardly be denied. Contemporary researchers in behavior therapy need to investigate refinements and conceptual revisions which might add to the power and comprehensiveness of their perspective. Devotion to theory, technique, or paradigm must be replaced by a simpler and inherently more empirical fidelity—a devotion to data.

REFERENCES

Bandura, A. *Principles of behavior modification*. New York: Holt, Rinehart & Winston, 1969.

Campbell, D. T., & Stanley, J. C. *Experimental and quasi-experimental designs for research*. Chicago: Rand McNally, 1963.

Kazdin, A. E. Methodological and assessment considerations in evaluating reinforcement programs in applied settings. *Journal of Applied Behavior Analysis*, 1973, 6, 517–531.

Lazarus, A. A. *Behavior therapy and beyond*. New York: McGraw-Hill, 1971.

Lazarus, A. A., & Davison, G. C. Clinical innovation in research and practice. In A. E. Bergin & S. L. Garfield (Eds.), *Handbook of psychotherapy and behavior change*. New York: Wiley, 1971, pp. 196–213.

Mahoney, M. J. *Cognition and behavior modification*. Cambridge, Mass.: Ballinger, 1974.

Mahoney, M. J., Kazdin, A. E., & Lesswing, N. J. Behavior modification: delusion or deliverance? In C. M. Franks and G. T. Wilson (Eds.), *Annual review of behavior therapy theory and practice*, Vol. 2. New York: Brunner/Mazel, 1974.

Paul, G. L. Behavior modification research: design and tactics. In C. M. Franks (Ed.), *Behavior therapy: appraisal and status*. New York: McGraw-Hill, 1969, pp. 29–62.

Thoresen, C. E. The intensive design: an intimate approach to counseling research. Paper presented at the American Educational Research Association, Chicago, 1972.

12 DISCUSSION: Behavior Therapy. Some General Comments and a Review of Selected Papers

DAVID C. RIMM

Since some readers of this volume may be rather unfamiliar with behavioral approaches, a description or definition of behavior therapy may be of some value. This is not as easy as it may sound because, in reality, there are many behavior therapies, just as there are many psychotherapies. It is possible to define behavior therapy in terms of what we *do* (for example, relaxation, systematic desensitization, assertive training, use of modeling procedures, operant approaches, aversive conditioning, implosive therapy and flooding, behavioristic approaches to self-control, etc.) or in terms of our basic assumptions: in contrast with dynamic approaches, we assume that for a great many psychological disorders it is generally better to deal with the problem behavior itself, defined in a situation-specific manner, than with presumed deep-seated causes (e.g., psychosexual conflicts). Operant conditioners tend to remain on a purely behavioral level relative to those of us who also assume that it is useful to deal with constructs such as anxiety and implicit verbalizations.[1]

Our orientation is very much in the "here and now." We tend to assume that learning is an important etiological factor, and our treatment methods emphasize learning. A very fundamental assumption is that our methods are to be subjected to experimental investigation. The basic assumptions of behavior therapy are discussed at length in a variety of texts (for example, Bandura, 1969; Kanfer & Phillips, 1970; Rimm & Masters, 1974).

David C. Rimm, Ph.D., Associate Professor of Psychology, Southern Illinois University, Carbondale.
The author wishes to express his gratitude to Dr. Sol L. Garfield, Department of Psychology, Washington University; to Dr. William T. McReynolds, Department of Psychology, University of Missouri; and to Dr. Thomas R. Schill, Department of Psychology, Southern Illinois University, for their helpful comments on an earlier draft of this paper.

The term "behavior modification" is sometimes used as a synonym and sometimes is not, which has made for confusion (see Franzini & Tilker, 1972). In the United States the term behavior modification is often identified with the operant approaches, with behavior therapy the more inclusive label. I use the term behavior therapy in this manner.

IS BEHAVIOR THERAPY A FAD?

Mahoney, in the present volume, has indicated that it is not a fad. Let me now attempt to convince you that Mahoney is correct. In terms of present usage the term behavior therapy was introduced independently by Lazarus and by Eysenck in 1959 (see Lazarus, 1971). In 1963 the first behavior therapy journal (*Behavior Research and Therapy*) was founded. A second, *Journal of Applied Behavior Analysis*, was founded in 1968. Two additional journals appeared in 1970 (*Behavior Therapy* and *Behavior Therapy and Experimental Psychiatry*). Articles pertinent to behavior therapy are by no means restricted to these journals and appear with undiminished frequency in "traditional" journals (for example, in the *Journal of Abnormal Psychology* and the *Journal of Consulting and Clinical Psychology*). The *Journal of Abnormal Psychology* is highly respected and, as much as any journal, ought to reflect trends in the field of clinical psychology. As a matter of curiosity I counted the number of behavior therapy articles appearing in this journal in 1969 and compared this with the number appearing in 1973 (excluding the April, 1973, issue, which was devoted to cigarette smoking, and including the December, 1972 issue). In both years the number was ten. Keep in mind that two additional behavior therapy journals appeared in 1970. Were it not for this, I suspect that the number of articles appearing in the *Journal of Abnormal Psychology* in 1973 would have been greater.

Further evidence that behavior therapy is not a fad is seen in the large number of behavior therapy texts appearing in the past six years (Bandura, 1969; Krumboltz & Thoresen, 1969; Franks, 1969; Kanfer & Phillips, 1970; Yates, 1970; Lazarus, 1971, 1972; Graziano, 1971; Franks & Wilson, 1973; Schwitzgebel & Kolb, 1974; Rimm & Masters, 1974; Wolpe, 1974; Mahoney & Thoresen, 1974; Thoresen & Mahoney, 1974). This list is not exhaustive.

Benassi and Lanson (1972) graphically indicate how course offerings in behavior therapy have increased sharply, especially since 1967, with no indication (through the date of their survey) of any leveling off. Of the 290 departments of psychology in the United States responding to their query, 180 indicated they offered courses in the area; 110 indicated that they did not. Given existing trends, it must be assumed that course offerings will have increased considerably by the time this volume appears.

By definition, fads have two characteristics. They are of relatively brief duration and they are marked by over-zealousness. From what I've said it should be obvious that behavior therapy does not qualify as a fad, as per the durability criterion. As far as over-zealousness is concerned, I can provide only an impressionistic reaction, which is that among behavior therapists the ratio of messianics to non-messianics has gone down considerably over the years, probably in direct proportion to the degree to which behavior therapy has become an acceptable discipline. Fifteen years ago it was possible to horrify almost any psychological or psychiatric audience with pronouncements that direct "symptomatic" treatment might be advantageous or that symptom substitution was a rather rare phenomenon. Without implying that the basic assumptions of behavior therapy are now universally accepted (obviously, this is far from the truth), the principal impetus for messianism, which is very widespread and rabid opposition, has diminished considerably.

The fact that behavior therapy is not a fad doesn't imply that it is therefore a good thing. Given my orientation, it isn't surprising that my enthusiasm for psychoanalysis is less than overwhelming. But who in his right mind (excuse me: right behavior) would argue that psychoanalysis and its derivatives constitute a fad? Obviously I do believe behavior therapy as a whole is a very worthwhile enterprise, among other reasons because of its "self-conscious" attitude (Kanfer & Phillips, 1970) in relation to empirical validation of its techniques. Historically, at least, this is a characteristic notably lacking among dynamic approaches (see Astin, 1961).[2]

Let me illustrate what I mean by self-consciousness, using systematic desensitization as an example. The same case can be made for the other behavior therapies, although the literature, except that for operant methods, is considerably less extensive. It is likely that Wolpe's initial impact (Wolpe, 1958) was more a function of his impressive array of case history data (much involving desensitization) than of his animal research, or even his theoretical formulations. Nevertheless he *did* offer animal data which tended to provide some support for his reciprocal inhibition therapy and he *did* provide a general theoretical groundwork which many found quite plausible. Thus, in the early 1960's we had clinical case histories, some animal data, and a theoretical rationale, all tending to suggest the value of systematic desensitization. Perhaps for some this constituted a sufficient basis for employing desensitization with a client. Others, however, felt the need for additional supporting data in the form of investigations having some manner of control. Among the earlier studies looking at the efficacy of desensitization, that is, the total "treatment package," to use Paul's term (Paul, 1969b), were those of Lazarus (1961) and Lang and Lazovik (1963). Subsequently, efforts at providing better controls appeared, in particular dealing with the so-called non-specifics of treatment (e.g., Lang, Lazovik, & Reynolds, 1965; Paul, 1966). Shortly thereafter Davison (1968) presented results suggesting counter-conditioning as the process underlying desensitization (in support of Wolpe). For a more complete review of this literature, see Paul, 1969b and 1969c.

Since the late 1960's and continuing through the present day, there have been a very large number of investigations dealing with a variety of issues relevant to desensitization. The following are but a few examples: the role of relaxation (see Nawas, Welsch, & Fishman, 1970; Miller & Nawas, 1970; also, see Schubot, 1966); the importance of an ascending hierarchy (Krapfl, 1967); and the role of non-specifics, especially subject expectancies (a topic dealt with later in this paper). In addition, a sizable number of studies have compared desensitization with other behavior therapy techniques (e.g., Bandura, Blanchard, & Ritter, 1969; McReynolds, 1969; Barrett, 1969; Richardson & Suinn, 1973; Armstrong & Rimm, 1974).[3]

In addition, there have been experiments examining a variety of important methodological variables (for example, the effects of repeated measurement on avoidance of phobic subjects; whether the subjects are "true" volunteers versus undergraduates fulfilling course requirements [see Bernstein & Nietzel, 1974]; the effects of arousal manipulations on avoidance behavior [see Rimm, Kennedy, Miller, & Tchida, 1971]).

I should mention that the above investigations (and other related research) do not uniformly support systematic desensitization as the treatment of choice for phobic subjects. Some suggest that desensitization may be inferior to other methods, under certain circumstances, while others raise important theoretical and methodological questions concerning those components of the desensitization treatment package which are truly necessary for improvement. The major point is that with very few exceptions, those who carry out such research either call themselves "behavior therapists" or have some clear identification with this area. This is to say that the continuing activities aimed at correcting and improving techniques and theory pertinent to the behavior therapies are carried out almost exclusively from within. To quote W. McReynolds (personal communication), and I don't think this is an overstatement, "We alone seem to be able to come up with worthy opponents for ourselves." This is what I mean by "self-consciousness."

BEHAVIOR THERAPY AND CLINICAL SKILL

In reading certain of the behavior therapy literature, it is easy to get the impression that the behavior therapist interacts with his client in a cold, almost mechanical fashion, rather in the manner in which an experimental psychologist might relate to a laboratory rat. This simply is not true (see Lazarus, 1971; Rimm & Masters, 1974). At least, if there is a behavior therapist who relates to his clients in this way, I haven't met that person. The behavior therapist, if he expects to make a reasonable livelihood, must possess a fair amount of "clinical skill." I admit this is a term not easy to define, but I'm referring to behaviors associated with making the client believe that the therapist cares about him and is sensitive to his needs. One could "fake" these qualities, I suppose, but it is a lot easier if the behavior therapist does truly care about his clients and is genuinely sensitive to their needs, as is the case, I believe, with most behavior therapists.

But what about operant conditioners running token economies in mental hospitals? It is true that their direct interaction with patients may be quite minimal. But, as anyone who has ever been involved in such a program knows, it is absolutely necessary to obtain staff cooperation if the program is to work (see Atthowe, 1973). If the operant conditioner emits cues to the effect that he does not care about, or is insensitive to, the needs of either the staff or the patients, I don't think he would get very much cooperation.

BEHAVIOR THERAPY AND "CONTROL"

About six years ago, we were interviewing a job candidate (at another university); it was not for a clinical position, but, as a matter of curiosity, I asked him what he thought about behavior therapy. "It's fine," he replied, "if you want to turn people into vegetables." This sort of mindless comment (it is a pity that he will probably never read this) is most often directed at operant conditioners. The implication is that operant conditioners want to control behavior in a kind of "police state" manner. Let me provide a not very original, but reasonable, rebuttal. If the operant principles are in the main *invalid* (i.e., stimulus events and reinforcers do not have an important and lawful effect on human behavior), there can be no issue of unethical control because there *is* no control. However, if their assumptions have reasonable validity, and there are hundreds of experiments which suggest they do (the reader is referred to any issue of the *Journal of Applied Behavior Analysis*), then this clearly implies that human behavior is, to an important degree, under the control of stimulus and consequent events. To ignore this fact does not make our behavior any less controlled. Instead, it is to defer to control by fortuitous factors which may not be beneficial (e.g., inadvertently reinforcing that very psychotic behavior which led to a patient's hospitalization). It makes more sense to *confront* the issue by systematically using what we know about behavioral control to the advantage of the patient. I admit that an operant conditioner running a token economy could use his knowledge of behavioral control in a self-serving or unethical fashion, but I think he would lose his job in relatively short order. As far as turning people into "vegetables" goes, the evidence is quite to the contrary (e.g., King, Armitage, & Tilton, 1960). As I indicate in a later section, this study may not be the fairest comparison of operant procedures and psychotherapy, but, viewed as a controlled assessment of operant conditioning, its results with withdrawn schizophrenics are impressive.

COMMENTS ON SELECTED PAPERS

Luborsky, Singer, and Luborsky. Before commenting on the specifics of this paper, I'd like to make a few observations concerning difficulties inherent in comparing behavior therapy with psychotherapy approaches. Some of these are also discussed by Luborsky et al. The first has to do with *dependent measures* (i.e., outcome measures). The behaviorist is concerned with rather specific treatment goals, while the psychotherapist typically aims at effecting changes more global in nature. This does not necessarily present serious tactical problems, but can lead to conflicting interpretations. If the client (subject, since these comments apply equally to analog and clinical studies) shows a marked decrease in, for example, specific phobic behavior, but not an increase in, let us say, ego strength, the behaviorist would view treatment as a success, while the psychotherapist might see it as a failure. Obviously, the converse of this is also true. On the other hand, changes in neither type of measure would be interpreted by both as indicative of failure, and changes in both would be taken as an indication of success. The second, which presents a more serious problem, pertains to *duration of therapy*. This is because usually behavior therapies are considerably more brief than psychotherapies. If duration for both is brief, this would bias the results in favor of the behavioral treatment. If the duration of the behavioral treatment is lengthened so as to correspond to the length of psychotherapy, one is no longer comparing the behavioral treatment as it is actually employed in a clinical setting. A more natural solution would seem to be to conduct the behavior therapy over that period of time which is typically prescribed (i.e., until the specific goals are met), following the same procedure for the psychotherapy treatment. However, unless the behavior therapist completely discounts the importance of "nonspecifics," he may view this as biasing the results in favor of psychotherapy. Here is another problem. Given the greater duration of psychotherapy, extraneous external factors are more likely to play a role. This could bias the results in either direction.

Before leaving the issue of treatment duration, I would like to raise a practical matter. To say that the behavior therapies in general require fewer treatment sessions than the psychotherapies is to say that the former are more efficient. It can be argued that this brevity stems partly from the fact that behavior therapists treat very specific disorders, which happens to be true. But this is almost entirely a matter of conceptualization (as opposed to client selection). Thus, if a client's presenting complaint is "general unhappiness," the behavior therapist will attempt to determine the specific environmental cues (and the client's responses to them) which led to his personal discomfort. For example, perhaps the client is unhappy because he is lonely, which is a result of a lack of certain social skills; rather than attempting to deal with the unhappiness at some global level, the behavior therapist would attempt to enhance those specific social skills (e.g., by employing assertive training).

The third issue which I would like to discuss pertains to *therapist experience*. Certain behavior therapies can be taught to an intelligent novice in a relatively short period of time. I would not think this would be the case with most forms of psychotherapy (the Patterson, Levene, & Breger 1971 study supports this position). In the extreme, psychoanalysts typically do not begin full-fledged practice until their thirties. On the other hand, one can easily conceive of an undergraduate performing operant conditioning or systematic desensitization after a two-month crash course. If our comparison is between a thirty-three-year-old analyst and a nineteen-year-old "behavior therapist," this age discrepancy could bias the results in either direction, depending on the nature of the patient population. We could standardize for age (for example, requiring that all therapists be between thirty-five and forty). But the odds are high that the behaviorist will have treated a good many more patients than the psychotherapist because psychotherapy usually requires substantially more time to complete (ergo, fewer completed psychotherapies). In the interest of equating for age, we have sacrificed one important dimension of experience.

The aforementioned difficulties associated with attempting to compare psychotherapy with behavior therapy are by no means trivial. I am able to offer no ready-made solutions. By raising these issues I am not suggesting that one not attempt such comparisons. I am suggesting that anyone who does should be prepared to live with a fair amount of ambiguity.

In examining "box scores" such as those presented by Luborsky et al., it is essential to keep in mind that neither behavior therapy nor psychotherapy represents some unitary set of behaviors emitted by proponents of each of these points of view. As we have indicated, there are many behavior therapies and psychotherapies, and it would be erroneous to assume that they are equally effective. Obviously it depends on the nature of the problem and on the patient. But even for those techniques which supposedly deal with the same problem, it is a mistake to assume that they are equally effective, a priori. As cases in point, Bandura et al. (1969)

found that modeling plus guided participation was superior to standard desensitization in treating snake phobics, and Rimm and Mahoney (1969) provided evidence that this same procedure was superior to an operant procedure in overcoming snake avoidance.

Now I would like to provide my own evaluation of the studies presented by Luborsky et al. As a matter of convenience, I'll cite them in chronological order.

King et al. (1960) represents a fairly well-controlled comparison between psychotherapy and an operant approach with withdrawn schizophrenics. Since both groups were given about 22 hours of treatment, the bias is in favor of behavior therapy, which was found to be superior (with some evidence of improvement maintained at a six-month followup). Given bias resulting from the brevity of treatment, I would rate this as indicating a *slight* advantage for operant conditioning.

The Lazarus (1961) study compared desensitization with brief therapy with a variety of phobics. His results, while impressively in favor of desensitization, are subject to bias since he was the therapist in both treatments. While his adherence, wherever possible, to stringent behavioral assessment of improvement is commendable, and while his followup data generally support the behavioral approach, the brevity of the insight approach (approximately twenty-two sessions), coupled with possible inadvertent bias on the part of the therapist, suggests only a *slight* advantage for desensitization.

Two studies (Cooper, Gelder, & Marks, 1965; Marks & Gelder, 1965) are retrospective; that is, they had to rely on a variety of indirect historical sources of information as well as direct interviews when possible. They are seriously contaminated by lack of control (see Paul, 1969b), including use of drugs and supportive interviews in behavior therapy, psychosurgery in some cases, etc. As tests of the effects of psychotherapy, they are quite unfair. For instance, only a small portion of the "psychotherapy" patients in Cooper et al. received intensive psychotherapy, and apparently the same is true for Marks and Gelder. I fail to see how *any* conclusions can be drawn from either of these studies.

The Gelder and Marks 1966 study is a vast improvement over the two above investigations; Paul's (1969b) criticisms notwithstanding, I would take this as providing some evidence that, for severe agoraphobia at least, behavior therapy (graduated retraining, desensitization, and sometimes, assertive training) was not superior to psychotherapy.

In the Gelder, Marks, and Wolff (1967) investigation, the biases seem to favor analytically oriented therapy; only one of the five therapists administering behavior therapy had any prior experience. The number of sessions (about 60 for individual analytic therapy and 80 for group analytic therapy) I would judge as more or less adequate, although Gelder et al. do not share this view. I interpret the relatively more positive results with their behavioral approach as providing some degree of support for its superiority over the analytically oriented psychotherapy.

The Levis and Carrera (1967) study, while it can be taken as providing some support for implosive therapy, suffers from major weaknesses. First, the sole measure of improvement was MMPI performance. Second, one of their control groups involved a mere 10 hours of conventional therapy (another retrospective control group apparently involved 37 hours). Both are relatively brief; the second control, were it not retrospective, would have served as a basis for a fairer comparison. In relation to the comparison at hand, I view these results as inconclusive.

The McReynolds (1969) experiment, although well controlled from the patient aspect, also suffers from certain weaknesses. There were four treatments, two relaxation conditions, a desensitization condition, and an insight therapy condition. For our purposes, the most relevant comparison is between the last two treatments, although it might be pointed out that while all tended to reflect some improvement, a significant treatment effect was not found. The same therapists, whose orientation emphasized "insight and affective awareness," treated both insight and desensitization patients. Although the desensitization training procedure appears adequate, apparently none of the therapists had prior experience with this method. This clearly biases the results against behavior therapy. On the other hand, the limited treatment (8 to 12 sessions) would tend to favor desensitization. The author cogently points out that with a sample of neurotics in such a hospital setting, brief treatment is often necessary. However, given the design biases, the results relative to the desensitization-psychotherapy comparison are inconclusive.

The Patterson et al. study (1971), while interesting in its own right, indicates mainly that novice therapists can be taught a behavior therapy method more readily than a psychoanalytically oriented therapy. While Luborsky et al. cite this study as favoring behavior therapy, the overall results do not favor either. One might be tempted to view this as a "tie." However, given the obvious effect of therapist experience on outcome, there is certainly the possibility that even at the conclusion of the study therapists were not functioning maximally with either mode of therapy. The marked brevity of treatment (about 6 sessions) is hardly a fair test of either method. With respect to the behavior therapy-psychotherapy comparison, these results are quite inconclusive.

I am unable to evaluate Sloane et al. (in preparation) since I do not have their report.

I should add that, given their ground rules, the Luborsky et al. compilation appears to be comprehensive. They might have included Obler's (1973) comparison of a variant of systematic desensitization with insight-oriented psychotherapy in the treatment of clients suffering from a variety of sexual dysfunctions. Although the results of desensitization were vastly superior, the brevity of the psychotherapy renders this an unfair comparison. Obler quite correctly describes the psychotherapy treatment as a *control*.

My conclusions may be summarized as follows. Among the studies which Luborsky et al. view as relevant (excluding Sloane et al.) three seem to me to suggest some superiority of behavior therapy over psychotherapy. Five I see as inconclusive. One I would judge as a "tie." Perhaps this evaluation reflects my behavior therapy bias. I should mention, however, that whereas Luborsky et al. conclude that six studies support behavior therapy over psychotherapy, I have halved that number. More importantly, in my view at least, none of the studies suggesting an advantage of a behavior therapy approach provides a test of conventional psychotherapy which, from the vantage point of most conventional psychotherapists, would be viewed as truly fair. From their comments, I assume that Luborsky et al. would agree with this statement. In two of the three studies favoring behavior therapy, I don't believe the comparison is without bias. What can be concluded regarding the relative merits of behavior therapy versus psychotherapy, given the studies reviewed by Luborsky et al., is, in my opinion, very little.[4]

What I am saying, in effect, is that at this stage the data are simply "not in." As I've suggested, I have no quarrel with anyone wishing to make a legitimate comparison between a particular behavior therapy and a particular psychotherapy. However, I must add that relative to the type of comparison which Luborsky et al. wish to make, I doubt that the data will ever be in. The majority, perhaps all of the investigators cited by Luborsky et al., would seem to have more of an identification with behavior therapy than with the more traditional psychotherapies. If indeed the best predictor of future behavior is past behavior, then the kinds of comparisons with which Luborsky et al. concern themselves will be carried out by behavior therapists rather than psychotherapists. But if one examines the behavior therapy literature over the past several years, it is clear that behavior therapists are showing little inclination to demonstrate that any of the behavior therapies are superior to any of the more traditional psychotherapies. Instead we are more interested in "doing our own thing," which means comparing different forms of behavior therapy, attempting to extract essential components of any existing behavior therapy, and validating new behavior therapies.

I would like to make a few comments about analog research which, given their concerns, the Luborsky et al. survey ignored. The fact is that most of the research supporting the many behavior therapies, and there is a great deal, is of the analog variety. The exception is the small *n* or single

n experiments performed by operant conditioners in *clinical* settings? In the typical analog, subjects are a relatively homogeneous group of volunteers (usually students) who share the same problem (usually a source of inconvenience rather than a major disability). The advantages of analog research are discussed in detail elsewhere (see Paul, 1969a). The major disadvantage is that one cannot be certain that the results can be generalized to an actual clinical population. For this reason, relatively convincing evidence that a particular behavior therapy "works" involves a combination of well-controlled analog experiments and a reasonably large number of well-documented clinical case histories. Obviously, when feasible, well-controlled experimentation in a clinical setting adds a sizable increment of credibility to the treatment in question.

A Comment on the Applicability of Behavior Therapies. Luborsky et al. have intimated that behavior therapy may not be suited for severe phobias. It is true that almost all analog studies use persons as subjects who at worst could be described as moderately phobic. This is merely a matter of convenience, inasmuch as really severe phobics are harder to come by (I freely admit this is not the best of all reasons). However, that behavior therapy (certain behavior therapies) can deal quite effectively with severe phobic reactions is seen in the study by Bandura et al. (1969). Many of their snake-phobic subjects (volunteers who responded to an advertisement in the city newspaper) were quite incapacitated; for example, the plumber whose livelihood was in jeopardy because he refused to crawl under a house and the real estate salesman who was unable to show a house in a rural area.[6] That severe and/or complex cases do respond to behavior therapy is pointed out by Wolpe (1969), although as he indicates, such individuals typically require a greater number of treatment sessions.

Assuming that certain behavior therapies are effective in eliminating severe phobic reactions, this in itself has rather broad therapeutic implications. Wolpe's (1958) view that anxiety is the core of most, if not all, "neurotic" behavior is not an original one. It is a view that has been espoused in almost every textbook on abnormal psychology or psychopathology (Ullman & Krasner, 1969, is an exception). If this is the case, and if we further assume (as almost all behavior therapists do assume) that anxiety is situation-specific, then *any* techniques which are effective in alleviating such anxiety reactions have potential applicability to virtually any person labeled "neurotic." Thus, from our vantage point, a critic who argues that the behavior therapies are only effective in dealing with circumscribed phobias is, in fact, paying us quite a compliment, although he is vastly underestimating our capabilities.

For the present, let us consider the value of dealing with anxiety in a situation-specific manner. While Masters and Johnson (1970) may not view themselves as behavior therapists, their approach in the main is behavioral. Without suggesting that they derived their highly successful treatment techniques from the behavior therapy literature, or that they are in any way indebted to Joseph Wolpe, I would point out that they do tend to view most sexual dysfunctions as mediated by situation-specific anxiety. While it is true that they stress sexual re-education and communication between the dysfunctional couple (and I don't think any behavior therapist would take issue with this, when presented with the same problem), their techniques typically involve a sequence of graded, non-anxiety-eliciting behavioral tasks. They stress the importance of removing the debilitating pressure to "perform" as they encourage the couple to go through several stages of "sensate focusing," followed by a graduated sequence of behaviors leading to sexual consummation. When I say that this procedure may well be characterized as a form of very skillfully programmed in vivo desensitization, again I am not suggesting that the discipline of behavior therapy deserves credit for their impressive success rate. I am saying that it is in the main a behavioral approach and it works! That a somewhat more "traditional" behavior therapy approach may be effective in dealing with similar dysfunctions is seen in the Obler (1973) study.

In addition to sexual dysfunction, behavioral approaches aimed at dealing with specific anxiety reactions have been shown to be effective in dealing with fear of public speaking (e.g., Paul, 1966; Woy & Efran, 1972), examination anxiety (e.g., Johnson, 1966), and even asthmatic attacks (Moore, 1965). My purpose is not to provide a comprehensive review of the literature dealing with behavioral approaches to anxiety reduction (which is vast), but rather to provide the reader with some notion of the degree to which such approaches have relevance to a very broad spectrum of important clinical phenomena.

Another major behavior therapy technique, assertive training (Wolpe, 1958, 1969), has been used by therapists for a good many years, although controlled studies (and there are several—see Rimm & Masters, 1974) have appeared only relatively recently. Assertive training, which stresses behavioral rehearsal and modeling on the part of the therapist, aims at teaching the client to express his feelings, both positive and negative, in a socially appropriate and rewarding fashion. While it may be viewed as an anxiety-inhibiting procedure (see McFall & Marston, 1970; Rimm, Hill, Brown, & Stuart, 1974), it also involves the enhancement of important social skills (how to ask a person for a date or the boss for a raise; how to inform an in-law in a non-hurtful fashion that his behavior is interfering with one's marriage). Obviously, assertive training is applicable to a wide variety of clinical problems.

The data supporting the efficacy of the operant techniques in dealing with a great diversity of socially relevant behavioral problems are voluminous, to say the least. For example, these techniques have been used successfully in dealing with anorexia (Bachrach, Erwin, & Mohr, 1965), refusal of a child with a severe visual deficit to wear glasses (Wolf, Risely, & Mees, 1964), withdrawn behavior in hospitalized schizophrenics (King et al., 1960; Sherman, 1965), aggression in delinquent adolescents (Horton, 1970), the removal of litter in the natural environment (Powers, Osborne, & Anderson, 1973), modification of verbal behavior in mentally retarded children and adolescents (Baer, Peterson, & Sherman, 1967; Keilitz, Tucker, & Horner, 1973), attention deficits in retarded children in a classroom setting (Kazdin & Klock, 1973), chronic lack of punctuality in industrial workers (Hermann, de Montes, Dominguez, Montes, & Hopkins, 1973), and enuresis (Foxx & Azrin, 1973).

The Wilson paper (in the present volume) illustrates the potential value of the use of punishment procedures in the treatment of alcoholism (I discuss this issue later in this paper). Reports by Feldman and MacCulloch (1965, 1971) point to the value of aversive conditioning procedures in the treatment of homosexuality, as do reports by Marks and Gelder (1967) and Gelder and Marks (1969) in the treatment of fetishism and transvestism. The above studies all employed electric shock as the aversive stimulus. Barlow, Leitenberg, and Agras (1969) employed covert sensitization, wherein the aversive stimulus—typically, nausea—is imagined. They obtained promising results with a pedophilic and a homosexual. Positive results, using this technique in the treatment of obesity, have been reported by Janda and Rimm (1972). Again, this review is not comprehensive but is presented merely to provide a kind of overview of the sorts of problems to which aversive control procedures may be applied.

In recent years, evidence pointing to the effectiveness of behaviorally based self-control procedures has been accumulating. Some of the findings are rather impressive, as in Stuart (1967), Harris (1969), Wollersheim (1970), and Mahoney, Moura, and Wade (1973), all dealing with obesity, and Sachs, Bean, and Morrow (1970), concerning the treatment of cigarette smoking. The interested reader is referred to Thoresen and Mahoney (1974) and Mahoney and Thoresen (1974), both dealing with this topic.

In the above paragraphs I have attempted to make two points which I consider to be very important: (1) certain behavior therapies have been shown to be effective in alleviating phobic behaviors of a non-trivial nature, and that is saying a great deal for the general applicability of those treatment methods; (2) other behavior therapies have been shown to be effective for a very broad spectrum of clinically important problems. If the aforementioned "self-consciousness" of behavior therapists is one reason why I am partial to these approaches, the second is that there are so many positive findings in the literature. Clearly, with respect to the behavior therapies themselves, the data are not "in," by any stretch of the imagination; we have a great deal to learn, and I hope that we will have the openmindedness and integrity which will enable our knowledge to grow. I do maintain that at this stage there is a legitimate basis for enthusiasm regarding the behavior therapies. And I am enthusiastic.

Frank. Before commenting on the substance of Dr. Frank's paper, I'd like to respond to two statements which he has made which I believe are somewhat misleading; my remarks do not in any sense detract from the thrust of his observations and are offered only as points of clarification. Frank states that behavior therapies (e.g., desensitization, flooding) are based, not on gaining mastery of one's fears through insight, but rather "on the realization that one can endure such feelings" (see p. 48). But this is but one interpretation and by no means the "standard" view (see Wolpe, 1958, 1969; Bandura, 1969; Rimm & Masters, 1974). From my prior comment it should be clear that the far more prevalent view is that the behavior therapies, rather than teaching the client to withstand or tolerate the anxiety, are able to effect a reduction or elimination of the anxiety. That is to say, the formerly phobic person is now non-avoidant, not because he has learned to tolerate aversive levels of anxiety, but because he is no longer afraid. Frank (p. 48) goes on to suggest that therapies which "deny altogether the importance of subjective experiences . . . often stress assertiveness training." In fact, therapists engaging in assertiveness training typically stress very strongly the importance of subjective states, especially anxiety (see Wolpe, 1969; Lazarus, 1971; Rimm & Masters, 1974).

The thrust of Frank's paper is that successful therapy involves two important ingredients. One involves the provision of a "coherent conceptual framework" (for instance, a behavior therapist might tell his agoraphobic client that he is fearful in crowds not because he is insane or a weak person but because he has *learned* to feel this way). While this in itself may have some temporary curative effects, I doubt that in general it would account for much in the way of long-term improvement. I've known many phobics who were able to point to learning experiences which they felt, quite plausibly, were responsible for their present fears, but who continued to remain phobic. As a case in point, I treated a World War II bombardier who, some twenty years later, was still fearful of high places and loud sounds resembling antiaircraft fire. He came to therapy with the "appropriate" conceptual structure, which he had had for many years (to no apparent avail). He did experience a marked reduction in both fears following systematic desensitization. I am not suggesting that phobics can always point to precipitating traumas which then serve to provide a conceptual framework which allows them to "understand" the origins of their difficulties (Lazarus, 1971, provides data to the contrary). The point is that when they can, they are not necessarily freed of their phobias. Frank's assertion that "to name something is to gain power over it" (p. 49) can easily be overinterpreted.

The second ingredient of successful therapy, the *provision of success*, is, in my view, the far more important component. Frank's discussion of the several variables related to the experiencing of success, especially in relation to task difficulty, is highly cogent. As Frank notes, it is especially applicable to the therapies which involve structured hierarchies. This certainly applies to systematic desensitization, participant modeling, and implosive therapy (here it is not as obvious as in desensitization, although the ordering becomes clear if one examines an implosive protocol; see Hogan, 1969). The same basic principle is fundamental to the operant techniques which involve successive approximations or shaping and to the behavioristic approaches to self-control (see Thoresen & Mahoney, 1974).

Assuming the importance of success experiences in therapy, I would like to deal with a very fundamental question: to what extent is the origin of that success experience (i.e., the manner in which it is programmed) related to long-term therapeutic benefit? What are some of the ways in which the therapist provides his client with the success experience? One of the more obvious ways would be to provide him with experiences or skills which really do have a subjective and/or external "payoff." As an illustration, consider assertive training. If, indeed, being assertive reduces anxiety and increases interpersonal effectiveness (and empirical findings tend to be supportive; see Rimm & Masters, 1974), the payoff is rather obvious, and enhanced assertion should be maintained by in vivo consequences.

A second way is to structure things so the client perceives he has had a success experience, especially if the success can be viewed as emanating from within rather than from some external source. Frank's own study and that of Davison, Tsujimoto, and Glaros (1973) follow this approach, as does an experiment by Davison and Valins (1969) involving pain tolerance. Valins and Ray (1967) provided evidence that subjects fed a "bogus" heart rate indicating that they were relatively fearless in the presence of slides of snakes showed greater snake-approach behavior than control subjects. However, this study, which stressed the value of a success experience vis-à-vis snakes in effecting a reduction in snake fear, has not been successfully replicated. Borkovec, Wall, and Stone (1974) used a related approach with speech-anxious subjects. Their main finding was that subjects who were fed a bogus increased heart rate during a speech showed greater anxiety on a subsequent speech than those who had been fed back a decreased heart rate or a heart rate indicating no change. This suggests that, indeed, phobic behavior may be modified using procedures of this nature (they fall under the rubric of "attribution theory"), and the observation by Davison and Wilson (1973) that such experimentation is of "doubtful relevance" to the modification of severe, long-standing phobias may be somewhat premature. However, much additional research is needed before statements strongly supportive of this approach can be justified. One serious shortcoming of much of this research (Frank's study is an exception) is the lack of a reasonable followup. Artificially induced success (or failure) may lead to short-term behavior changes. Whether these changes typically endure is open to question.

A third way to attempt to induce success is to program the subject or client to expect success. There is a rather sizable literature dealing with precisely this issue, especially in relation to systematic desensitization. A review of this literature is beyond the province of this paper (but see Wilkins, 1971, 1972; Davison & Wilson, 1972, 1973). However, a few comments are in order.

First, rather than assuming that the effectiveness of a particular treatment is simply the sum of the impact of the specifics of treatment and the so-called "non-specifics," it makes more sense to think in terms of an interaction of the two. I would think this would be especially true with respect to the client's expectations. Borkovec (1973) has also suggested the importance of expectancies interacting with "active ingredients" of a treatment. Assuming the traditional (i.e., Wolpian) view of what is necessary for successful desensitization, it is clear that a great deal is required of the subject. He must learn to relax, participate in hierarchy construction, generate and hold specific visual images, and signal when he experiences anxiety. If, for any reason, he believes that the treatment is unlikely to help him (e.g., if he is told that it is an untested procedure or that it is lacking in surface validity), it seems likely that he will engage in some or all of these activities in a less effective manner; to the extent that the traditional assumptions regarding desensitization are valid, one would expect a reduction in the effectiveness of treatment. There have been studies (e.g., McGlynn & Mapp, 1970; McGlynn, 1971) wherein negative expectations fed to desensitization subjects did not lead to a significant reduction in treatment efficacy. One possibility is that in such instances the surface validity of the technique tended to counteract the initial negative expectancy.

After reviewing the literature on the role of expectancy in the behavioral treatment of phobias, Borkovec (1973) was led to hypothesize that such effects were more likely to influence overt behavior among subjects relatively less fearful (among the analog phobic population). Perhaps the more phobic subjects are more likely to involve themselves in treatment, irrespective of what they are led to expect, because they are more concerned about their fears (i.e., they are more likely to cooperate in a "therapeutic" venture even when led to believe its value is questionable). This is, of course, mere speculation.

As in the case of attribution research, one of the problems in evaluating the expectancy literature is that in most instances followups are lacking. There are exceptions (e.g., Miller, 1972; Borkovec, 1972; Steinmark & Borkovec, 1974). The last study is instructive in that it demonstrates how "legitimate" behavioral treatments (relaxation, and desensitization in insomnia) can be effective in the face of negative externally imposed expectancies, how a placebo treatment can be effective, given positive expectations, and how at a one-month followup differences favoring the treatment over the placebo appear to emerge. Those who received the behavioral treatment continued to improve significantly, whereas the placebo subjects showed a slight decrement in reported sleep latency. In both Miller, 1972, and Borkovec, 1972, there was no indication of a weakening of the expectancy effects, although in the former study the followup results are presented in incomplete detail. Additional research is required before definitive conclusions can be reached, especially regarding durability of behavior change resulting from expectancy manipulations.

One final comment. Frank cites four psychotherapy studies in which improvement was correlated with a shift of perceived "locus of control" towards internality. Rimm et al. (1974) in an analog study found that subjects receiving assertive training for the treatment of antisocial aggression showed significant increases in assertiveness (i.e., decreases in aggressiveness) and comfort level and a significant decrease in reported anger relative to placebo subjects, who received an essentially nondirective approach.[7] In terms of Rotter's I. E. measure, experimental subjects showed a very slight (nonsignificant) change in the external direction. Controls showed no change. I mention this study because the subjects were respondents to a newspaper ad who were genuinely concerned about their inability to control their anger. We provided them with a treatment which seemed to help them in this regard, but we obtained no change on the locus of control variable. Obviously, one such result proves nothing, but it would be of interest to see this measure included in other behavior therapy studies.

The Menninger Project. My comments regarding Dr. Kernberg's paper will be brief, for several reasons. First, Dr. McNair has already provided a critique. Second, certain of the data-handling procedures are rather unique and I am not in a position to assess their relevance or utility. Third, many of their constructs (e.g., Ego Strength) are not part of my "construct system" and many of the constructs (e.g., reinforcement) which

I hold dear to my heart appear to be ignored. This is in no sense a criticism. It is merely an affirmation of a point made by Wiest (1967): different systems are built on different constructs, and it is not the responsibility of a proponent of one system to account for what is going on in another system in terms of his own constructs.

Although many of Dr. McNair's criticisms seem to me to be cogent, I find myself positively impressed by the effort put into the project, by the fact that some functional relationships have emerged which seem to be of practical value to the analytically oriented clinician, and by the fact that this study has apparently modified the behavior of the Menninger Clinic therapists.

Wilson. The results of the Wilson study (Experiment 4, involving contingent punishment), in concert with the results of other investigations referred to in his paper, do indeed provide a basis for optimism in relation to dealing with alcoholism. I am surprised that covert sensitization was not more successful, for precisely the reasons given by Wilson. Attempting to eliminate drinking by negatively valencing alcohol-related cues via electric shock has never made a great deal of sense to me (I'm not referring to Wilson's punishment procedure), for the following reason: assuming that the conditioning technique has been successful, most alcoholics will not then experience terror or panic when confronted with alcohol-related cues. Mild to moderate anxiety is a more likely response. But it is a reasonable presumption that the alcholic's modal response to anxiety is to drink. If in walking by a bar or liquor store he experiences some anxiety, he *knows*, I would think, that a few drinks will take care of this quite nicely. On the other hand, if, as a result of covert sensitization, an intense nausea response has been conditioned (strong enough to cause vomiting if he does imbibe), this is an entirely different matter. Wilson's findings notwithstanding, at this stage I think it would be premature to ignore covert sensitization as part of a broader treatment regimen for alcoholics.

I don't think that any conditioning procedure in isolation can, in general, be expected to have long-term positive effects (I don't think Wilson would take issue with this). After all, the alcoholic knows that in the real world, painful shock is not going to follow his taking a drink. As far as the conditioning of nausea and vomiting is concerned, the following case history illustrates how this response can be overcome, given the proper level of motivation and skill. A Veterans Administration Hospital patient, in his early forties, had been a heavy drinker for many years. He subsequently underwent treatment involving pairing an emetic with alcohol, which, from his report, was successful. Following a period of abstinence, one day, for reasons unclear to the patient, he decided he wanted to be able to drink again. His self-administered treatment involved mixing ever-increasing amounts of vodka with orange juice. If my memory serves me correctly, the "cure" required but one day and was lasting! Obviously this is merely anecdotal, but it does suggest the need for actual contingencies in the real world, such as are exemplified in the Hunt and Azrin (1973) study. I am not partial to the Alcoholics Anonymous approach, mainly because of its insistence on total abstinence, which is not always necessary, as the work of Sobell and Sobell (1973) suggests, and which, in many cases, may be self-defeating. But A.A. does make the point that the alcoholic will improve when, and only when, the reasons for change outweigh the reasons for not changing. Substitute "contingencies" for "reasons," and this is the essence of the behavioristic philosophy. The very major difference, of course, is that whereas A.A. must depend on naturally occurring contingencies, behavioral approaches (such as that of Hunt & Azrin, 1973) systematically program important contingencies into the alcoholic's environment.

O'Leary and Kent. The results of this study are certainly suggestive of the value of a behavioral approach. The treatment and control children were well matched, and the treatment, although not described in great detail in the paper, appears to be high on "surface validity." However, there are problems with every experiment, and this one is no exception. First, no reliability data are presented. This criticism would be far more telling had the authors failed to obtain significant treatment effects, since lack of reliability would be expected to attenuate group differences. That they obtained significant differences on three major measures implies some reasonable level of reliability.

Second, a placebo control would have helped us interpret their results. I am aware of the problems inherent in attempting to include such a condition in a clinical setting (it may have been impossible). From the report, two of the three measures were based upon teacher ratings (I assume that the experimenters evaluated classroom disruption). Now, it is clear from their questionnaire data that the teachers saw the therapists as likable, committed, capable persons. Could this very positive view of the therapists have biased the teacher ratings in favor of the treatment subjects? I can't answer this question, but when you consider that the CAT, a measure which should not have reflected any such bias, revealed no significant treatment effect, such a possibility cannot be totally discounted. Finally, I wish there had been a followup reported. Perhaps one will be forthcoming.

Marks. Dr. Marks presents a very useful and timely review of an important literature. I would see it as especially valuable to American therapists, inasmuch as many of these studies are published in journals not ordinarily read by many Americans (this is in no way an expression of any chauvinistic sentiment; to attempt to keep up with all of the literature pertinent to therapy published in the United States and abroad, would be to invite insanity).

I found the diazepam (Valium) studies especially interesting, mainly because this drug is widely prescribed in the United States. As a psychologist (who cannot prescribe drugs), I am certain that I would experience no difficulty in finding a physician who would prescribe Valium for use in connection with any legitimate psychological therapy. For two of the three controlled diazepam studies the results suggest that the drug facilitated the effects of the behavioral treatment. Marks discusses factors which might have masked drug effects in the third study. Obviously, more research of this nature is needed.

NOTES

1. Among certain behavior therapists implicit verbalizations are seen as an important source of behavioral control. This view is apparent in the work of Meichenbaum and his associates (e.g., Meichenbaum & Goodman, 1969a, 1969b; Meichenbaum & Cameron, 1973). Rimm (1973) and Rimm, Saunders, and Westel (in press) also reflect this approach. The roots of such an approach are to be found in Rational-Emotive Therapy (Ellis, 1963), "thought stopping" (popularized by Wolpe; see Wolpe, 1969), and perhaps in the covariant control formulation of Homme (see Homme, 1965).

2. Much as I would like to believe that this self-consciousness is shared by other contemporary approaches, I don't believe this is entirely true. Gestalt psychotherapy is a good case in point. Personally, I find some Gestalt techniques very exciting and of considerable possible therapeutic value. But if there is a research literature of any magnitude in this area, I've not been able to find it. From my point of view, this is unfortunate, given the increasing popularity of Gestalt therapy.

3. See W. McReynolds (in press) for a review of much of this literature; I should mention that I'm not entirely in agreement with all of McReynolds' conclusions.

4. Just for the sake of argument, assume that the Luborsky et al. evaluation of these studies is more valid than mine. I presented seven of my clinical colleagues and six graduate students with their results, identifying behavior therapy as treatment X and psychotherapy as treatment Y. I posed the following question: "given only this information, if you had to choose one of the two modes of treatment, which would it be?" All 13 indicated "X," most without hesitation ($p < .0003$). That is, if all one had was the Luborsky et al. compilation, the logical choice would be behavior therapy, even though there were twice as many studies indicating a "tie" than indicating that behavior therapy was superior.

5. Mahoney, in the present volume, has dealt briefly but adequately with the scientific validity of the small n approach. I should simply like to add that this experimental strategy, the ABA design being the simplest version, is not to be confused with the standard clinical case history, which is lacking in experimental control.

6. Mahoney (1971) treated a female who had volunteered for a study but was so fearful that she was unable to participate. Just to illustrate the degree to which this woman was afraid of snakes, according to Mahoney (personal communication) "when her husband's boss and wife came over for dinner, they sat quietly at the table watching the last few minutes of the news on television. The announcer made some reference to a snake [Mahoney does not recall whether one was actually shown] at which point she panicked, screamed, and turned the table upside down, literally spilling its contents all over the guests and floor." This very severe phobic successfully underwent a sequential treatment involving desensitization, symbolic modeling, live modeling, and participant modeling.

7. If the reader is disturbed at our referring to nondirective treatment as a placebo, please keep in mind that the treatment was brief (8 hours) and therefore hardly a fair test of nondirective therapy. The use of some form of psychotherapy as a placebo is common in behavior therapy analog research. Because of the brevity of treatment such investigations are not presented as comparisons of behavior and psychotherapy, which would be manifestly unfair.

REFERENCES

Armstrong, D., & Rimm, D. C. A comparison of thought stopping-covert assertion and systematic desensitization in the treatment of snake phobics. Unpublished M.A. thesis, Southern Illinois University at Carbondale, 1974.

Astin, A. W. The functional autonomy of psychotherapy. *American Psychologist*, 1961, **16**, 75–78.

Atthowe, J. M., Jr. Token economies come of age. *Behavior Therapy*, 1973, **4**, 646–654.

Bachrach, A. J., Erwin, W. J., & Mohr, J. P. The control of eating behavior in an anorexic by operant conditioning techniques. In L. P. Ullmann & L. Krasner (Eds.), *Case studies in behavior modification*. New York: Holt, 1965, pp. 153–163.

Baer, D. M., Peterson, R. F., & Sherman, J. A. The development of imitation by reinforcing behavioral similarity to a model. *Journal of the Experimental Analysis of Behavior*, 1967, **10**, 405–416.

Bandura, A. *Principles of behavior modification*. New York: Holt, 1969.

Bandura, A., Blanchard, E. B., & Ritter, R. The relative efficacy of desensitization and modeling approaches for inducing behavioral, affective, and attitudinal changes. *Journal of Personality and Social Psychology*, 1969, **13**, 173–199.

Barlow, D. H., Leitenberg, H., & Agras, W. S. Experimental control of sexual deviation through manipulation of the noxious scene in covert sensitization. *Journal of Abnormal Psychology*, 1969, **74**, 596–601.

Barrett, C. L. Systematic desensitization versus implosive therapy. *Journal of Abnormal Psychology*, 1969, **74**, 587–592.

Benassi, V., & Lanson, R. A survey of the teaching of behavior modification in colleges and universities. *American Psychologist*, 1972, **27**, 1063–1069.

Bernstein, D. A., & Nietzel, M. T. Behavioral avoidance tests: the effects of demand characteristics and repeated measures of two types of subjects. *Behavior Therapy*, 1974, **5**, 183–192.

Borkovec, T. D. Effects of expectancy on the outcome of systematic desensitization and implosive treatments for analogue anxiety. *Behavior Therapy*, 1972, **3**, 29–40.

Borkovec, T. D. The role of expectancy and physiological feedback in fear research: a review with special reference to subject characteristics. *Behavior Therapy*, 1973, **4**, 491–505.

Borkovec, T. D., Wall, R. L., & Stone, N. M. False physiological feedback and the maintenance of speech anxiety. *Journal of Abnormal Psychology*, 1974, **83**, 157–163.

Cooper, J. E., Gelder, M. G., & Marks, I. M. Results of behaviour therapy in seventy-seven psychiatric patients. *British Medical Journal*, 1965, **1**, 1222–1225.

Davison, G. C. Systematic desensitization as a counterconditioning process. *Journal of Abnormal Psychology*, 1968, **73**, 91–99.

Davison, G. C., Tsujimoto, R. N., & Glaros, A. G. Attribution and the maintenance of behavior change in falling asleep. *Journal of Abnormal Psychology*, 1973, **82**, 124–133.

Davison, G. C., & Valins, S. Maintenance of self-attributed and drug-attributed behavior change. *Journal of Personality and Social Psychology*, 1969, **11**, 25–33.

Davison, G. C., & Wilson, G. T. Critique of "desensitization: social and cognitive factors underlying the effectiveness of Wolpe's procedure." *Psychological Bulletin*, 1972, **78**, 28–31.

Davison, G. C., & Wilson, G. T. Processes of fear-reduction in systematic desensitization: cognitive and social reinforcement factors in humans. *Behavior Therapy*, 1973, **4**, 1–21.

Ellis, A. *Reason and emotion in psychotherapy.* New York: Lyle Stuart, 1963.

Feldman, M. P., & MacCulloch, M. J. The application of anticipatory avoidance learning to the treatment of homosexuality: I. theory, technique and preliminary results. *Behaviour Research and Therapy,* 1965, **2**, 165–183.

Feldman, M. P., & MacCulloch, M. J. *Homosexual behavior: therapy and assessment.* Oxford: Pergamon, 1971.

Foxx, R. M., & Azrin, N. H. Dry pants: a rapid method of toilet training children. *Behaviour Research and Therapy,* 1973, **11**, 435–442.

Franks, C. M. (Ed.) *Behavior therapy: appraisal and status.* New York: McGraw-Hill, 1969.

Franks, C. M., & Wilson, G. T. (Eds.) *Annual review of behavior therapy: theory and practice.* New York: Brunner/ Mazel, 1973.

Franzini, L. R., & Tilker, H. A. On the terminological confusion between behavior therapy and behavior modification. *Behavior Therapy,* 1972, **3**, 279–282.

Gelder, M. G., & Marks, I. M. Severe agoraphobia: a controlled prospective trial of behaviour therapy. *British Journal of Psychiatry,* 1966, **112**, 309–319.

Gelder, M. G., & Marks, I. M. Aversion treatment in transvestism and transsexualism. In R. Green and J. Noney (Eds.), *Transsexualism and sex reassignment.* Baltimore: Johns Hopkins Press, 1969.

Gelder, M. G., Marks I. M., & Wolff, H. H. Desensitization and psychotherapy in the treatment of phobic states: a controlled inquiry. *British Journal of Psychiatry,* 1967, **113**, 53–73.

Graziano, A. M. (Ed.) *Behavior therapy with children.* Chicago: Aldine, 1971.

Harris, M. B. Self-directed program for weight control: a pilot study. *Journal of Abnormal Psychology,* 1969, **74**, 263–270.

Hermann, J. A., de Montes, A. I., Dominguez, B., Montes, F., & Hopkins, B. L. Effects of bonuses for punctuality on the tardiness of industrial workers. *Journal of Applied Behavior Analysis,* 1973, **6**, 536–570.

Hogan, R. A. Implosively oriented behavior modification: therapy considerations. *Behaviour Research and Therapy,* 1969, **7**, 177–184.

Homme, L. E. Perspectives in psychology: XXIV. Control of coverants, the operants of the mind. *Psychological Record,* 1965, **15**, 501–511.

Horton, L. E. Generalization of aggressive behavior in adolescent delinquent boys. *Journal of Applied Behavior Analysis,* 1970, **3**, 205–211.

Hunt, G. M., & Azrin, N. H. A community-reinforcement approach to alcoholism. *Behaviour Research and Therapy,* 1973, **11**, 91–104.

Janda, H. L., & Rimm, D. C. Covert sensitization in the treatment of obesity. *Journal of Abnormal Psychology,* 1972, **80**, 37–42.

Johnson, S. M. The effects of desensitization and relaxation in the treatment of test anxiety. Unpublished M.A. thesis, Northwestern University, 1966.

Kanfer, F. H., & Phillips, J. S. Learning foundations of behavior therapy. New York: Wiley, 1970.

Kazdin, A. E., & Klock, J. The effect of nonverbal teacher approval on student attentive behavior. *Journal of Applied Behavior Analysis,* 1973, **6**, 643–654.

Keilitz, I., Tucker, D. J., & Horner, R. D. Increasing mentally retarded adolescents' verbalizations about current events. *Journal of Applied Behavior Analysis,* 1973, **6**, 621–630.

King, G. F., Armitage, S. G., & Tilton, J. R. A therapeutic approach to schizophrenics of extreme pathology: an operant-interpersonal method. *Journal of Abnormal and Social Psychology,* 1960, **61**, 276–286.

Krapfl, J. E. Differential ordering of stimulus presentation and semi-automated versus live treatment in the systematic desensitization of snake phobia. Unpublished Ph.D. dissertation, University of Missouri, 1967.

Krumboltz, J. D., & Thoresen, C. E. (Eds.) *Behavioral counseling: cases and techniques.* New York: Holt, Rinehart and Winston, 1969.

Lang, P. J., & Lazovik, A. D. Experimental desensitization of a phobia. *Journal of Abnormal and Social Psychology,* 1963, **66**, 519–525.

Lang, P. J., Lazovik, A. D., & Reynolds, D. J. Desensitization, suggestibility, pseudotherapy. *Journal of Abnormal Psychology,* 1965, **70**, 395–402.

Lazarus, A. A. Group therapy of phobic disorders by systematic desensitization. *Journal of Abnormal and Social Psychology*, 1961, **63**, 505–510.

Lazarus, A. A. *Behavior therapy and beyond*. New York: McGraw-Hill, 1971.

Lazarus, A. A. (Ed.) *Clinical behavior therapy*. New York: Brunner/Mazel, 1972.

Levis, D. J., & Carrera, R. Effects of ten hours of implosive therapy in the treatment of outpatients; a preliminary report. *Journal of Abnormal Psychology*, 1967, **72**, 504–508.

Mahoney, M. J. Sequential treatments for severe phobia. *Journal of Behavior Therapy and Experimental Psychiatry*, 1971, **2**, 195–197.

Mahoney, M. J., Moura, N. G. M., & Wade, T. C. The relative efficacy of self-reward, self-punishment, and self-monitoring techniques for weight loss. *Journal of Consulting and Clinical Psychology*, 1973, **40**, 404–407.

Mahoney, M. J., & Thoresen, C. E. *Self-control: power to the person*. Monterey, Calif.: Brooks/Cole, 1974.

Marks, I. M., & Gelder, M. G. A controlled retrospective study of behaviour therapy in phobic patients. *British Journal of Psychiatry*, 1965, **111**, 561–573.

Marks, I. M., & Gelder, M. G. Transvestism and fetishism: clinical and psychological changes during faradic aversion. *British Journal of Psychiatry*, 1967, **113**, 711–729.

Masters, W. H., & Johnson, V. E. *Human sexual inadequacy*. Boston: Little, Brown, 1970.

McFall, R. M., & Marston, A. R. An experimental investigation of behavior rehearsal in assertive training. *Journal of Abnormal Psychology*, 1970, **76**, 295–303.

McGlynn, F. D. Experimental desensitization following three types of instructions. *Behaviour Research and Therapy*, 1971, **9**, 367–369.

McGlynn, F. D., & Mapp, R. H. Systematic desensitization of snake-avoidance following three types of suggestion. *Behaviour Research and Therapy*, 1970, **9**, 197–201.

McReynolds, W. T. Systematic desensitization, insight-oriented psychotherapy and relaxa-·ion therapy in a psychiatric population. Unpublished Ph.D. dissertation, University of Texas at Austin, 1969.

McReynolds, W. T. An empirical reappraisal of systematic desensitization. In McReynolds, W. T. (Ed.), *Behavior therapy in review*. New York: Jason Aronson, in press.

Meichenbaum, D., & Cameron, E. Training schizophrenics to talk to themselves: a means of developing attentional controls. *Behavior Therapy*, 1973, **4**, 515–534.

Meichenbaum, D., & Goodman, J. The developmental control of operant motor responding by verbal operants. *Journal of Experimental Child Psychology*, 1969, **7**, 553–565. (a)

Meichenbaum, D., & Goodman, J. Reflection-impulsivity and verbal control of motor behavior. *Child Development*, 1969, **40**, 785–797. (b)

Miller, H. R., & Nawas, M. M. Control of aversive stimulus termination in systematic desensitization. *Behavior Research and Therapy*, 1970, **8**, 57–61.

Miller, S. B. The contribution of therapeutic instructions to systematic desensitization. *Behaviour Research and Therapy*, 1972, **10**, 159–169.

Moore, N. Behavior therapy in bronchial asthma: a controlled study. *Journal of Psychosomatic Research*, 1965, **9**, 257–276.

Nawas, M. M., Welsch, W. V., & Fishman, S. T. The comparative effectiveness of pairing aversive imagery with relaxation, neutral tasks, and muscular tension in reducing snake phobia. *Behaviour Research and Therapy*, 1970, **6**, 63–68.

Obler, M. Systematic desensitization in sexual disorders. *Journal of Behavior Therapy and Experimental Psychiatry*, 1973, **4**, 93–101.

Patterson, V., Levene, H., & Breger, L. Treatment and training outcomes with two time-limited therapies. *Archives of General Psychiatry*, 1971, **25**, 161–167.

Paul, G. L. *Insight vs. desensitization in psychotherapy: an experiment in anxiety reduction*. Stanford, Calif.: Stanford University Press, 1966.

Paul, G. L. Behavior modification research: design and tactics. In C. M. Franks (Ed.), *Behavior therapy: appraisal and status*. New York: McGraw-Hill, 1969, pp. 29–62. (a)

Paul, G. L. Outcome of systematic desensitization. I: background and procedures, and uncontrolled reports of individual treatments. In C. M. Franks (Ed.), *Behavior therapy: appraisal and status*. New York: McGraw-Hill, 1969, pp. 63–104. (b)

Paul, G. L. Outcome of systematic desensitization. II: controlled investigations of individual treatment, technique variations, current status. In C. M. Franks (Ed.), *Behavior therapy: appraisal and status*. New York: McGraw-Hill, 1969, pp. 105–159. (c)

Powers, R. B., Osborne, J. G., & Anderson, E. G. Positive reinforcement of litter removal in the natural environment. *Journal of Applied Behavior Analysis*, 1973, **6**, 579–586.

Richardson, F. C., & Suinn, R. M. A comparison of traditional systematic desensitization, accelerated massed desensitization, and anxiety management training in the treatment of mathematics anxiety. *Behavior Therapy*, 1973, **4**, 212–218.

Rimm, D. C. Thought stopping and covert assertion in the treatment of phobias. *Journal of Consulting and Clinical Psychology*, 1973, **41**, 466–467.

Rimm, D. C., Hill, G. A., Brown, N. N., & Stuart, J. E. Group-assertive training in treatment of expression of inappropriate anger. *Psychological Reports*, 1974, **34**, 791–798.

Rimm, D. C., Kennedy, T. D., Miller, H. L., Jr., & Tchida, G. R. Experimentally manipulated drive level and avoidance behavior. *Journal of Abnormal Psychology*, 1971, **78**, 43–48.

Rimm, D. C., & Mahoney, M. J. The application of reinforcement and participant modeling procedures in the treatment of snake-phobic behavior. *Behaviour Research and Therapy*, 1969, 7, 369–376.

Rimm, D. C., & Masters, J. C. *Behavior therapy: techniques and empirical findings.* New York: Academic Press, 1974.

Rimm, D. C., Saunders, W. D., & Westel, W. Thought stopping and covert assertion in the treatment of snake phobics. *Journal of Consulting and Clinical Psychology*, 1975, **43**, 92–93.

Sachs, L. B., Bean, H., & Morrow, J. E. Comparison of smoking treatments. *Behavior Therapy*, 1970, **1**, 465–472.

Schubot, E. D. The influence of hypnotic and muscular relaxation in systematic desensitization of phobic behavior. Unpublished Ph.D. dissertation, Stanford University, 1966.

Schwitzgebel, R. K., & Kolb, D. A. *Changing human behavior: principles of planned intervention.* New York: McGraw-Hill, 1974.

Sherman, J. A. Use of reinforcement and imitation to reinstate verbal behavior in mute psychotics. *Journal of Abnormal Psychology*, 1965, 7, 155–164.

Sloane, R. B., Wolpe, J., Cristol, A. H., Yorkston, J. J., Freed, H., Whipple, K., & Stables, F. R. Short-term psychoanalytically oriented psychotherapy versus behavior therapy. In preparation, 1974.

Sobell, M. B., & Sobell, L. C. Evidence of controlled drinking by former alcoholics: a second year evaluation of individualized behavior therapy. Paper presented at the American Psychological Association, Annual Convention, Montreal, Canada, 1973.

Steinmark, S. W., & Borkovec, T. D. Active and placebo treatment effects on moderate insomnia under counter-demand and positive demand instructions. *Journal of Abnormal psychology*, 1974, **83**, 157–163.

Stuart, R. B. Behavioral control over eating. *Behaviour Research and Therapy*, 1967, **5**, 357–365.

Thoresen, C. E., & Mahoney, M. J. *Behavioral self-control.* New York: Holt, Rinehart and Winston, 1974.

Ullmann, L. P., & Krasner, L. *A psychological approach to abnormal behavior.* Englewood Cliffs, N.J.: Prentice-Hall, 1969.

Valins, S., & Ray, A. Effects of cognitive desensitization on avoidance behavior. *Journal of Personality and Social Psychology*, 1967, 7, 345–350.

Wiest, W. Some recent criticisms of behaviorism and learning theory with special reference to Breger and McGaugh and to Chomsky. *Psychological Bulletin*, 1967, **67**, 214–225.

Wilkins, W. Desensitization: social and cognitive factors underlying the effectiveness of Wolpe's procedure. *Psychological Bulletin*, 1971, **76**, 311–317.

Wilkins, W. Desensitization: getting it together with Davison and Wilson. *Psychological Bulletin*, 1972, **78**, 32–36.

Wolf, M. M., Risely, T., & Mees, H. L. Application of operant conditioning procedures to the behavior problems of an autistic child. *Behaviour Research and Therapy*, 1964, **1**, 305–312.

Wollersheim, J. P. Effectiveness of group therapy based upon learning principles in the treatment of overweight women. *Journal of Abnormal Psychology*, 1970, **76**, 462–474.

Wolpe, J. *Psychotherapy by reciprocal inhibition.* Stanford, Calif.: Stanford University Press, 1958.

Wolpe, J. *The practice of behavior therapy.* Oxford: Pergamon, 1969; New York: Pergamon, 1974.

Woy, J. R., & Efran, J. S. Systematic desensitization and expectancy in the treatment of speaking anxiety. *Behaviour Research and Therapy*, 1972, **10**, 43–49.

Yates, A. J. *Behavior Therapy.* New York: Wiley, 1970.

GENERAL DISCUSSION

DR. JOSEPH ZUBIN:* I am not a behavior therapist, although some people in our unit are working in this area, and I have been struck by two particular questions.

One. Science develops in two ways, through observation and theory. You have to develop models for making theory mesh with observation and then develop some hypotheses which can be tested for their tenability by observing experimentally whether the data fit the model or not. In this way we seesaw between the hypothesis and the model to see if they fit. Since facts cannot be altered, the model must be modified if the fit is not satisfactory.

Behavior therapy began with a learning theory based on animal experimentation and was gradually applied to humans. As a result, because it began with a theory, observations were needed in order to establish or disestablish it. Consequently, we have had a plethora of facts, but thus far there has been no one able to integrate these new facts into a theoretical structure. This is what is now lacking—a comprehensive structure to contain the data.

Two. Since a mental disorder is an emotional experience, we know that it consists of two aspects, a cognitive component and a physiological component. We know full well that physiology alone cannot give rise to an emotion, nor will a euphoric frame of mind alone produce an emotion. Unless the physiological component for euphoria is present, a true emotional experience will not occur.

If this model is tenable, the purpose of therapy is to separate the components of the emotional experience. By breaking up this compound of physiological and cognitive components the disorder should gradually disappear. If this is the basis for improvement, can it be accomplished experimentally? How, in the light of this model, does it happen that a great percentage of neurotics improve spontaneously? This is my challenge to the participants.

QUESTION: Dr. O'Leary, what is your experience with the use of drugs in the treatment of children?

DR. K. DANIEL O'LEARY:† As far as I know there have been no factorial experiments with hyperactive children evaluating medication and behavior modification singly or in combination. Actually last year a

*Biometrics Research Unit, New York State Department of Mental Hygiene.
†State University of New York, Stony Brook.

157

physician, Dr. Jacob, and I were quite quite interested in doing such a study with hyperactive children, but Dr. Jacob was reluctant to use medication with the children referred to us. Instead, we did a behavioral intervention study, and we were quite surprised at our ability to produce positive effects with the children.

There is some suggestive evidence from a study published this past year by Christensen and Sprague that the combination of medication and behavior modification is superior to either alone in reducing seat movements, but the study was a laboratory study, and consistent significant differences favoring the combined treatment were not shown. In fact, Dr. Klein with Dr. Gittleman at Hillside is conducting a study of hyperactive children comparing behavioral intervention with medication, and I would presume they will have some comparative results within a year.

I think it is particularly useful to do a comparative study with hyperactive children, and one reason why I am interested myself is that in a number of instances teachers are reluctant to use behavioral procedures with a child, either because of the extra effort involved or because of some philosophical disagreement with the general approach. My hope would be that in many instances the combination would be superior and that short trials of medication might make it much easier to achieve strong behavioral effects, allowing the teacher to introduce a behavioral program more readily.

DR. DONALD F. KLEIN:* We are fortunate in having Dr. O'Leary as a consultant in setting up a study of behavior modification with medication on hyperactive children. He mentioned his own study on the use of classroom observation. I would like to underscore this as something people might not think of. If you use the teacher to treat the patient, the objective report of behavior in the classroom becomes somewhat compromised. Therefore, it becomes mandatory to use an independent observation team within the classroom and maintain proper blind recordings. It turns out not to be easy to get a high degree of independent inter-rater reliability within a classroom. It has taken us a good part of the year to get this for several observers. So training for reliability is an important issue in making such observations.

We mention both data and theory and I would agree that, on the whole, we need more data, rather than more theory, but I think that theory is helpful.

With regard to Dr. Wilson's extremely interesting experience, the bottom line, as I see it, is that the contingency treatment for alcoholism lacks promise. There was nothing there that made it look like a useful behavioral technique. I wonder if that result is not predictable on

*Long Island Jewish-Hillside Medical Center.

theoretical grounds. As I understand it, the classical conditioning theory holds that by continually matching the stimulus with pain you develop an expectant anxiety. Therefore in conditions like impulsive gambling, where the behavior can be understood as a defective self-regulation due to defective development of the anxious state, pain conditioning can engender a moderate ability to develop an anxious response. Unfortunately, in alcoholism the development of anxiety leads the patients to self-medicate with a fine pharmacological treatment for anxiety—alcohol. So I think this anxiety-inducing procedure is unlikely to help the alcoholic.

DR. ISAAC MARKS:* I think there is an interesting relationship between anxiety and the results of aversion. I don't know the data on alcoholism, but in sexual deviations outcome has been correlated with patient's anxiety level; the higher the patient's anxiety before treatment the worse he did with aversion. I would agree with the comments made. We might have to think about it in cognitive terms, although this is simply a vague way of indicating which haystack to search for the needle.

QUESTION: Dr. Marks, do you mean to conclude that we cannot really measure the activity of the brain? Also, would your study not have been more effective if you had used multiple small doses of diazepam over several days?

DR. MARKS: One difficulty we have had is that so far EEG patterns have correlated rather poorly with behavior. Although they sometimes reach statistical significance, they haven't been large enough to be convincing indicators of what is happening in the anxious patient.

Questions arise about which variables we should measure and for how long beforehand we should give the drug. I think you are absolutely right that we need to complete studies of different dosages and different periods of exposure for treatment. It is necessary to point out, however, that each of the two studies I have described so far occupied the full-time resources of one psychiatrist for two years. That is a total of four years of work, and these studies alone have raised enough additional questions to keep someone busy for a decade. When there are so many possible questions each taking so long to answer, we must try to ensure that the ones we actually study are good questions, questions that are likely to lead somewhere.

What I am saying is that in this complicated field the therapeutic payoff is not going to be quick. It will be several decades before we understand how to combine these drugs and psychological maneuvers in optimum fashion. Our knowedge of the physiological mechanisms and of the psychological procedures involved is so far tenuous, but obviously we must move towards remedying these deficiencies.

*Institute of Psychiatry, University of London.

There is one disheartening clinical observation that makes me wonder whether we yet have the right end of the stick. Of the addicted phobic patients we have treated, quite a few who have been on and off high doses of diazepam for months or years have been treated successfully by being taken into hospitals and taken off drugs, after which they are exposed to the real phobic situation without the help of any drugs. There is something happening here which we do not understand. If these drugs are anxiolytic, why should people on these high doses have remained phobic before they were treated by exposure in vivo?

DR. ARTHUR K. SHAPIRO:* I have two points I would like to make. The first involves possible confusion that may occur in interpretation of experimental and clinical data involving benzodiazepines. They are often considered mysterious compounds that reduce anxiety without sedation and have little effect on cognition. This concept often obfuscates interpretation of data which would be readily understandable if benzodiazepines were considered antianxiety-sedative-hypnotic drugs similar to barbiturates. The formulas, dose response curves, effect on the EEG, addiction potential, withdrawal effects, and other neuropharmacologic effects are the same for barbiturates and benzodiazepines. The only difference is the larger toxic-to-therapeutic ratio for the benzodiazepines compared with barbiturates, which can be understood by considering pharmacologic properties such as lipid solubility, distribution, dose response curve, half-life of various metabolic compounds, and so on. This concept has been alluded to by Goth, Elliott, the AMA Council on Drugs, and Myers et al., and is described in greater detail in a chapter on psychochemotherapy in a forthcoming book edited by Grenell and Gabay, entitled *Biological Foundations of Psychiatry*.

The problems concerning interpretation of the data presented by Drs. Marks and Lipman can be more readily understood if diazepam were considered an antianxiety-sedative-hypnotic drug like barbiturates.

The papers on behavior therapy presented today seemed to avoid the main theme of this conference, namely, the comparative efficacy of the psychotherapies. What is the evidence that behavior therapy is a therapeutic breakthrough and not the latest fad? Most of the data on behavior therapy presented today were for the most part browsing, retrospective, inadequately controlled reports, primarily involving non-clinical conditions. The designs are largely subject to the *post hoc, ergo propter hoc* fallacy. Designs using the patient as his own control are generally inadequate to control for the placebo effect of treatment. The crucial question for the behavior therapies is whether therapeutic response is specifically associated with the specific procedures, as defined by the

*New York Hospital-Cornell Medical Center.

theory, or whether the procedures are another placebo therapy in the history of medical treatment. Lessons from that history, which is largely the history of the placebo effect, indicate that elegant theory, clinical reports, great numbers of reported successfully treated patients, testimonials by insightful and gifted clinicians, and so on, are no guarantee of clinical efficacy. Only carefully controlled studies, including control for the placebo effect of treatment, can yield reliable and valid data about clinical efficacy.

DR. MARKS: I am reminded of the British leader of the Flat Earth Society who was interviewed by the BBC the day after America sent up spacemen who encircled the earth and photographed the globe. They asked him what was going to happen to his society. He replied "It will continue, as I believe in promoting the spirit of skepticism."

DR. MAHONEY: I would like to comment briefly on the question raised by Dr. Shapiro as to whether there is any evidence to indicate that behavior therapy is more than a placebo effect. His question, I think, illustrates some of the unfortunate isolation which often characterizes specialized sciences. A researcher frequently limits his exposure to a select few journals and a restricted theme of interests. The issue of placebo effects has been addressed in numerous studies over the last half decade —many of them using elaborate double-blind designs and multiple control groups. Their findings have been relatively consistent: (1) placebo and expectancy effects appear to play a role in some behavior therapy procedures; (2) the magnitude of that effect varies widely from one procedure to another; and (3) arguments about behavior therapy being "nothing but" placebo effects have failed to receive empirical support. I might add that even if the opposite were true—that is, that behavioral strategies derived most of their power from placebo sources—we would still be faced with the task of explaining the relatively consistent superiority of behavior therapy over non-behavioral therapies. Is the behavior therapist simply better skilled at capitalizing on placebo influences? I doubt it.

The placebo controversy illustrates an interesting chronology in criticisms of behavior therapy. Early arguments claimed that it simply didn't work. As supporting evidence on clinical effectiveness accumulated, the argument changed slightly. It was then contended that behavior therapy works, but only on superficial and circumscribed responses. Moreover, symptom substitution was said to be a frequent byproduct. When broader realms of performance fell under the behavioral purview and the data failed to reveal symptom substitution, the argument again shifted. Two of the more contemporary claims are that when behavior therapy works, it works for reasons other than those suggested by behavioral theory. The placebo argument is one illustration. A second argument states that—

even if behavior therapy is effective—it is unethical. The cogency of this latter contention has been evaluated in the review I mentioned earlier. Suffice it to say that the critiques have run an interesting route in the last two decades. If the tenacity and mutability of its critics are any index, then behavior *theory* has generated almost as much responding as its principles.

DR. HEINZ E. LEHMANN:* A comparison occurs to me. When the question of broad-spectrum or broad-band behavior modification therapy and its justification was discussed, it occurred to me that this rang a bell somewhere. I am thinking of orthomolecular therapy. This therapy —which is supposed to have just about those characteristics of a broad-spectrum drug therapy, or whatever you want to call it—started out from a clearly defined theory, or several theories, about the beneficial effects of high doses of vitamins—much higher than the normal requirements. The theories didn't work and appeared to be faulty. Clinically the treatment gives very controversial results. Anecdotal reports are enthusiastic; controlled studies turn out negative.

Now, behavior therapy is different. It can be experimentally and clinically proved, but one has to be careful about what new indications are added to it. All of the factors and procedures that are recommended for use in broad-band, multifaceted behavior therapy should be checked out, one by one. However, in the enthusiasm over behavior therapy having worked so well, I am afraid that sometimes some of the newly added broad-spectrum factors are not checked out very carefully, and anecdotal claims of therapeutic results overtake articulate theory and experimental controls.

*Douglas Hospital, Montreal.

PART III:
COMBINED DRUG AND
PSYCHOLOGICAL THERAPIES

13

THE EFFICACY OF PSYCHOTHERAPY IN DEPRESSION:
Symptom Remission and Response to Treatment

MYRNA M. WEISSMAN, GERALD L. KLERMAN,
BRIGITTE A. PRUSOFF, BARBARA HANSON,
and EUGENE S. PAYKEL

Psychotherapy combined with drugs is a common course of treatment for outpatient depressives. However, the value of combination therapy rests on slim research evidence.

While the efficacy of drugs alone in the treatment of acute depression has been established (Klerman & Cole, 1965), the efficacy of psychotherapy through research studies has been particularly difficult to establish (Segal, 1972; Fisher, 1973; Luborsky, Chandler, Auerbach, Cohen, & Backrach, 1971). This difficulty has been attributed to problems in design and in the selection of appropriate outcome measures (Fiske, Hunt, Luborsky, Orne, Parloff, Reiser, & Tuma, 1970; Strupp & Bergin, 1969).

There exists some debate about the value of combining the treatments and of their potential interactions (Uhlenhuth, Lipman, & Cori, 1969). This debate about drug/psychotherapy interactions tends to be polarized. The antagonists say that pill-taking has a negative effect on psychother-

Myrna M. Weissman, Ph.D. (Epidemiology), Associate Professor in Psychiatry, and Brigitte A. Prusoff, M.P.H. (Biometry), Assistant Professor in Psychiatry, Yale University School of Medicine.

Gerald L. Klerman, M.D., Professor of Psychiatry, Harvard University Medical School.

Barbara Hanson, M.S. (Social Work), Foxborough State Hospital, Foxborough.

Eugene S. Paykel, M.D., Consultant Psychiatrist, St. George's Hospital, London.

The work was supported by National Institute of Mental Health Research Grants MH-13738, MH-15650, and MH-17728. Alberto DiMascio, Ph.D., was Principal Investigator of the Boston State Hospital study. Clinical care was provided in Boston by Abram Chipman, Ph.D., David Haskell, M.D., Eva Deykin, M.S., and Shirley Jacobson, M.S., and in New Haven by the late Mason de la Vergne, M.D., Clive Tonks, M.D., Ruth Bullock, M.S.W., and Effie Geanakoplos, M.S.W. Data analyses were carried out by Janis Tanner. Merck Sharp & Dohme supplied the special tablets of amitriptyline and placebo. Address for reprints: Myrna M. Weissman, Yale University School of Medicine, Depression Research Unit, 904 Howard Ave., Suite 5, New Haven, Conn.

apy by reducing patient motivation for change and by increasing passivity and compliance. The proponents, on the other hand, argue that drugs facilitate patient accessibility to psychotherapy and contribute to optimism and confidence (Klerman, unpublished).

Findings from the New Haven-Boston Collaborative Depression Project allow for a partial resolution of the conflicting models and a test of the efficacy of psychotherapy.[1] In this study, 150 depressed female outpatients were treated with drugs and psychotherapy in a prophylactic trial to determine the appropriate treatment following recovery from an acute depression.

This paper will explore the complexities of drug/psychotherapy studies and will give a rationale for combined treatment. We will show that psychotherapy effects require sufficient timing, symptom reduction, appropriate outcome measures, and appropriate statistical analysis.

METHODS

Subjects. Subjects for this study were 150 moderately depressed women between the ages of twenty-five and sixty, who responded to acute treatment with amitriptyline. Criteria for entrance into acute treatment was a definitive depression of at least two weeks' duration, reaching a total score rating of seven or more on the Raskin Depression Scale (range 3-15) (Raskin, Schulterbrandt, Reatig, & McKeon, 1969). Patients were excluded if their depression was secondary to another predominant syndrome or if they were alcoholics, drug addicts, of subnormal intelligence, had serious physical illnesses, were receiving psychotherapy, or had failed to respond to an adequate course of tricyclic antidepressants in the last six months. Patients who met these criteria were treated with amitriptyline, most as outpatients. Those who showed at least a 50 percent improvement on the Raskin Depression Scale at the end of four to six weeks were assigned to the experimental maintenance treatment design.

Design. The study took the form of a 2 × 3 balanced factorial design, stratified further by the two clinics (see Fig. 1). On a randomized basis, one-half of the patients began once- to twice-weekly psychotherapy with a psychiatric social worker (psychotherapy). All patients also saw the initial psychiatrist monthly in brief interviews for assessments and prescribing. For the second half of the patients, these brief interviews comprised the only continuing contact (low contact). All patients continued to receive amitriptyline for two more months and then were further randomized as to drug. Within each contact group, one-third of the patients continued on amitriptyline, one-third withdrew double-blind onto placebo, and one-third withdrew overtly onto no medication. Treatment continued in these

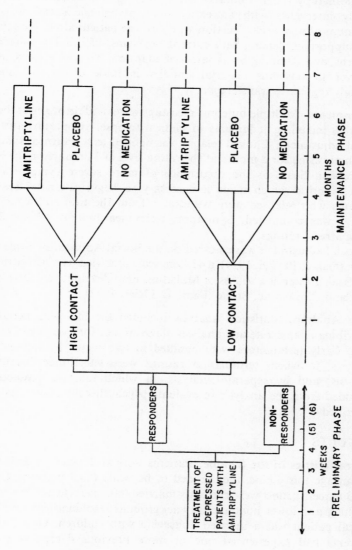

FIG. 1. Design of study.

six treatment cells for a further six months to a total of nine months (eight months in maintenance and one month in acute treatment).

Psychotherapy (High Contact). Psychotherapy consisted of one or two weekly interviews with an experienced psychiatric social worker; a minimum of one weekly session was with the patient alone. The therapy was supportive, dealing with current problems, identifying maladaptive patterns, and attaining better levels of adaption. No attempt was made to uncover unconscious material, modify infantile drives, or induce a strongly regressive transference.

Assessments. Multiple outcome measures were used throughout the eight months, including judgments of clinical relapse, symptom return, and social adjustment. Clinical relapse was defined as a return of symptoms which persisted for a month at the rating level of 7 or more on the Raskin Depression Scale or the occurrence of more severe symptoms for a shorter period which made it necessary to begin alternate treatment. Patients who relapsed were withdrawn from the trial and a full set of ratings was completed. Symptoms were measured by self-report and psychiatrists' ratings.

Social adjustment was assessed on the Social Adjustment Scale (SAS) (Weissman & Paykel, 1974), a 42-item scale modified from the Structured and Scaled Interview to Assess Maladjustment developed by Dr. Gurland (Gurland, Yorkstone, Stone, Fank, & Fleiss, 1972).

Data Analysis. Statistical analysis included the life table method for describing relapse rate and analysis of covariance for assessment of rating data. Early terminators were handled in two ways: by the end point analysis, in which termination ratings were substituted in the final analysis, and by separate analysis, in which relapsed patients were excluded from the analysis to evaluate psychotherapy effects, as will be described.

RESULTS

Characteristics of the Sample. Patients were all females in their thirties (mean age thirty-nine; they tended to be white (83.3 percent), Catholic (55.3 percent); most were currently married (60.0 percent); they were from working and lower middle class backgrounds (Hollingshead, 1957). The modal patient was a married housewife with children. Over half (59.0 percent) had experienced one or more previous depressive illnesses. Patients were predominantly neurotic depressives; 87 percent received a diagnosis of depressive neurosis and 13 percent a diagnosis of affective psychosis. Only 3.8 percent of the patients had a documented history of elation. There were no significant differences in a variety of sociodemographic and initial clinical characteristics between the patients completing the study and those who relapsed.

Completion Rates. One hundred fifty patients completed at least two months of maintenance treatment and were not replaced in the study. Of this total, 44 patients dropped out of the study between the second and eighth month (33 because of clinical relapse and 11 because of noncooperation), leaving a total of 106 patients who completed, without relapse, the one-month acute treatment and the eight-month maintenance treatment. These 106 patients can be considered the treatment successes in terms of symptomatic improvement and absence of relapse.

Summary of Therapeutic Effects. Table 1 presents a summary of the therapeutic effects of eight months of maintenance treatment on the major outcome measures: clinical relapse, symptom return, and social adjustment. The factorial design allowed for examining the drug and psychotherapy effects separately. In each case, amitriptyline was compared to placebo and no pill, and psychotherapy was compared to low contact. No formal treatment or clinic interactions were found. The relapse rates were calculated by the life table method for describing survival experiences over time. The other statistical analysis involved analysis of covariance for assessment of rating data. These data have been published elsewhere by Drs. Klerman, Paykel, and DiMascio, and Mrs. Prusoff, who have described details of the statistical analysis and full results (Klerman, DiMascio, Weisman, Prusoff, & Paykel, 1974; Paykel, DiMascio, Haskell, & Prusoff, 1974; and Weissman, Klerman, Paykel, Prusoff, & Hanson, 1974).

Table 1. Summary of Therapeutic Effects during Eight-Month Maintenance Treatment of Depression

Treatment Group	Sample Size	Effect on Various Outcome Criteria		
		Relapse	Symptom Return	Social Adjustment
Amitriptyline[a]	150	reduced	prevented	no effect
Psychotherapy[b]				
total patient sample	150	no effect	no effect	no effect
patients completing study only	106[c]	—	—	improved

[a] Amitriptyline is in all cases compared to placebo and no pill. No treatment or clinic interactions were found.
[b] Psychotherapy is in all cases compared to low contact.
[c] Forty-four patients were excluded, thirty-three due to clinical relapse and eleven due to noncooperation.

As can be easily seen in the summary table, eight months of maintenance amitriptyline reduced the relapse rate and prevented symptom return but had no effect on social adjustment. Alternately, psychotherapy did not prevent relapse or symptom return and showed no effect on social adjustment when the full sample, including the end-point analysis for early terminators, was used. However, psychotherapy did enhance social adjustment in those patients who completed the eight-month trial and did not relapse. Taken together, these results show a clear differential treatment response which has been repeatedly stressed. Drugs largely affected symptoms, and psychotherapy enhanced social adjustment. Furthermore, the efficacy of psychotherapy was related to the patient's remaining symptom-free and not relapsing, even though the psychotherapy itself did not prevent the relapse.

Psychotherapy Effects on Social Adjustment. We will next look at the psychotherapy effects in greater detail in those patients who completed the eight-month trial to see how long it took for effects to become apparent and what areas of social adjustment were effected. Figures 1–4 compare the social adjustment of psychotherapy and low contact patients after four months and after eight months of treatment. The mean of all 42 social adjustment items, the evaluation of overall adjustment, and the six factor scores will be presented.

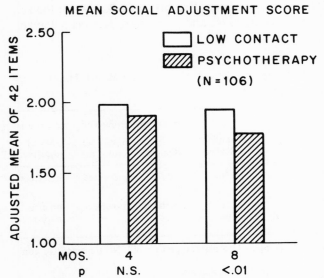

FIG. 2. Comparison between psychotherapy and low contact after four and eight months of treatment.

Overall Evaluations of Adjustment. These next two figures give a summary of the patients' adjustment. Figure 2 shows the mean of all 42 social adjustment items and indicates no treatment effects at four months but significant effects at eight months, with the psychotherapy patients less impaired.

Figure 3 shows the raters' global evaluation of the patients' overall adjustment. This, essentially, repeats the other finding: no therapeutic effect at four months and a psychotherapy effect at eight months.

Work Performance as a rating reflects the patients' actual performance, attendance, or days completing work and their interest and feelings of adequacy in work, either outside the home or in household tasks.

As can be seen (Fig. 4), there is no treatment effect at four months, but at eight months the psychotherapy patients have significantly better work performance.

Interpersonal Friction described patterns of overt friction, arguments, and resentment, extending across all roles. Again, at four months there is no treatment effect (Fig. 4), but at eight months psychotherapy patients have significantly less interpersonal friction.

Inhibited Communication involved reticence and withdrawal from marital and extended family and friends. At four months (Fig. 4) there are

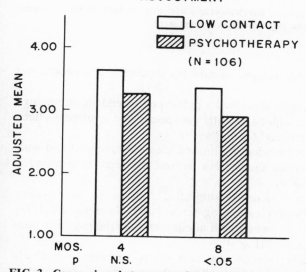

FIG. 3. Comparison between psychotherapy and low contact after four and eight months of treatment.

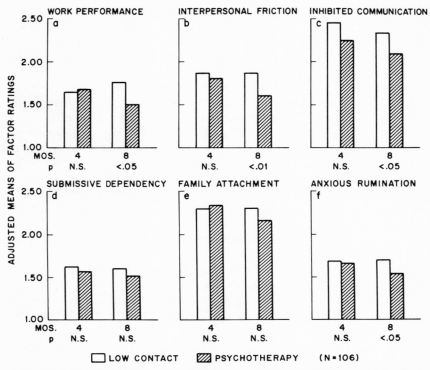

FIG. 4. Comparisons between psychotherapy and low contact on social adjustment factors after four and eight months of treatment.

no treatment effects, but at eight months the psychotherapy patients are less reticent.

Submissive Dependency described a pattern of dependent, submissive, nonassertive behavior, especially with the spouse. No treatment effects were found at four or at eight months (Fig. 4).

Family Attachment included diminished social interactions and withdrawal from the extended family. No treatment effects were found at either time period (Fig. 4).

Anxious Rumination denoted subjective feelings of overconcern, distress, and dissatisfaction, extending across roles. No treatment differences were found at four months, but at eight months the psychotherapy patients were less impaired (Fig. 4).

Overall, these results show no treatment differences after four months and positive psychotherapy effect after eight months of treatment in patients who completed the trial and did not relapse.

DISCUSSION

These findings have substantive implications about psychotherapy and its relationship to symptom remission, its timing and outcome, as well as methodologic implications about the analysis of long-term trials.

Psychotherapy and Prior Symptom Remission. The most important substantive finding is that psychotherapy is effective in enhancing adjustment for those patients who remain in symptomatic remission. While psychotherapy did not itself prevent relapse, drugs did, and, of course, many patients remained well who were not on medication after the acute episode had subsided. The result was a kind of synergistic effect of two effective treatments (drug and psychotherapy) that did not produce any formal interactions, since the treatments affected different areas at different times. These findings suggest that the effectiveness of psychotherapy in depression may require that the patients' symptomatic status be handled adequately and independently. Previous reports, which have commented that psychotherapy may make some patients better and some worse, might not have taken into account symptomatic worsening. The inclusion of patients who clinically relapsed might have negated a psychotherapy effect. Taken together, these findings are a strong argument for combined treatments to maximize the therapeutic effect.

Timing. It was quite clear in these data that psychotherapy required six to eight months before effects were apparent. It is not clear, however, whether this was due to the design of the study or whether, in fact, an extended length of time is required for psychotherapy to show an effect. In regard to the study, this was not an ideal design to test out psychotherapy. Psychotherapy began after the patient had showed a marked symptomatic response to amitriptyline. This timing may have delayed the psychotherapy effect, since recovering patients are less interested in treatment than acutely ill patients. Patients were initially treated with medication without psychotherapy and were clear drug responders. They attributed their improvement to the medication and often did not feel an immediate need for psychotherapy, which was a supplemental approach. Similarly, at the initiation of psychotherapy, therapists may have been careful not to undermine the patients' recent symptomatic recovery and, therefore, may have proceeded cautiously. The introduction of psychotherapy meant the introduction of a new therapist in addition to the psychiatrist who prescribed the medication, and it took time for a new therapeutic alliance to form. In future research we would like to introduce psychotherapy into the acute as well as the maintenance treatment phase and determine whether the early introduction of psychotherapy decreases the response time.

On the other hand, the delayed psychotherapy effect may be independent of the design. It is consistent with the results of Hogarty, Goldberg, & The Collaborative Study Group (1973). While their data demonstrated the importance of long-term psychotherapy in a study of maintenance rehabilitative treatment of schizophrenics, a positive psychotherapy effect took one year to develop. The negative psychotherapy findings in previously reported studies may be related to inadequate timing of followup.

Social Adjustment as an Outcome of Psychotherapy. The importance of suitable outcome criteria for psychotherapy studies has been repeatedly stressed (Fiske, et al., 1970). Frank (1961), as we have often noted, emphasized the distinction between symptom comfort and social effectiveness and showed that the effects of group psychotherapy were most marked on the latter. This distinction has since been made by many others (Park & Imboden, 1970; Goldman & Mendelson, 1969; Malan, Bacal, Heath, & Balfour, 1968; Cawley, 1971). Our findings underscore the need for appropriate outcome criteria for psychotherapy. Had symptomatic improvement, relapse rate, or hospitalization been the sole outcome measures, or had treatment been shorter, we would not have demonstrated a psychotherapy effect. Social adjustment appears to be an appropriate outcome measure.

Attention should be paid, however, to the social adjustment assessment used, which was a rater judgment based on what the patient told the interviewer. The lack of independently validated behavior measures, such as a relative rating, may have influenced ratings. For example, psychotherapy, unlike drug treatment, could not be blinded. Even though raters were independent of treatment, the raters' preconceptions about psychotherapy could possibly have colored the ratings. Alternately, patients receiving psychotherapy may have felt more comfortable with the raters and, therefore, appeared better adjusted at assessment interviews. The fact that psychotherapy effects were not consistent, either at both time periods or on all variables, however, argues against this possible influence. Two ways of reducing bias might be through the use of patients' self-report rather than interviewer ratings and through independent ratings by relatives. None of the techniques alone (patient self-report, relatives' ratings, or patient interviews) is ideal. If this study were replicated, we would use independent assessments of the patients' adjustment through interviews with relatives, using the Katz Adjustment Scale (Katz & Lyerly, 1963) and, possibly, a patient self-report as well.

The Analysis of Maintenance Trials: Total Sample vs. Subsets. The psychotherapy effect in this study was found when only patients who completed the study were included in the analysis, and when the subset of relapsers was excluded. The end-point analysis of the total sample did not show a psychotherapy effect. This raises an important and unresolved issue about the handling of dropouts in a long-term clinical trial, an issue frequently mentioned in publications dealing with the design of clinical trials in psychiatry (Levine, Schiele, & Bouthilet, 1971). This problem, of course, is not unique to studies of psychotherapy, combined therapies, or psychiatry. For example, heated debate still emerges in the literature on the diabetes clinical trial, where the effectiveness of tolbutamide rests partially on such issues as the handling of attrition (Schor, 1971).

About a decade ago, in the analysis of psychopharmacologic trials of acute disorders, the end-point analysis was adopted as a solution. This is the method by which early terminators are rated at the point of termination and this rating is included in all subsequent analysis in their original treatment group (Goldberg, 1972). The rationale behind this approach is that the best predictor of the patient's clinical status at the termination of the trial is his status at dropout. This method is an effective resolution of the attrition problem in a short-term acute trial where patients are recovering from an episode. There is now some evidence reached independently by Hogarty, Goldberg, and their associates and by our study that this method may not always be appropriate in prophylactic trials (Hogarty et al., 1973). In maintenance trials, the end-point analysis may obscure an important process in which some patients are getting better and some are getting worse.

In our study an end-point analysis was appropriate for symptoms, since symptom return was the main criterion for termination. A sample of completers would have been biased in the direction of not showing a therapeutic effect on symptoms. Social adjustment, however, was not a criterion for termination, so that the same bias did not necessarily apply. Since psychotherapy effects on social adjustment were slow to develop, an analysis of patients completing the study was necessary to show therapeutic effects. Both forms of analysis, end-point and completers, may be appropriate, depending on the circumstances. Considerably more attention to the analysis of maintenance trials is required.

CONCLUSIONS

This study supports the value of weekly maintenance psychotherapy over a period of six to eight months in enhancing the social adjustment of recovering depressed female outpatients. However, the efficacy is contingent on the patient's remaining symptomatically well, either by antidepressants or natural remission. Therefore, psychotherapy is not an alternative to antidepressant treatment and does not prevent relapse or the recurrence of symptoms. Alternately, maintenance amitriptyline has no effect on social adjustment and is no better or worse than a placebo or no pill. A study of these patients following termination from treatment is now under way; it will provide data on any enduring effects of treatment. This information is necessary before any conclusions about long-term preventive effects can be drawn. Methodologically, these data indicate that psychotherapy studies should pay attention to the timing of treatment, the patients' symptomatic status, the outcome measure, and the analytic problem of attrition.

NOTE

1. A preliminary report of these results was presented at the American Psychopathological Association Meeting in 1972 (Paykel, Klerman, DiMascio, Weissman, & Prusoff, 1973).

REFERENCES

Cawley, R. The evaluation of psychotherapy. *Psychological Medicine*, 1971, 1, 101–103.

Fisher, J. Is casework effective? A review. *Social Work*, 1973, 18(1), 5–20.

Fiske, D. W., Hunt, H. F., Luborsky, L., Orne, M. T., Parloff, M. B., Reiser, M. F., & Tuma, A. H. Planning of research on effectiveness of psychotherapy. *Archives of General Psychiatry*, 1970, 22, 22–32.

Frank, J. D. *Persuasion and healing*. Baltimore: Johns Hopkins Press, 1961.

Goldberg, S. Dealing with dropout in the analysis of the experiment. Paper presented at the Tenth Annual American College of Neuropsychopharmacology Association Meeting, San Juan, Puerto Rico, 1972.

Goldman, R. K., & Mendelsohn, G. A. Psychotherapeutic change and social adjustment: a report of a national survey of psychotherapists. *Journal of Abnormal and Social Psychology*, 1969, 74, 164–172.

Gurland, B. J., Yorkstone, M. J., Stone, A. R., Frank, J. D., & Fleiss, J. L. The structured and scaled interview to assess maladjustment (SSIAM): description, rationale, and development. *Archives of General Psychiatry*, 1972, 27, 259–264.

Hogarty, G. E., Goldberg, S. C., & The Collaborative Study Group. Drugs and sociotherapy in the aftercare of schizophrenic patients. *Archives of General Psychiatry*, 1973, 28, 56–64.

Hollingshead, A. Two factor index of social position. New Haven: Yale University, 1957.

Katz, M. M., & Lyerly, S. B. Methods of measuring adjustment and social behavior in the community: rationale, description, discriminative validity and scale development. *Psychological Reports*, 1963, 13, 503–535.

Klerman, G. L. Issues in the relationship between the pharmacotherapy and psychotherapy of depression. Unpublished manuscript.

Klerman, G. L., & Cole, J. O. Clinical pharmacology of imipramine and related antidepressant compounds. *Pharmacological Reviews*, 1965, 17, 101–141.

Klerman, G. L., DiMascio, A., Weissman, M. M., Prusoff, B. A., & Paykel, E. S. Treatment of depression by drugs and psychotherapy. *American Journal of Psychiatry*, 1974, 131, 186–190.

Levine, J., Schiele, B. C., & Bouthilet, L. (Eds.) *Principles and problems in establishing the efficacy of psychotropic agents*. Public Health Service Publication 2138. Washington, D.C.: U.S. Public Health Service, 1971.

Luborsky, L., Chandler, M., Auerbach, A., Cohen, J., & Backrach, H. M. Factors influencing the outcome of psychotherapy: a review of quantitative research. *Psychological Bulletin*, 1971, 75, 145–185.

Malan, D. H., Bacal, H. A., Heath, E. S., & Balfour, F. H. G. A study of psychodynamic changes in untreated neurotic patients. *British Journal of Psychiatry*, 1968, **114**, 525–551.

Park, L. C., & Imboden, J. B. Clinical and heuristic value of clinical drug research. *Journal of Nervous and Mental Disease*, 1970, **151**, 322–340.

Paykel, E. S., DiMascio, A., Haskell, D., & Prusoff, B. A. The effects of maintenance amitriptyline and psychotherapy on symptoms of depression. Submitted for publication, 1974.

Paykel, E. S., Klerman, G. L., DiMascio, A., Weissman, M. M., & Prusoff, B. A. Maintenance antidepressants, psychotherapy, symptoms and social function. In J. Cole, A. Friedhoff, & A. Freedman (Eds.), *Psychopathology and psychopharmacology*. Baltimore: Johns Hopkins University Press, 1973.

Raskin, A., Schulterbrandt, J., Reatig, N., & McKeon, J. J. Replication of factors of psychopathology in interview, ward behavior and self report ratings of hospitalized depressives. *Journal of Nervous and Mental Disease*, 1969, **148**, 87–98.

Schor, S. The university group diabetes program: a statistician looks at the mortality results. *Journal of the American Medical Association*, 1971, **217**, 1671–1675.

Segal, S. P. Research on the outcome of social work therapeutic interventions: a review of the literature. *Journal of Health and Social Behavior*, 1972, **13**, 3–17.

Strupp, H. H., & Bergin, A. E. Some empirical and conceptual bases for coordinated research in psychotherapy: a critical review of issues, trends, and evidence. *International Journal of Psychiatry*, 1969, **7**, 18–90.

Uhlenhuth, E. H., Lipman, R. A., & Covi, L. Combined pharmacotherapy and psychotherapy. *Journal of Nervous and Mental Disease*, 1969, **1**, 52–64.

Weissman, M. M., Klerman, G. L., Paykel, E. S., Prusoff, B., & Hanson, B. Treatment effects on the social adjustment of depressed outpatients. *Archives of General Psychiatry*, 1974, **30**, 771–778.

Weissman, M. M., & Paykel, E. S. *The depressed woman: a study of social relationships*. Chicago: University of Chicago Press, 1974.

14 OUTPATIENT TREATMENT OF NEUROTIC DEPRESSION: Medication and Group Psychotherapy

RONALD S. LIPMAN and LINO COVI

At the time the present study was initiated, 1969, the efficacy of the tricyclic antidepressants such as amitriptyline and imipramine were reasonably well established. Studies by such investigators as Hare, McCance, and McCormick (1964), Overall, Hollister, Johnson, and Pennington (1966), Hollister, Overall, Shelton, Pennington, Kimbell, and Johnson (1967), Rickels, Raab, De Silverio, and Eternad (1967), and Wheatley (1969) raised real questions, however, about the potential role of the tranquilizer-sedatives in the treatment of depression. It was suggested that the therapeutic mechanism of action in treating depression was mediated by the sedative properties of psychotropic medication. The work of Overall and Hollister and their associates, however, suggested a differential pattern of efficacy, with the tricyclic antidepressants most beneficial in the treatment of retarded-withdrawn depressions and the tranquilizers most effective in depressions characterized by high levels of coexisting anxiety.

Ronald S. Lipman, Ph.D., Chief, Clinical Studies Section, Psychopharmacology Research Branch, National Institute of Mental Health.

Lino Covi, M.D., Associate Professor of Psychiatry, Johns Hopkins University School of Medicine.

This work was supported by National Institute of Mental Health Grant MH-15720.

The authors wish to thank Joseph H. Pattison, M.D., and James J. Smith, M.D., who served as therapists. Leonard Derogatis, Ph.D., provided valuable statistical consultation. Shashi K. Pande, M.D., and Renato D. Alarcon, M.D., helped in patient selection and with clinical monitoring. Albert P. Cohen, M.Ed., and Nathan Miller, M.S.S.W., served as observers in group psychotherapy and conducted interviews with the husband/husband-equivalent of the patient. John Serio and Darryl Bertolucci provided programming assistance. Margaret B. Winogrodzki, Laura Koblish, Julia Martin, and Lena L. Fones provided technical assistance. We are particularly grateful to Robert R. Rawlings, M.S., Division of Computer Systems, ADAMHA, for his statistical advice and help, and to Virginia K. Smith, Johns Hopkins, who provided the bulk of the analyses reported in this paper. The authors also wish to acknowledge the assistance of Dr. Edgar Grunwaldt, formerly Associate Director of Research, Geigy Pharmaceuticals, who arranged the manufacture of the experimental capsules, and of Dr. Lee Gordon, formerly of Hoffmann-La Roche.

Unlike the pharmacotherapy literature, where treatment efficacy had clearly been demonstrated, the psychotherapy of depression is much more ambiguous (cf. Bednar & Lawlis, 1971; Fiske, Hunt, Luborsky, Orne, Parloff, Reiser, & Tuma, 1970). Along these lines, Meltzoff and Kornreich (1970), in their extensive review of the psychotherapies, conclude that "individual or collective treatment, or combinations of the two, are all equally effective or ineffective as the case may be" (p. 184). In any event, group psychotherapy and psychotropic medication are frequently combined in treating depressed outpatients, and this particular treatment combination had not heretofore been studied in a controlled manner. Indeed, the only controlled study in the literature at the time this research was initiated (Daneman, 1961) involved the double-blind comparison of imipramine and placebo within the context of individually oriented psychoanalytic therapy. The more recent literature, however, contains two somewhat relevant studies. Klerman, DiMascio, Weissman, Prusoff, and Paykel (1974) have evaluated the relative efficacy of amitriptyline and psychotherapy in preventing the relapse of depressed female outpatients, and Friedman (1972) has compared the effectiveness of marital therapy and amitriptyline in the acute phase of outpatient depression. Both studies employed placebos as the control for active medication and brief contact with the treating psychiatrist as the control for the more extensive psychotherapeutic contact.

METHODS AND PROCEDURE

The design of this outpatient depression trial involved the double-blind comparison of three medications: diazepam, a minor tranquilizer of the benzodiazepine series; imipramine, a tricyclic antidepressant; and placebo, prepared in capsules of identical appearance. Two types of psychotherapy were employed: brief supportive contact, involving individual interviews of roughly twenty minutes' duration, held biweekly after the initial three visits; and psychodynamically oriented weekly group psychotherapy sessions of ninety minutes' duration. It should be noted that group therapy patients were also seen individually by the treating doctor to check medication, side effects, etc. This was done on a biweekly basis after group meetings so that, in effect, group patients were also receiving brief supportive contact. The main thematic focus of group psychotherapy was on current reality-oriented problems, i.e., family relationships and working and living arrangements. Because groups were open-ended and membership was continually in flux, the therapist tended to participate actively in the group discussions. Dynamic interpretations were offered when appropriate. Discussions of medication, dosage, side effects, etc., were deferred for individual sessions with the doctor after the regular group meeting. In order to collect a sufficiently large patient sample, two Baltimore clinics, the Gundry Hospital Outpatient Department and the Outpatient Department of the Henry Phipps Psychiatric Clinic of The Johns Hopkins Hospital, participated.

Patients were treated at these clinics by one of two experienced psychiatrists (one with ten years of post-residency experience and the other with eighteen years) who participated in both treatment modalities at both settings. This procedure of employing the same two physicians for both individual and group therapy at each clinic was thought to be a promising way of reducing "nonspecific" clinic variance; i.e., physicians were constant across clinics. The study design involved psychiatric screening, followed by a two-week placebo washout period and sixteen weeks of active treatment. All patients completing this phase were then carefully screened to determine whether or not they were sufficiently improved to enter a twelve-month, minimal contact, maintenance medication phase. Those patients not sufficiently improved to enter maintenance were removed from the study and treated openly by doctor's choice. The initial month of the twelve-month maintenance phase was used to reduce medication dosage and to switch patients, at random, to placebo. Half the placebo group was to continue on pill and half on no pill.

The full design of the study is shown in Figure 1. Initial screening was followed by two evaluation visits during which prior medication was withdrawn and placebo substituted. Patients were then randomly assigned to one of the six combinations of three drugs and two types of therapy. Psychotherapy groups had been constituted by the study doctors prior to the start of the study, using similar non-study patients. Thus, study patients could be directly assigned to an appropriate ongoing group ("core group"), thereby avoiding the difficulties inherent in using a waiting list. Throughout the course of the study, use was made of depressed non-study patients to maintain the continuity of active groups and to maintain group size within reasonable limits. Both group and supportive therapy patients were seen weekly for dosage adjustment for the first two weeks on active medication (visits 4 and 5). All dosage adjustments were then made on a biweekly basis. After sixteen weeks of active treatment (visit 19) patients were screened and, when appropriate, assigned to maintenance therapy after two biweekly visits; patients were seen once a month to complete the twelve-month course of treatment. Only brief supportive contact with the original psychiatrist was given during maintenance.

Medication was started at two pills a day following the placebo washout period. This corresponded to 100 mg/d of imipramine and 10 mg/d of diazepam. The following week, dosage was increased by one pill to reach the modal dose of 15 mg/d of diazepam and 150 mg/d of imipramine.

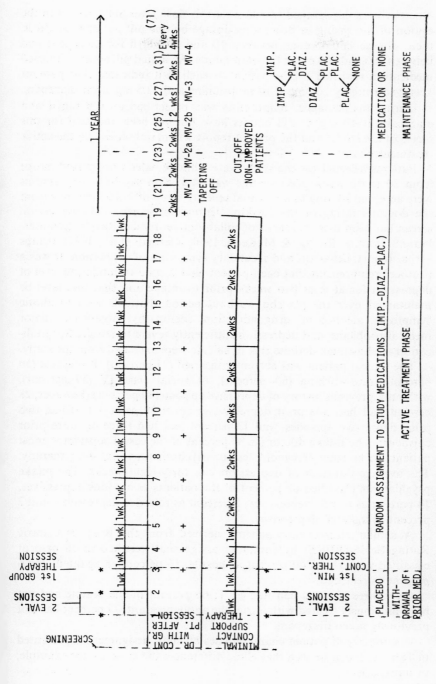

FIG. 1. NIMH-PRB outpatient treatment of depression: study flow chart.

Doctors were encouraged to maintain this dose level but were given the option of increasing or decreasing dosage by one pill per day. In effect, then, dosage could range between 10 and 20 mg/d for diazepam and between 100 and 200 mg/d for imipramine. An actual pill count of unused medication returned by the patient at each visit indicated that patients averaged roughly 125 mg/d of imipramine and 12.5 mg/d for diazepam.

During maintenance, imipramine was prescribed at 100 mg/d and diazepam at 10 mg/d. Pill counts have not yet been analyzed for this phase of the study, and the present report will mainly focus on the active treatment phase.

Patients selected for the study were white females who ranged in age from 20 to 50 years. Average age was 34.4. Non-psychotic depressions were accepted so long as a minimal severity score of 7 was obtained from the doctor's rating of the Raskin Depression Screen. This depression screen has been used in a series of collaborative studies (Raskin, Schulterbrandt, Boothe, Reatig, & McKeon, 1970; Klerman et al., 1974); it taps verbal report, behavior, and secondary symptoms of depression. It was a protocol requirement that each patient have a mild to moderate level of depression for at least two weeks prior to intake and that that level be maintained over the placebo washout period. Patients with psychotic symptoms, alcoholism, drug addiction, sociopathy, organicity, major medical problems, and depression sufficiently severe to require hospitalization or showing a definite risk of suicide were excluded from the study.

The typical patient was currently married (71 percent), Protestant (50 percent), non-working (60 percent), of social class IV (39 percent), without a previous history of depressive episode (40 percent) (however, 28 percent had had one prior depressive episode; 19 percent had had two prior depressive episodes; and 13 percent had had three or more prior episodes). The intake doctor (in 80 percent of the cases) considered most patients to be suitable candidates for psychotherapy and drug therapy. The average duration of depression was forty-eight weeks. The intake psychiatrists classified 67 percent of the patients as anxious depressives, 14 percent as hostile depressives, 5 percent as retarded depressives, and 2 percent as agitated depressives.

A similar classification schema derived from the Brief Psychiatric Rating Scale (BPRS) by computer assignment[1] resulted in 38 percent classified as anxious, 40 percent as hostile, 16 percent as agitated, and 6 percent as retarded.

Only three patients had had ECT; 66 percent of the sample had not been previously treated with a tricyclic antidepressant; 73 percent had not previously taken diazepam.

A summary of patient characteristics by clinic assignment is presented in Table 1. It can be seen that clinic differences did exist, as, for example, in social class.

Table 1. Demographic and Illness-Related Patient Characteristics

Characteristics	Phipps[a]	Gundry[b]
Therapy assignment		
minimal	54	54
group	51	53
Drug assignment		
placebo	34	36
imipramine	35	35
diazepam	36	36
Religion		
Catholic	38	39
Protestant	47	52
Jewish	5	9
other	6	1
no affiliation	9	6
Marital status		
never married	15	13
currently married	65	79
formerly married	25	15
Head of household (.10)[d]		
patient	36	23
husband/husband-equivalent	69	84
Social class (.01)[d]		
I	2	5
II	5	14
III	20	27
IV	39	43
V	39	18
Employment		
full-time	33	28
over half-time	5	4
half-time	3	2
under half-time	2	6
unemployed	56	57
Peak of present illness (relative to screening)		
less than 1 week	34	34
1 week to less than 1 month	34	26
1 month to less than 6 months	25	29
6 months to less than 12 months	6	7
1 year or more	6	11
Immediate precipitants		
none	35	36
previous episode not precipitating	4	3
previous episode uncertain	32	34
previous episode predominant precipitant	34	33
Previous ECT		
none	105	101
bad effect	0	2
uncertain effect	0	0
good effect	0	4

Table 1. (Continued)

Characteristics	Phipps[a]	Gundry[b]
Previous tricyclic		
none	72	69
bad effect	5	5
uncertain effect	12	15
good effect	16	17
Previous Valium		
none	78	75
bad effect	3	6
uncertain effect	15	10
good effect	6	13
Prior relevant drug experience by drug class		
minor tranquilizers, barbiturates	31	39
antidepressants	17	19
antipsychotic Compazine	4	5
analgesics, aspirin	4	2
amphetamines, diet pills	1	4
antihistamines	0	1
multiple drugs	7	6
sleep medication	0	3
Patient's main treatment goal		
resolution of inner conflicts	58	55
relief of psychological symptoms	27	41
relief of somatic symptoms	1	0
help with reality problem	10	7
seeks treatment as results of outside pressure	2	2
ambiguous	7	2
Treatment patient expected (.10)[d]		
psychotherapy	51	43
guidance or advice	23	19
medication	9	20
none	19	25
combinations	3	0
Treatment recommended		
drug therapy	11	8
psychotherapy	11	12
both	80	81
specific guidance	2	4
Overall clinical syndromes (physician classification)		
anxious	65	72
hostile	11	16
retarded	5	4
agitated	0	4
no agreement	24	10
Occupation of head of household		
higher executive	2	6
business manager	6	12
administrative person	17	19
clerical	31	25

Table 1. (Continued)

Characteristics	Phipps[a]	Gundry[b]
Occupation of head of household (cont.)		
skilled manual	31	22
machine operator	10	16
unskilled, unemployed	13	6
Education of head of household		
graduate degree	3	6
college degree	8	17
partial college	17	21
high school	32	29
partial high school	17	14
junior high school	20	14
under 7 years	7	5
Occupation		
higher executive	0	2
business manager	3	4
administrative	4	5
clerical	35	28
skilled manual	6	3
machine operator	10	9
unskilled, unemployed	44	55
Patient's attitude toward drug (.05)[d]		
very eager	10	21
somewhat eager	28	33
neither eager nor reluctant	47	34
somewhat reluctant	14	16
very reluctant	3	0
Patient's attitude toward therapy		
very eager (toward group)	5	10
somewhat eager	22	22
neither eager nor reluctant	52	50
somewhat reluctant	19	20
very reluctant	4	3
Age (years)	32.1[f]	33.6[f]
Longest period of continuous employment (months)[c]	38.9	49.8
Duration of present illness (weeks)	42.5	54.4
Previous episodes	1.3	1.4
Previous depressive episodes	1.2	1.3
Duration of medication in year prior to study (days)[c]	14.2	22.0
SCL factors (week 3)[e]		
General sample		
depression	1.22	1.15
anxiety	1.23	1.23
somatization	.73	.72
obsessive-compulsiveness	1.08	1.02
interpersonal sensitivity[c]	1.12	.96

Table 1.   (Continued)

---

[a] Size of Phipps sample, 105.
[b] Size of Gundry sample, 107. Totals do not always add to 105 (Phipps) and 107 (Gundry) because of missing data.
[c] $p < .05$.
[d] Chi square significant at the level indicated in parentheses.
[e] Means are for patients who completed sixteen weeks of active treatment.
[f] Numbers here and below represent means.

It was hypothesized that active medications would be better than placebo, that group therapy plus some individual doctor contact would be better than minimal contact alone, and that medications would be found to interact with subtypes of depression as defined by the BPRS in keeping with the earlier reports of Overall and Hollister (1966). Thus, we expected diazepam to be most effective in the anxious depressions and imipramine to be the drug of choice for the more retarded depressions.

Improvement measures were provided independently by three classes of raters: the patient, the treating psychiatrist, and the patient's husband or husband-equivalent. The patient contributed the most extensive ratings, followed, in this order, by the physician and the husband or husband-equivalent. Our major dependent measures have been culled from two outpatient self-rating scales which have proved quite sensitive to drug effects. The mood scale is a minor adaptation of the Psychiatric Outpatient Mood Scale (POMS) developed by McNair and Lorr (1964), and its ten factors are presented in Table 2. The treating physician made a global rating for eight of these ten factors. Our main study hypotheses were, of course, related to the depressed mood factor, although all these factors are of clinical interest.

The second major measuring instrument is the Symptom Distress Checklist (SCL) which had its roots in the Cornell Medical Index, in early work of Frank, Gliedman, Imber, Nash, and Stone (1957) and Parloff, Kelman, and Frank (1954) at Hopkins, and more recently in the research of Lipman and his associates (Lipman, Rickels, Covi, Derogatis, & Uhlenhuth, 1969; Derogatis, Lipman, Rickels, Uhlenhuth, & Covi, 1974). A general factor solution for this instrument is presented in Table 3; a factor structure derived from a depressed sample is given in Table 4. It should be noted that two anxiety factors, somatic anxiety and phobic anxiety, were present in the structure derived from the depressed sample.

As with the mood scale, our main focus, vis-a-vis hypothesis testing, lies with the symptom factor of depression.

Additional measures include global improvement (7-point scale), BPRS total scores, and dimensions of the Barrett-Lennard Relationship

Table 2.   Depression Study: Factor Composition of Mood Scale

I.   Depression
      1. sad
      9. confused
    11. downhearted
    17. worthless
    22. unhappy
    28. useless
    32. depressed
    39. blue
    43. troubled
    48. worried
    50. lonely

II.   Friendliness
      6. good-natured
    16. friendly
    27. kind
    31. efficient
    35. dependable
    38. alert
    46. warm-hearted
    49. pleasant
    52. considerate

III. Anxiety
      2. tense
    12. on edge
    23. anxious
    24. impatient
    33. restless
    40. nervous
    44. jittery

IV.   Guilt
    36. troubled by conscience
    42. sorry for things done
    47. ashamed

V.   Hostility
      3. angry
    13. irritable
    34. annoyed
    41. rude
    45. sarcastic

VI.   Activity
      8. full of pep
    14. carefree
    19. active
    30. lively

VII. Fatigue
      7. tired
    18. sleepy
    29. worn-out
    37. weary
    20. forgetful

Table 2. (Continued)

VIII. Well-Being
       4. happy
       5. relaxed
     15. at ease
     25. cheerful
     26. satisfied

IX.   Cognitive
     10. able to think clearly
     21. able to concentrate

X.   Carefree[a]
       4. happy
       5. relaxed
       8. full of pep
     14. carefree
     15. at ease
     19. active
     25. cheerful
     26. satisfied
     30. lively

---

[a]"Carefree" factor from Raskin's analysis.

Inventory (Barrett-Lennard, 1962). Sample items defining the dimensions of Level of Regard, Empathetic Understanding, Unconditionality of Regard, and Congruence are given in Table 5.

RESULTS

Completion Rate. In Table 6, the total flow of patients through the study is presented for each clinic. The table indicates that a total of 346 patients were screened for inclusion in the study, more at Phipps than at Gundry. Of the 279 patients who were accepted for the study at intake, 149 completed the 16-week active treatment phase with reasonable adherence to protocol (46.6 percent attrition rate). It should be noted that roughly half (47 percent) of this patient attrition took place during the 2-week placebo washout period prior to the actual assignment of patients to medication. Of these early attritions 25 percent represented no-shows, 7 percent represented scores on the Raskin screen below the cut-off of 7, 37 percent represented patient decisions covering a spectrum of reasons ranging from logistical problems in keeping regular clinic appointments to rejection of the need for treatment. Roughly one-quarter (23 percent)

Table 3. SCL General Factor Solution (GSCL)

I. Somatization
1. headaches
4. faintness or dizziness
12. pains in the heart or chest
14. feeling low in energy or slowed down
27. pains in the lower part of your back
42. soreness of your muscles
48. trouble getting your breath
49. hot or cold spells
52. numbness or tingling in parts of your body
53. a lump in your throat
56. weakness in parts of your body
58. heavy feelings in your arms or legs

II. Depression
5. loss of sexual interest or pleasure
15. thoughts of ending your life
19. poor appetite
20. crying easily
22. a feeling of being trapped or caught
26. blaming yourself for things
29. feeling lonely
30. feeling blue
31. worrying or stewing about things
32. feeling no interest in things
54. feeling hopeless about the future

III. Obsessive-Compulsiveness
9. trouble remembering things
10. worried about sloppiness or carelessness
28. feeling blocked or stymied in getting things done
38. having to do things very slowly in order to be sure you were doing them right
45. having to check and double check what you do
46. difficulty making decisions
51. your mind going blank
55. trouble concentrating

IV. Interpersonal Sensitivity
6. feeling critical of others
11. feeling easily annoyed or irritated
24. temper outbursts you could not control
34. your feelings being easily hurt
36. feeling others do not understand you or are unsympathetic
37. feeling that people are unfriendly or dislike you
41. feeling inferior to others

V. Anxiety
2. nervousness or shakiness inside
17. trembling
23. suddenly scared for no reason
33. feeling fearful
39. heart pounding or racing
50. having to avoid certain things, places, or activities because they frighten you
57. feeling tense or keyed up

Table 4.   SCL Factors Derived from Depressed Sample (DSCL)

I.   Somatization
        1. headaches
        4. faintness or dizziness
        12. pains in the heart or chest
        27. pains in the lower part of your back
        39. heart pounding or racing
        40. nausea or upset stomach
        42. soreness of your muscles
        48. trouble getting your breath
        49. hot or cold spells
        52. numbness or tingling in parts of your body
        53. a lump in your throat
        56. weakness in parts of your body
        58. heavy feelings in your arms or legs

II.   Depression
        14. feeling low in energy or slowed down
        15. thoughts of ending your life
        22. a feeling of being trapped or caught
        26. blaming yourself for things
        28. feeling blocked or stymied in getting things done
        29. feeling lonely
        30. feeling blue
        31. worrying or stewing about things
        32. feeling no interest in things
        35. having to ask others what you should do

III.   Hostility
        11. feeling easily annoyed or irritated
        24. temper outbursts you could not control
        63. having impulses to beat, injure, or harm someone
        67. having impulses to smash things

IV.   Anxiety: 1 (somatic)
        2. nervousness or shakiness inside
        3. being unable to get rid of bad thoughts or ideas
        17. trembling
        44. difficulty in falling asleep or staying asleep
        57. feeling tense or keyed up

IV.   Anxiety: 2 (phobic)
        23. suddenly scared for no reason
        33. feeling fearful
        50. having to avoid certain things, places, or activities because they frighten you

V.   Sleep Disturbance
        44. difficulty in falling asleep or staying asleep
        64. awakening in the early hours of the morning and unable to fall asleep again
        66. sleep that is restless and disturbed

Table 5. Sample Items Defining the Categories of the Barrett-Lennard Relationship Inventory

---

1. Level of Regard
    He respects me as a person.
    He feels a true liking for me.
    I feel appreciated by him.
    He cares for me.

2. Empathetic Understanding
    He wants to understand how I see things.
    He nearly always knows exactly what I mean.
    He usually senses or realizes what I am feeling.
    He realizes what I mean even when I have difficulty in saying it.

3. Unconditionality of Regard
    Whether I am feeling happy or unhappy with myself makes no real difference to the way he feels about me.
    His feeling toward me doesn't depend on how I feel toward him.
    I can (or could) be openly critical or appreciative of him without really making him feel any differently about me.
    How much he likes or dislikes me is not altered by anything that I tell him about myself.

4. Congruence
    He is comfortable and at ease with me.
    I feel that he is real and genuine with me.
    He does not avoid anything that is important for our relationship.
    He expresses his true impressions and feelings with me.

---

of the patients took non-prescribed psychotropic medication during the placebo washout period, and a few patients (4 percent) required immediate treatment because of an exacerbation of their depression.

Of the 218 patients who entered the active treatment phase, 69 (31.7 percent) did not fully comply with the study protocol for the full 16 weeks of treatment. These deviating patients were not reliably disproportionate as a function of type of therapy or clinic but approached disproportionality as a function of medication ($\chi^2 = 3.90$; df $= 2$; $.20 > p > .10$). In this regard, the non-compliance rate for placebo patients (40.3 percent) was somewhat higher than the deviation for imipramine- (29.2 percent) and diazepam- (25.7 percent) treated patients.

Of the 212 patients who completed at least two weeks of active treatment, 32 (51 percent) became no-shows, while 31 were classified as attritions for other reasons—primarily because the patient worsened and required other treatment ($N = 14$) or because the patient became a major medication deviation ($N = 14$) due to missed visits, taking other medication, taking less than the prescribed amount of medication, or some combination of these reasons. The major reason for no-shows was treatment-related ($N = 20$) and ranged from sufficient improvement as

Table 6. Description of Patient Flow

Category	Phipps	Gundry	Total
Active treatment phase			
1. patients screened	200	146	346
2. rejected or declined at intake	56	11	67
3. accepted at intake	144	135	279
4. no show at visit 1	1	4	5
5. attrition prior to medication	33	23	56
6. active medicated patients	110	108	218
7. attrition, early (visit 4)	5	1	6
(sub-total patients remain)	105	107	212
8. attrition, middle (visits 5–12)	22	17	39
(sub-total patients remain)	83	90	173
9. attrition, late (visits 13–19)	11	13	24
10. completed active treatment	72	77	149
Maintenance medication phase			
11. not assigned to maintenance	23	18	41
12. assigned to maintenance	49	59	108
13. attrition between visits 19 and 2A	4	5	9
14. entered maintenance 2A	45	54	99
15. attrition, early (visits 2B–6)	16	18	34
16. attrition, middle (visits 7–10)	6	7	13
17. attrition, late (visits 11–13)	4	4	8
18. completed maintenance	19	25	44

defined by the patient ($N = 5$) to lack of improvement ($N = 5$) to dissatisfaction with the treatment given ($N = 9$). One-third of the no-shows were nontreatment-related and involved problems with scheduling visits arising from the patient moving, changing jobs, baby sitter difficulties, illness in other family members, etc. It should be noted here that of the 19 patient attritions because of worsening, 9 were on diazepam, 9 on placebo, and 1 on imipramine ($\chi^2 = 6.92, p < .05$).

Side Effects. In assessing side effects, the physician recorded those effects spontaneously reported by the patient, provided they could be reasonably attributed to medication. No patients were terminated because of side effects, and, in general, most side effects were of a very low incidence of occurrence, 4 percent or less, with only three side effects found to be reliably medication related. In this regard, drowsiness and fatigue were more frequently noted in diazepam patients ($\chi^2 = 10.01, p < .01$), while dry mouth occurred more frequently in imipramine patients ($\chi^2 = 8.63, p < .02$). The incidence of dry mouth was slightly higher in imipramine non-completers (16 percent) than in imipramine completers (12 percent) and this same pattern was also noted with regard to drowsiness: non-completers on diazepam were characterized by a 28 percent incidence vs. an 18 percent incidence of drowsiness in diazepam completers. The next two figures display the time course of dry mouth and drowsiness for the full sample of patients. As can be seen in Figures 2 and 3, the incidence of these side effects builds over the first few weeks of treatment and then tends to decrease over time.

The differential occurrence of dry mouth with imipramine reflects the most typical autonomic atropine-like side effect of the tricyclics, while the differential incidence of drowsiness and fatigue with diazepam represents the typical sedative side effect of the minor tranquilizers. In essence, these side effect data are reassuringly predictable from the literature (cf. Rickels, Chung, Feldman, Gordon, Kelly, & Weise, 1973). It should be noted, in passing, that the occurrence of side effects was not related to either the type of therapy given or to clinic setting.

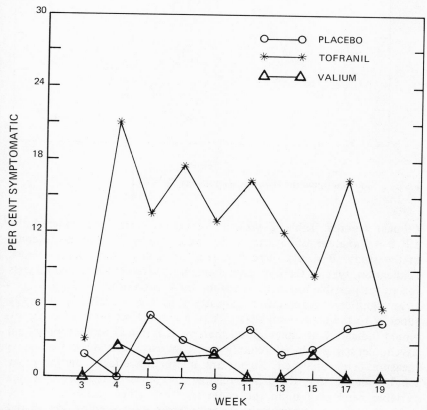

FIG. 2. Side reactions: dry mouth, all patients (N = 212).

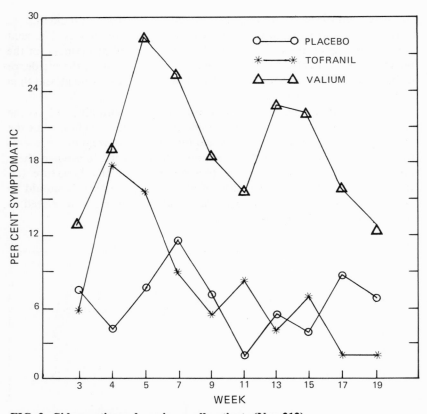

FIG. 3. Side reactions: drowsiness, all patients (N = 212).

Clinical Results. Table 7 presents the effect terms that entered the $3 \times 2 \times 2$ analyses of covariance that were employed to test the outcome of the study. Basically there is a test for each of three main effects: medication, type of therapy, and clinic, and there are also separate tests for all the possible interactions among these variables.

A significant main effect indicates that one variable is generally superior to the other variable(s). Thus, a main effect for psychotherapy would indicate that either group therapy or minimal contact individual psychotherapy produced reliably more improvement on the outcome measure being analyzed. Significant interaction effects, on the other hand, indicate that there is a reliable difference in the effect of one variable depending upon the context of the other variable(s) in the interaction. Thus, for example, the prior findings reported by Overall and Hollister (1966) were indicated by a medication by depression subtype

Table 7.   Effects Examined by Analyses of Covariance

Main effects

1. drug (D)
   imipramine
   placebo
   diazepam

2. psychotherapy (Rx)
   group therapy
   minimal contact

3. clinic (C)
   Phipps
   Gundry

Interaction effects

4. drug by psychotherapy (D by Rx)
5. drug by clinic (D by C)
6. psychotherapy by clinic (Rx by C)
7. drug by psychotherapy by clinic (D by Rx by C)

---

interaction. Thus, the effectiveness of tricyclic vs. tranquilizer medication was found to vary reliably as a function of the subtype of depression involved; tranquilizers were more effective with anxious depressions while antidepressants were more effective with retarded depressions.

Table 8 presents the outcome analyses after 16 weeks of treatment for that subgroup of patients who adhered to protocol (N = 146) and for the entire sample of patients who completed at least 2 weeks of active treatment (N = 207). The data at visit 19, week 16, were used as the variate for the "completers." An end-point score corresponding to the patient's score at the last valid treatment visit (i.e., before medication deviation, no-show, etc.) was used as the variate for the "end-point" analyses.

In order to determine the exact visit at which the patient's data was still valid, each study record was carefully reviewed, at least twice, by the study technicians and by the principal investigator (L. C.). The following information was used: the treating doctor's clinical notes; the technicians' reports regarding medication deviation (pill counts); missed visits; reasons for missed visits; reasons for treatment termination; etc. The principal investigator, blind to medication assignment, made the final classification of the last visit at which the patient had conformed to protocol requirements. It should be noted that this procedure was particularly important since many patients were continued in treatment (some were reassigned as "core-group" patients), and they continued to complete study forms exactly as did regular experimental study patients.

Table 8. *P* Values for Analysis of Covariance on Patient Self-Rated Outcome Measures (Week 19)

Criterion Measures	Completers Only[a]			End-Point Analysis[b]		
	Drug	D by C	Additional	Drug	D by C	Additional
SCL factors						
General sample						
Somatization	.05	.05		.05	.05	
Depression	.001	.001		.001	.01	
Anxiety	.05	n.s.		n.s.	n.s.	
Obsessive-Compulsiveness	.001	.05		.001	n.s.	
Interpersonal Sensitivity	.001	.05		.001	.05	
Depressed sample						
Depression	.001	.001		.001	.01	
Anxiety 1 (somatic)	.05	n.s.		.05	n.s.	D by Rx (.05)
Anxiety 2 (phobic)	.05	n.s.		n.s.	n.s.	
Hostility	.05	.05		.05	.05	
Sleep Disturbance	n.s.	n.s.	D by Rx (.05)	n.s.	n.s.	D by Rx (.01)
Modified POMS factors						
Depression	.001	.01		.001	.05	
Friendliness	.05	n.s.	D by Rx by C (.01)	.05	n.s.	
Anxiety	.001	.01		.001	.05	
Guilt	n.s.	n.s.		.05	n.s.	
Hostility	.001	.01		.001	.01	
Activity	.001	n.s.	C (.05)	.001	n.s.	
Fatigue	.001	.001		.001	.01	
Well-Being	.05	n.s.		.01	.05	
Cognitive	.01	n.s.	D by Rx (.05)	.05	n.s.	D by Rx (.05)
Carefree	.01	n.s.	C (.05)	.001	.05	
Patient global improvement	.01	n.s.				

[a] Number, 146.
[b] Number, 207.

Visit 3 scores were used as the covariate for these analyses. It should be noted that while the results of the analyses for the 146 patients completing the 16-week active treatment phase can only be generalized to patients who showed reasonable adherence to protocol requirements, the results of the end-point analyses can be generalized to the larger sample of patients who completed at least two weeks of active treatment.

The reliable main effects and interactions for these covariance analyses are given in Table 8. There were no reliable main effects for psychotherapy and only two for clinic setting. The only consistently reliable main effects were for medication.

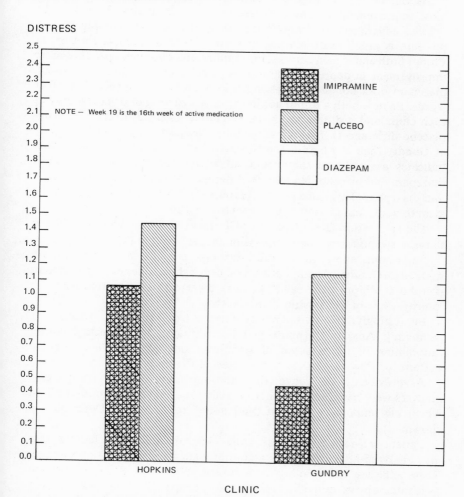

FIG. 4. **Adjusted mean distress levels, week 19, RMS Depression.**

As can be seen in Table 8, the outcome pattern is very similar for the "completing" and the end-point analyses. Both sets of data indicate a very strong and very consistent main drug effect in the presence of a somewhat weaker but consistent drug by clinic interaction. Figure 4 for mood Depression indicates visually the main drug effect and the drug by clinic interaction.

The closely cross-hatched, diagonally lined, and empty white bars represent, respectively, average distress levels for imipramine, placebo, and diazepam. Results are shown separately for each clinic.

As can be seen in Figure 4, imipramine is the drug which produces most improvement in mood depression at both clinics. However, the relative advantage for imipramine, as contrasted with diazepam and placebo, is much more marked at Gundry than at Phipps. Further, at Phipps both active medications, imipramine and diazepam, produce more improvement in depression than does placebo. At Gundry, by contrast, diazepam does not produce as much improvement as placebo. In other words, there is both a difference in the rank ordering of drug response at each clinic and a difference in the magnitude of drug effects (i.e., drug-placebo differences) from clinic to clinic. Drug effects are much stronger at Gundry than at Phipps. The Newman-Keuls range test (Winer, 1962) indicates a significant therapeutic advantage for imipramine vs. both diazepam and placebo. No reliable difference was found between placebo and diazepam. This same general pattern was found for almost all of the symptom and mood factors as presented in Table 9.

The Depression factor from the SCL shows an almost identical pattern to the corresponding mood Depression factor from the POMS (Figure 5).

Imipramine shows an overall advantage but one that is particularly marked at Gundry. Again, both active drugs show a better response than placebo at Phipps, whereas at Gundry diazepam is associated with less improvement in Depression than placebo.

Interestingly, the two Anxiety factors from the SCL (Anxiety 1 [Somatic]; Anxiety 2 [phobic]) reflected main drug effects favoring imipramine in the absence of significant interactions. This outcome pattern for Phobic Anxiety is displayed in Figure 6.

As previously mentioned, the end-point and 16-week "completers" analyses were remarkably similar. This can be seen visually in Figure 7, in which the outcome pattern at "end point" for symptom Depression is shown.

Patient self-ratings on these same symptom and mood factors were also analyzed after two weeks and after eight weeks of active treatment. These analyses, while failing to reveal any differential efficacy for group psychotherapy vs. individual brief psychotherapy, did reveal reliable main drug effects and the presence of drug by psychotherapy, drug by clinic, and drug by psychotherapy by clinic interactions.

Table 9. Summary of *P* Values for Newman-Keuls Multiple Range Tests of Patient (Completers Only) Self-Rated Outcome Measures (Week 19)

Criterion Measures	Imipramine vs. Placebo	Imipramine vs. Diazepam	Diazepam vs. Placebo
SCL factors			
General sample			
Depression	.01	.01	n.s.
Anxiety	.05	.10	n.s.
Obsessive-Compulsiveness	.01	.01	.10
Interpersonal Sensitivity	.01	.01	n.s.
Somatization	.05	.01	n.s.
Depressed sample			
Depression	.01	.01	n.s.
Anxiety 1 (somatic)	.05	.05	n.s.
Anxiety 2 (phobic)	.10	.05	n.s.
Hostility	.10	.05	n.s.
Modified POMS factors			
Depression	.01	.01	n.s.
Hostility	.01	.01	n.s.
Fatigue	.01	.01	n.s.
Friendliness	.05	.05	n.s.
Anxiety	.01	.01	n.s.
Activity	.01	.01	n.s.
Well-Being	.05	.05	n.s.
Cognitive	n.s.	.01	.10
Carefree	.01	.01	n.s.

Note: data were missing for 7 of the 149 patients who completed sixteen weeks of active treatment.

In general, Table 10 suggests that the antidepressant effects of medication are already present after two weeks and become stronger and more general by eight weeks. The drug by clinic interactions are similar in pattern to those observed after 16 weeks of treatment, while the drug by therapy interactions indicate that drug effects, favoring impramine, are stronger under minimal therapy than under group psychotherapy. Pairwise contrasts among medications for the 8-week period are given in Table 11. It is clear from this table that imipramine is more effective than placebo but strikingly more effective than diazepam, which is actually showing reliably less efficacy than placebo on symptom and mood depression, obsessive-compulsiveness, and mood fatigue at this time period.

In order to synthesize the results of the patient ratings, a multivariate analysis of covariance approach was employed in which week 3 scores were employed as the covariate and weeks 7, 11, 15, and 19 as the variate scores. The program used is called the Multivariate General Linear Model

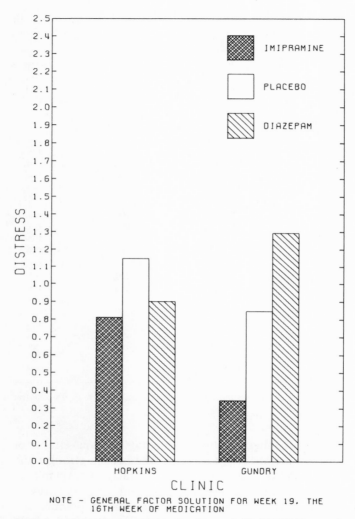

FIG. 5. Adjusted mean distress levels, week 19, HSCL Depression.

program as adopted from Anderson (1958) by Rawlings (personal communication). This program treats multiple time periods as other multivariate programs treat multiple variables. In essence, the program provides a single probability value for the main effects and for the interactions among variables over time. In this regard, however, the reader should keep in mind that drug effects generally became stronger over time.

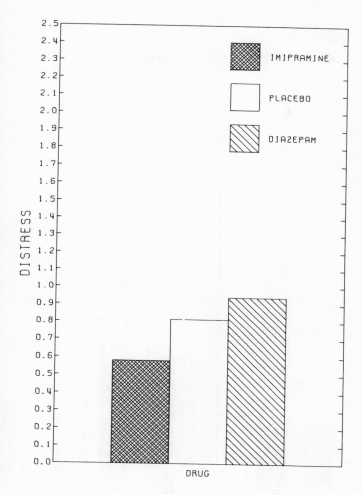

NOTE - SPECIAL FACTOR SOLUTION FOR WEEK 19. THE
16TH WEEK OF MEDICATION

FIG. 6. Adjusted mean distress levels, week 19, HSCL Anxiety 2 (Phobic).

An examination of Table 12 indicates, as anticipated, the presence of strong and fairly general main drug effects. No other main effects were found; i.e., no clinic differences or differences between group psychotherapy and individual supportive contact. Some interaction patterns, primarily between drug and clinic but also between drug and psychotherapy and between drug, clinic, and psychotherapy, were also identified. An examination of medication differences, as shown in Table 13, reveals an

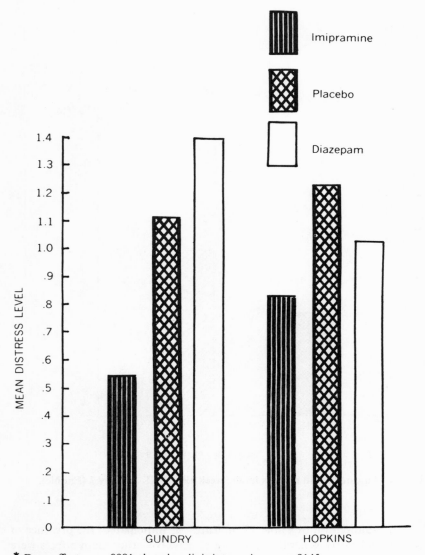

Main Drug Effect and Drug-by-Clinic Interaction for SCL Depression Factor at End Point*

* Drug effect: p < .0001: drug-by-clinic interaction: p < .0145.

FIG. 7. Adjusted mean distress levels, end point, DSCL Depression.

Table 10. *P* Values for Analysis of Covariance on Patient Self-Rated Outcome Measures

Criterion Measures	Completers Only,[a] Week 5		Completers Only,[b] Week 11		
	Drug	Additional	Drug	D by C	Additional
SCL factors					
General sample					
Somatization	n.s.	D by Rx (.05)	.01	n.s.	n.s.
Depression	.05	n.s.	.01	.05	D by Rx (.05)
Anxiety	n.s.	n.s.	.10	n.s.	D by Rx (.01)
Obsessive-Compulsiveness	.05	n.s.	.001	n.s.	n.s.
Interpersonal Sensitivity	.01	n.s.	.001	.05	D by C by Rx (.01)
Depressed sample					
Depression	.01	n.s.	.001	.01	n.s.
Anxiety 1 (somatic)	n.s.	D by Rx (.05)	n.s.	n.s.	D by Rx (.001)
Anxiety 2 (phobic)	n.s.	Rx by C (.05)	.05	n.s.	D by Rx (.02)
Hostility	.01	n.s.	n.s.	.01	n.s.
Sleep Disturbance	n.s.	D by Rx (.05)	n.s.	.05	D by Rx (.001)
Modified POMS factors					
Depression	.05	n.s.	.001	.05	n.s.
Friendliness	n.s.	Rx by C (.05)	n.s.	n.s.	D by C by Rx (.01)
Anxiety	n.s.	n.s.	.001	.05	D by Rx (.05)
Guilt	n.s.	C (.05)	n.s.	n.s.	n.s.
Hostility	.01	n.s.	.001	.001	n.s.
Activity	n.s.	n.s.	.01	n.s.	C (.05)
Fatigue	.001	n.s.	.001	.001	n.s.
Well-Being	n.s.	n.s.	.05	n.s.	D by C by Rx (.05)
Cognitive	n.s.	n.s.	n.s.	n.s.	n.s.
Carefree	n.s.	n.s.	.01	n.s.	n.s.

[a] Number, 146.
[b] Number, 142.

Table 11. Summary of P Values for Pair-Wise Contrasts among Medications on Patient Self-Rated Outcome Measures (Week 11)

Criterion Measures	Imipramine vs. Placebo	Imipramine vs. Diazepam	Diazepam vs. Placebo
SCL factors			
General sample			
Depression	.01	.001	.01
Interpersonal Sensitivity	.06	.001	n.s.
Obsessive-Compulsiveness	n.s.	.001	.02
Somatization	.05	.01	n.s.
Depressed sample			
Depression	.01	.001	.05
Anxiety 2 (phobic)	n.s.	.01	n.s.
Modified POMS factors			
Depression	.01	.001	.05
Hostility	.01	.001	n.s.
Anxiety	.01	.001	n.s.
Fatigue	.01	.001	.05
Activity	n.s.	.01	n.s.
Carefree	.05	.01	n.s.
Well-Being	.05	.01	n.s.

advantage for imipramine as compared with both placebo and diazepam. When the data for all time periods are examined by a multivariate synthesis, diazepam and placebo could not be reliably differentiated, although the pattern of p values clearly indicates that the relative rank ordering of medication is from imipramine to placebo to diazepam.

The typical medication by psychotherapy interaction is shown for Somatic Anxiety in Figure 8. As can be seen in this figure, drug effects are more apparent in minimal than in group therapy. In particular, the advantage for imipramine is much more marked in minimal than in group contact. Placebo patients, on the other hand, show more improvement in Somatic Anxiety under group psychotherapy than under individual brief supportive contact with the treating doctor.

The typical drug by clinic interaction pattern has already been illustrated earlier and, again, drug effects are much more pronounced at Gundry than at Phipps. A good example of the drug by clinic by psychotherapy interaction pattern can be seen in Figure 9 for the symptom factor of Interpersonal Sensitivity.

While imipramine always ranks as the most therapeutic medication, its therapeutic margin of superiority is most pronounced under minimal therapy at Gundry. It should be noted that the relative rank ordering of placebo and diazepam differs from Phipps to Gundry. At Gundry,

Table 12. Summary of *P* Values for Multivariate Analysis of Covariance on Patient Self-Rated Outcome Measures

Criterion Measures	Drug Effects	Additional Effects
SCL factors		
General sample		
Depression	.001	.05 D by C
Anxiety	n.s.	n.s.
Somatization	n.s.	.05 D by Rx by C
Obsessive-Compulsiveness	.01	n.s.
Interpersonal Sensitivity	.01	.05 D by Rx by C
Depressed sample		
Depression	.001	.01 D by C
Anxiety 1 (somatic)	n.s.	.05 D by Rx
Anxiety 2 (phobic)	.05	n.s.
Hostility	n.s.	.05 D by C
Sleep Disturbance	n.s.	.01 D by Rx
Modified POMS factors		
Depression	.001	.01 D by C
Anxiety	.005	.05 D by C
Well-Being	n.s.	n.s.
Friendliness	n.s.	.01 D by Rx by C
Cognitive	n.s.	n.s.
Activity	.01	n.s.
Guilt	n.s.	n.s.
Fatigue	.001	.001 D by C
Hostility	.001	.005 D by C
Carefree	.01	n.s.

Note: data were missing for 7 of the 149 patients who completed sixteen weeks of active treatment.

diazepam does worse than placebo, particularly under minimal contact. At Phipps, diazepam does better than placebo.

The last of the patient ratings to be presented here involves dimensions of interpersonal relationship that others have used to characterize the quality of the good therapist. In this context, however, these ratings represent the patient's rating of her husband or husband-equivalent. It was on these dimensions that we had particularly anticipated finding differences between group psychotherapy and minimal contact. The only significant effects, however, were for medication with imipramine producing the most positive change in the way the patient perceived her husband or husband-equivalent. This drug effect was particularly striking on the dimensions of Empathetic Understanding (see Table 14).

Doctor Ratings of Clinical Improvement. As with the patient self-rated improvement measures, doctor ratings were also analyzed for the main effects of psychotherapy, medication, clinic setting, and the interactions

Table 13. Summary of *P* Values for Pair-Wise Contrasts among Medications
on Patient Self-Rated Outcome Measures

Criterion Measures	Imipramine vs. Placebo	Imipramine vs. Diazepam	Diazepam vs. Placebo
SCL factors			
General sample			
Depression	.05	.001	n.s.
Obsessive-Compulsiveness	.10	.001	n.s.
Interpersonal Sensitivity	.10	.005	n.s.
Depressed sample			
Depression	.01	.001	n.s.
Anxiety 2 (phobic)	.05	.05	n.s.
Modified POMS factors			
Depression	.005	.001	n.s.
Anxiety	.01	.001	n.s.
Activity	.10	.005	n.s.
Fatigue	.01	.001	n.s.
Hostility	.05	.001	n.s.
Carefree	n.s.	.05	n.s.

Note: data were missing for 7 of the 149 patients who completed sixteen weeks of active
treatment.

among these variables. The outcome of these doctor ratings are presented
in Table 15.

As can be seen in the table, the most reliable effect on improvement is
that attributable to differences among the medications. We have not yet
analyzed doctor ratings for earlier time periods. When the main drug
effects at week 19 are analyzed more closely by the Newman-Keuls
multiple range test, the typical pattern is again seen, with imipramine
being more therapeutic than placebo and still more therapeutic than
diazepam.

The next three figures provide a visual display of the doctor ratings for
mood depression (main effect), mood hostility (main effect), and mood
anxiety (drug by psychotherapy interaction).

It is interesting to note that the drug by psychotherapy interaction
pattern seen in the doctor's rating of mood anxiety is quite similar to the
patients' interaction pattern seen for Somatic Anxiety (see Fig. 8).

Miscellaneous Analyses. In keeping with both doctor and patient global
improvement ratings, which showed reliable main drug effects favoring
imipramine, global improvement ratings by the patient's husband or
husband-equivalent (N = 102) also revealed a significant ($p < .05$) main

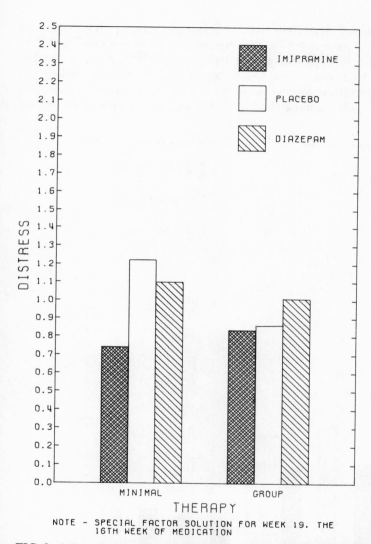

FIG. 8. Adjusted mean distress levels, week 19, Anxiety 1 (Somatic).

drug effect favoring imipramine. This week 19 rating failed to indicate any other reliable main effects or interactions, and again the relative rank ordering of the medications showed placebo to rank better than diazepam. An end-point analysis of covariance of the Brief Psychiatric Rating Scale ($N = 212$) data from the psychiatrists revealed a very reliable main drug effect ($p < .001$), with imipramine ranking best followed by placebo and diazepam. This analysis failed to reveal any interactions including the hypothesized patient profile type by medication interaction. It will be recalled that four patient profile types were identified for us by Dr. Overall: anxious depression; hostile depression; retarded depression; and agitated depression. At the outset of the study, it was postulated that diazepam would be most effective in the anxious subtype while imipra-

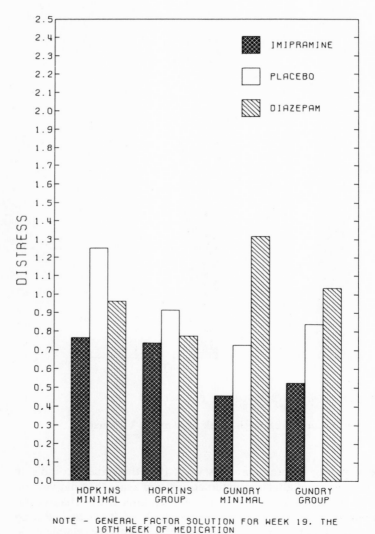

NOTE - GENERAL FACTOR SOLUTION FOR WEEK 19. THE 16TH WEEK OF MEDICATION

FIG. 9. Adjusted mean distress levels, week 19, HSCL Interpersonal Sensitivity.

Table 14. Summary of *P* Values for Covariance Analyses of Patient Ratings of Husband or Husband-Equivalent on Dimensions of the Barrett-Lennard Relationship Inventory

Criterion Measures	Drug Effects	Additional Effects
Level of Regard	.05	n.s.
Empathic Understanding	.005	n.s.
Unconditionality of Regard	.05	n.s.
Congruence	n.s.	n.s.
Total score	.05	n.s.

Note: data for 47 of the 149 patients who completed sixteen weeks of active treatment were not included in these analyses because they were not involved with a "significant" other (husband or husband-equivalent).

mine would be most effective in the retarded subtype of depression. This interaction pattern was not even remotely indicated by the analysis, using total BPRS scores as the dependent measure of change. It was also not found in a week 19 step-search multiple regression analysis (Uhlenhuth, Duncan, & Park, 1969) in which the Depression factor of the HSCL and the Depression factor of the POMS were used as the dependent variables. While it is beyond the focus of this publication to present the detailed results of these predictor analyses, it should be noted that a strong main

Table 15. Summary of *P* Values for Doctor Ratings of Patient Mood, Depression, Anxiety, and Global Improvement (Week 19)

Criterion Measures	Drug Effects	Additional Effects
Mood factors		
Depression	.05	n.s.
Hostility	.01	n.s.
Guilt	n.s.	n.s.
Anxiety	.05	.05 D by Rx
Carefree	n.s.	n.s.
Fatigue	.01	.05 C
Cognitive	.05	n.s.
Friendliness	.05	n.s.
Raskin (depression)	.05	n.s.
Covi (anxiety)	n.s.	n.s.
Global improvement	.05	n.s.

Note: 6 doctor ratings are missing (of a total of 149). Covariance analyses were done for all variables but global improvement (variance analysis).

Table 16. Summary of P Values for Newman-Keuls Multiple Range Tests of
Doctor Ratings of Patient Improvement (Week 19)

Criterion Measures	Imipramine vs. Placebo	Imipramine vs. Diazepam	Diazepam vs. Placebo
Mood factors			
Depression	.05	.05	n.s.
Hostility	n.s.	.01	n.s.
Anxiety	n.s.	.05	n.s.
Fatigue	.01	.01	n.s.
Cognitive	.05	.01	n.s.
Friendliness	n.s.	.05	n.s.
Raskin (depression)	.10	.05	n.s.
Global improvement	.05	.05	n.s.

Note: 6 doctor ratings are missing (of a total of 149).

drug effect and two interactive predictors were identified; i.e., clinic by medication and social class by medication. This later interaction emerged only when the clinic variable was not included in the predictor pool. Other variables which were examined but not found related to outcome either generally or in combination with medication were age, anxiety, attitude toward medication, length of illness, previous episodes, presence of precipitants, and prior medication classifications. In all predictor analyses, a highly reliable main drug effect ($p < .005$) favoring imipramine was present.

Of the 149 patients who completed the active medication phase of the study, 31 patients (per protocol) were not considered sufficiently improved to be assigned to the long-term maintenance phase in which placebo and no-pill groups were involved. These 31 patients were not randomly distributed as a function of treatment assignment ($\chi^2 = 10.80$, df $= 5$, $.10 > p > .05$). This disproportionality mainly reflects medication differences in which 11.3 percent of the imipramine group were not assigned to maintenance as contrasted with 21.7 percent of the placebo and 27.3 percent of the diazepam group ($\chi^2 = 3.11$, $.10 > p > .05$ for imipramine vs. combined diazepam and placebo).

Data from the maintenance phase of this study have not been fully analyzed. With this qualification, 43 imipramine patients entered maintenance; 24 were assigned to imipramine and 19 to imipramine-placebo. Only 20 of these 43 patients completed the full 11 months on the maintenance dosage regimen. Neither the number of dropouts nor the rate of dropping out of treatment during maintenance was different as a function of imipramine vs. imipramine-placebo. However, patient global improvement ratings did show a reliable ($t = 2.30, p < .05$) advantage for the 12 imipramine patients completing treatment as contrasted with the 8 imipramine-placebo patients completing treatment. This same trend held

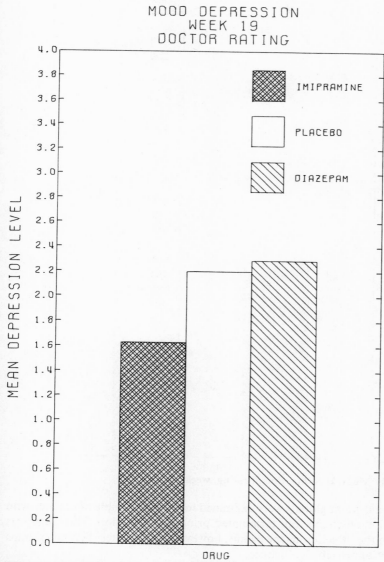

FIG. 10. Mood Depression, doctor rating, week 19.

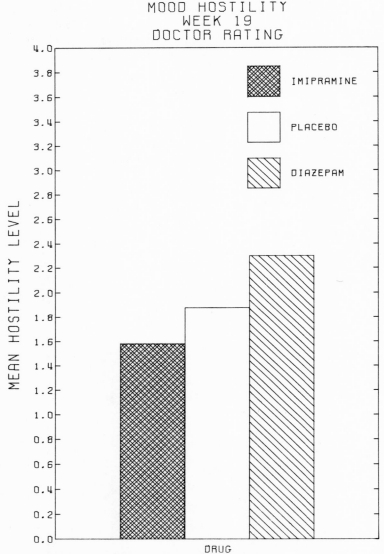

FIG. 11. Mood Hostility, doctor rating, week 19.

when end-point globals were examined for the full sample of patients who started maintenance but terminated prior to completion. This trend was only in the direction of the means, however, and the *t* test between groups did not approach significance.

Further analyses are obviously required, and the maintenance results reported here should be considered tentative.

DISCUSSION

The results of the present study provide consistent and dramatic support for the efficacy of the tricyclic imipramine in the treatment of non-psychotic depressed female outpatients. This therapeutic superiority for

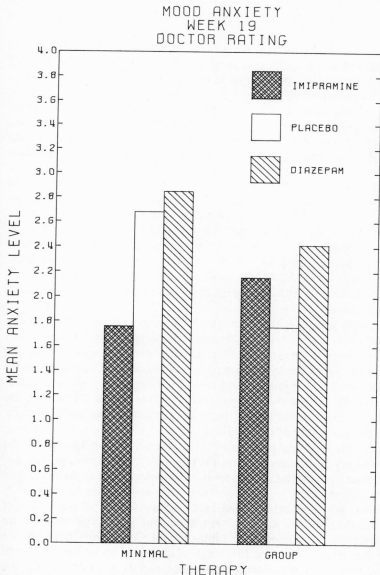

FIG. 12. Mood Anxiety, doctor rating, week 19.

imipramine with respect to placebo and particularly with respect to diazepam is seen in patient self-ratings, physician ratings, and ratings by the husband or husband-equivalent. It is seen in specific ratings of mood and symptom dimensions as well as in global judgments by the different raters. The magnitude of this effect is perhaps more impressive than the tabled p values would suggest since these were limited to three figures (e.g., .001) when in actuality many of these p values were of the order of .00003.

Estimates of the percentage of the variance in the reduction of symptom and mood depression attributable to medication range from 9.5 to 10.5 percent. This percentage is of the order of two to three times higher than comparable percentages reported by Raskin, Schulterbrandt, Boothe, Reatig, and McKeon (1970) for an inpatient depression study contrasting chlorpromazine, imipramine, and placebo. Viewed another way, mean pre-treatment depression symptom levels were roughly four standard deviations higher than the mean of a normative population (Uhlenhuth, Balter, Lipman, and Stern, 1972). After treatment, imipramine patients, on average, were only 1.5 S.D.s above the normative mean, while placebo patients were 3 S.D.s above the mean and diazepam patients were about 3.75 S.D.s above the mean. Sixty-nine percent of imipramine-treated patients reported themselves as very much better or quite a bit better after 16 weeks of medication, as contrasted with 40 percent of placebo patients and 36 percent of diazepam patients. Conversely, only 6 percent of imipramine patients reported themselves as worse, as compared with 12 percent of placebo patients and 20 percent of diazepam patients.

We would speculate that a number of factors may be responsible for the sensitivity of this trial: restriction of the sample to white women within the narrow age range of 20 to 50 years; use of a two-week placebo washout coupled with the requirement that patients maintain at least a moderate level of depression; and employing the same treating psychiatrists at both clinics and across both types of psychotherapy. These procedures, while undoubtedly reducing variance from many sources, restrict the generality of our findings.

We do not view our findings as being relevant to the question of the efficacy of psychotherapy. Our results may indicate that minimal supportive contact and individual group psychotherapy plus some individual physician contact are equally effective or, on the other hand, equally ineffective. While placebo served as an adequate control condition for active medication, we did not have a control group that received no psychotherapy. As Uhlenhuth, Lipman, and Covi (1969) indicate, the proper design to answer the full range of questions about the efficacy of psychotherapy and pharmacotherapy alone and in combination requires a group which receives psychotherapy alone, a group which receives pharmacotherapy alone, and a group which receives both together, and a group which receives none of these therapies. We did not have this type of design. It has also been pointed out by Luborsky, Singer, and Luborsky (in this volume) that psychotherapy effects typically take longer to be observed than do the effects of psychotropic drugs. In this regard, the maintenance depression study by Klerman et al. (1974) did not reveal any advantage for high social worker contact until the eight-month evaluation period. Strong drug effects favoring amitriptyline were seen much earlier. It might also be argued that our major dependent measures were not as appropriate for detecting differential psychotherapy effects as they were for detecting differential drug effects. Along these lines, the marital therapy study by Friedman (1972) suggested that antidepressant drug effects were readily apparent on symptoms and mood while psychotherapy differences were mainly observed on a few measures of social adjustment. In this regard, our measures of interpersonal perception, derived from the Barrett-Lennard Relationship Inventory, were probably the most relevant for the psychotherapy comparison. We were somewhat surprised not to find a differential effect favoring group psychotherapy on such measures as Empathetic Understanding and Level of Regard, and subsequent findings do show a differential effect.[2] The imipramine effect on these measures was not unanticipated because in early trials with anxious patients we found differential drug effects related to improved interpersonal perceptions (Lipman, Hammer, Bernades, & Park, 1965). Finally, we should comment that a more stable group composition might have provided a more therapeutic milieu than obtained in the present study, in which the frequent shifts in group membership were considered detrimental by many patients and by the treating psychiatrists.

Before closing, it should be mentioned that one of the more recent trends in the literature relevant to the pharmacotherapy of depression has been an increasing questioning of the general therapeutic superiority of the tricyclic antidepressants for the treatment of depressive disorders. In this regard, both the major and minor tranquilizers have been suggested as alternative treatments for depression, with a growing consensus that these classes of psychotropic drugs might be particularly effective for depressive disorders characterized by the presence of co-existing anxiety. Clearly, the data from the present study do not support this view. The drug effects, favoring imipramine over the four-month active medication phase, and the suggestive data from the twelve-month maintenance medication phase argue for the general superiority of the tricyclic antidepressants. Moreover, we could find no evidence to suggest any subgroup of patients for whom diazepam would be the drug of choice. This holds with regard to the Overall-Hollister subtypes of depression, to different configurations of symptom anxiety and depression as tested by our regression analyses, and to the observed interactions of medication with clinic, with psychotherapy, and with social class. In this regard, imipramine was always observed to be the most therapeutic drug although its therapeutic margin was most pronounced in the more socially advantaged, under minimal contact, and at Gundry Hospital. In the lower social class patient, drug effects were generally less apparent, a finding in agreement with the work of Downing and Rickels (1972). In the less socially advantaged, diazepam, although not as effective as imipramine, produced somewhat more benefit than did placebo on symptom depression. In the more middle class patient, diazepam was not as effective as placebo. It should be stressed, of course, that our present findings can only be generalized to comparable treatment situations and to comparable samples of non-psychotic depressed white women. It might be argued that our diazepam dosage was too low. This possibility must be seriously considered, although our diazepam dosage was sufficiently high to produce reliably more drowsiness than the other study medications, and study doctors did have the option of prescribing 20 mg/d of diazepam rather than the lower modal dose of 15 mg/d of diazepam. These findings argue against the therapeutic mechanism of action of thymoleptics being mediated by sedation.

It should also be stressed that the distribution of the Overall subtypes of depression in our outpatient sample contained only 5 or 6 percent of retarded depressions and therefore did not provide a real opportunity for replicating his inpatient findings.

NOTES

1. We wish to thank Dr. John Overall for performing the BPRS analyses for us.

2. Since the writing of this paper, a more refined analysis of these data, employing a somewhat larger sample of patients (N = 127), revealed a reliable main effect favoring group psychotherapy on the dimension of Empathetic Understanding ($p = .05$) and a trend ($p = .07$) on Congruence and the total score ($p = .06$) of the Barrett-Lennard Relationship Inventory. Patients receiving 16 weeks of group psychotherapy perceived their husband or husband-equivalent more positively than did patients receiving minimal physician contact. A reexamination of all analyses also revealed an error in not recording a main effect favoring group psychotherapy for the end-point analysis on the Hostility factor of the SCL ($p = .03$; Table 8) and the Anxiety factor of the POMS ($p = .02$; Table 8). Thus, these results do provide some support for the differential efficacy of group psychotherapy. These psychotherapy effects are, however, not as general nor as strong as the observed drug effects, and they do not occur as early in the treatment process.

REFERENCES

Anderson, T. W. *An introduction to multivariate statistical analyses.* New York: John Wiley and Sons, 1958.

Barrett-Lennard, G. T. Dimensions of therapist response as causal factors in therapeutic change. *Psychological Monographs*, 1962, **76**(43, Whole No. 562).

Bednar, R. L., & Lawlis, G. G. Empirical research in group psychotherapy. In A. E. Bergin & S. L. Garfield (Eds.), *Handbook of psychotherapy and behavior change.* New York: John Wiley and Sons, 1971, pp. 812–829.

Daneman, E. A. Imipramine in office management of depressive reactions (a double-blind study). *Diseases of the Nervous System*, 1961, **22**, 213–217.

Derogatis, L. R., Lipman, R. S., Rickels, K., Uhlenhuth, E. H., & Covi, L. The Hopkins Symptom Checklist (HSCL): a self-report symptom inventory. *Behavioral Science*, 1974, **19**, 1–15.

Downing, R. W., & Rickels, K. Predictors of amitriptyline response in outpatient depressions. *Journal of Nervous and Mental Disease*, 1972, **152**, 248–263.

Fiske, D. W., Hunt, H. G., Luborsky, L., Orne, M. T., Parloff, M. B., Reiser, M. F., & Tuma, A. H. Planning of research on effectiveness of psychotherapy. *Archives of General Psychiatry*, 1970, **22**, 22–32.

Frank, J. D., Gliedman, L. H., Imber, S. D., Nash, E. H., & Stone, A. Why patients leave psychotherapy. *Archives of Neurology and Psychiatry*, 1957, **77**, 283–299.

Friedman, A. S. The interactive effects of drug therapy and marital therapy with outpatient depressives. Paper presented at the annual meeting of the American College of Neuropsychopharmacology, San Juan, Puerto Rico, 1972.

Hare, E. H., McCance, C., & McCormick, W. O. Imipramine and "drinamyl" in depressive illness. *British Medical Journal*, 1964, **1**, 818.

Hollister, L. E., Overall, J. E., Shelton, J., Pennington, V., Kimbell, I., & Johnson, M. Drug therapy of depression: amitriptyline, perphenazine, and their combination in different syndromes. *Archives of General Psychiatry*, 1967, **17**, 486–493.

Klerman, G. L., DiMascio, A., Weissman, M., Prusoff, B., & Paykel, E. A. Treatment of depression by drugs and psychotherapy. *American Journal of Psychiatry*, 1974, **131**, 186–191.

Lipman, R. S., Hammer, H. M., Bernades, J. F., & Park, L. C. Patient report of significant life situation events. *Diseases of the Nervous System*, 1965, **26**, 586–590.

Lipman, R. S., Rickels, K., Covi, L., Derogatis, L. R., & Uhlenhuth, E. H. Dimensions of symptom distress in doctor ratings of anxious neurotic outpatients. *Archives of General Psychiatry*, 1969, **21**, 328–338.

McNair, D. M., & Lorr, M. An analysis of mood in neurotics. *Journal of Abnormal and Social Psychology*, 1964, **69**, 620–627.

Meltzoff, J., & Kornreich, M. *Research in psychotherapy.* New York: Atherton Press, 1970.

Overall, J. R., Hollister, L. E., Johnson, M., & Pennington, V. Nosology of depression and differential response to drugs. *Journal of the American Medical Association*, 1966, **195**, 946–948.

Parloff, M. B., Kelman, H. C., & Frank, J. D. Comfort, effectiveness, and self-awareness as criteria of improvement in psychotherapy. *American Journal of Psychiatry*, 1954, **111**, 343–351.

Raskin, A., Schulterbrandt, J. G., Boothe, H., Reatig, N., & McKeon, J. J. Treatment, social and psychiatric history variables related to symptom reduction in hospitalized depressions. In J. R. Wittenborn, S. C. Goldberg, & P.R.A. May (Eds.), *Psychopharmacology and the individual patient.* New York: Raven Press, 1970, pp. 135–159.

Rickels, K., Chung, H. R., Feldman, H. S., Gordon, P. E., Kelly, E. A., & Weise, C. C. Amitriptyline, diazepam, and phenobarbital sodium in depressed outpatients. *Journal of Nervous and Mental Disease*, 1973, **157**, 442–451.

Rickels, K., Raab, E., De Silverio, R., & Eternad, B. Drug treatment in depression: antidepressant or tranquilizer? *Journal of the American Medical Association*, 1967, **201**, 675–681.

Uhlenhuth, E. H., Balter, M. B., Lipman, R. S., & Stern, J. The demography of life stress. Paper presented at the eleventh annual meeting of the American College of Neuropsychopharmacology, 1972.

Uhlenhuth, E. H., Duncan, D. B., & Park, L. C. Some non-pharmacologic modifiers of the response to imipramine in depressed psychoneurotic outpatients: A confirmatory study.

In P. R. A. May & J. R. Wittenborn, (Eds.),*Psychotropic drug response: advances in prediction*. Springfield, Ill.: Charles C Thomas, 1969, pp. 155–197.

Uhlenhuth, E. H., Lipman, R. S., & Covi, L. Combined pharmacotherapy and psychotherapy. *Journal of Nervous and Mental Disease*, 1969, **148**, 52–64.

Wheatley, D. A comparative trial of imipramine and phenobarbital in depressed patients seen in general practice. *Journal of Nervous and Mental Disease*, 1969, **148**, 542–549.

Winer, B. J. *Statistical principles in experimental design*. New York: McGraw-Hill, 1962.

15

DISCUSSION:
Do Psychotherapeutic Interventions Really Influence the Drug Treatment of Depression?

SEYMOUR FISHER

The two preceding papers, each of which offers strong convergent support for the therapeutic usefulness of antidepressant drugs, have also sought to find evidence indicating that some form of psychotherapy (in its broadest sense), when added to a drug regimen, yields a better clinical response than simply the drug regimen with minimal interpersonal contact. In regard to this latter quest, perhaps the fairest conclusion to draw at present is that the proper role of "psycho-therapies" as adjuncts to chemotherapy remains highly uncertain.

In vivid contrast to the unequivocally clear therapeutic effects of the antidepressant drugs, the results of the psychotherapeutic interventions are much more ambiguous, inconsistent, and bewildering.

The Lipman and Covi paper reports generally similar outcomes for patients who received only minimal supportive contact and for those who received considerably more elaborate group therapy plus minimal supportive contact; they do note, however, a few scattered instances where group psychotherapy shows up as a main therapeutic effect or as interacting with the antidepressant medication. It is worth noting that their strongest results, dealing with drug effects, were the same regardless of whether patients completed sixteen weeks, or eight weeks, or only two weeks of treatment; the fragmentary psychotherapy effects, on the other hand, vary depending upon whether the results were based upon endpoint analyses or upon only those patients who actually completed a given period of treatment.

In the Weissman, Klerman, Prusoff, Hanson, and Paykel paper, evidence is adduced suggesting that although psychotherapy may have no effect on direct clinical criteria, certain measures of social adjustment are

Seymour Fisher, Ph.D., Professor of Psychiatry and Director, Psychopharmacology Laboratory, Division of Psychiatry, Boston University School of Medicine.

favorably influenced. The authors further argue that these psychotherapy effects are "latent" in the sense that they do not emerge until six to eight months after the initiation of maintenance treatment—a conclusion which derives from the fact that significant effects were seen only in the specially restricted group of patients who remained in the study for the entire eight months of treatment (survivors).

The confusing pattern of alleged psychotherapeutic effects can best be highlighted by the following thumbnail summaries.

Lipman and Covi do not find depressed mood or direct symptoms of depression being relieved by psychotherapy, although hostility and anxiety appear to be reduced in four months or less. Weissman et al. report their effects to be limited to certain measures of social adjustment, seen only after six to eight months.

Lipman and Covi find that, for symptomatic distress, the antidepressant drug effect is greater in magnitude for patients who do *not* receive group therapy;[1] Weissman et al. report finding no interactions between medication and psychotherapy.

Lipman and Covi find their psychotherapy effects on symptoms and mood only in end-point analyses; Weissman et al. find their effects only using survivors.

Since these two studies are concerned with the discrepancies seen between statistical analyses based upon survivors (at the end of treatment) and those based upon total patient sample, this immediately raises the familiar issue of how attrition can influence the interpretation of results. Although the Weissman et al. paper touches upon this crucial question, a few additional comments may be in order.

DROPOUTS AND SURVIVOR ANALYSES

There are several possible approaches to the problem of attempting to draw inferences about the effects of randomly assigned or matched treatments when the sample which survives at the end of an experiment is only a subset of the original sample. When an investigator analyzes the data from a moderately lengthy clinical trial, his primary fear is that the group comparisons made at the end of the trial may reveal something other than the effects of the treatments in which he is interested. A number of different statistical analyses are first generally undertaken to answer some basic questions. Using only the final survivors sample, are the results at the end of the trial the same as, for instance, those at two weeks? Were the different treatment groups within the survivor sample comparable prior to the beginning of treatment? Using all subjects available, are the results at two weeks the same as the two-week outcome from the survivor subsample? If for every dropout a "termination" score is estimated (i.e., "end-point analyses"), are the results for the complete original sample the same as for the different subsamples?

When the answer to each of these four questions is in the affirmative, the investigator breathes a sigh of relief and considers himself fortunate. He is probably getting a reasonably accurate picture of the true effects of treatments which are constant over time. However, when different analyses yield different outcomes, it may be extremely difficult to discern the true meaning of the trial.

While these considerations hold for any questions regarding a treatment effect at any point in time after some subjects have been lost, the problem becomes even more complex when the interpretation concerns the *emergence* of a treatment effect after some delayed period of time. The task of correctly identifying a "delayed" treatment effect is a particularly difficult one in any clinical trial, when a substantial number of dropouts is inevitable. Obviously, if the initial random (or matched) assignment of patients to treatment and control groups remains intact over the full treatment period, then a delayed treatment effect would be evident whenever its magnitude at a later time period is significantly greater than its magnitude at some earlier period.[2]

As soon as the reality of dropouts is recognized, however, the focus of the problem shifts to consideration of *other* possible meanings of different effects at different time periods. These other meanings can only be revealed by a fine analysis of the different groups of "surviving" patients compared to dropouts.

Effects which appear only in a survivor analysis (e.g., Weissman et al.) are quite consistent with a delayed-treatment hypothesis, since the survivors represent the purist group of homogeneously treated patients. However, an end-point analysis, while increasing the total number in the sample, does this by including patients who have not received the same experimental treatment as the survivors. In fact, when an end-point analysis indicates treatment effects which do *not* also appear in a survivor analysis (e.g., Lipman and Covi, p. 216, n. 2), this would seem to be inconsistent with any delayed-effect hypothesis: if four months of psychotherapy are required before effects are to be seen, then it is difficult to understand how the inclusion of patients who have received only one or two months of psychotherapy before dropping out can possibly clarify the picture.

On the other hand, an analysis based primarily upon a comparison of survivor subsamples can easily be misleading. "Survivor analysis" is tantamount to endorsement of an experimental design calling for infinite replacement of dropouts, a procedure which is rarely, if ever, advocated these days: the longer the duration of a clinical trial, the more likely that progressive deterioration of the original randomization or matching will occur, so that groups which are labeled as different "treatment" samples become systematically more and more different with respect to other factors as well. Thus, whenever a set of data seems to indicate a delayed treatment effect, it is the investigator's responsibility first to rule out the simpler hypothesis that differential attrition over time has resulted in a confounded comparison in which *different patient types* rather than different experimental treatments are responsible for the results.

If significant pretreatment differences on any variables are discovered between different subgroups of survivors,[3] this indirectly suggests that the experimental treatments have become confounded with patient types, and no number of covariance adjustments can perform the statistical wonders which are so often ingenuously expected of them.[4] While the absence of any significant differences on a large number of pretreatment scores would strengthen one's confidence that the surviving treatment subgroups remain unbiased, selective attrition on some unmeasured variables is still a distinct possibility.

A preferable solution (supplemental, not substitutive, to the above) is to seek information which will permit the planning of a better study to detect delayed treatment effects. If the hypothesis states that psychotherapy must be given for eight months before it begins to show an effect, then a first obvious requirement is to aim for a sample which will, as much as possible, be expected to survive eight months of treatment. Therefore, it becomes necessary to predict prior to the actual experiment which patients might be expected *not* to remain in treatment for the hypothesized time period and to exclude these patients from the trial.

True, this solution is considerably easier to suggest than to carry out. It does, however, imply that a clinical trial designed to detect real emergent treatment effects requires even more rigor and advance knowledge than a garden-variety trial which tests for an approximately constant treatment effect: attrition, which always increases with length of trial, must be kept to an absolute minimum. It is doubtful whether a study which anticipates a 40 to 60 percent attrition rate is capable of providing clear and persuasive answers to complex questions about delayed treatment effects.

When it is cautioned that, via selective attrition, a group of psychotherapy survivors might be composed of patients who are systematically different from a group of control patient survivors, it should be realized that the causes of these differences probably stem from treatment-related factors. As a hypothetical example, suppose that eventually only women remained in a psychotherapy group, while all women in the control group gradually sought treatment elsewhere. The final analysis of survivors would hopelessly confound treatment and sex. If sex had not been recorded, and if women could be expected to improve spontaneously more than men, any final differences on a clinical measure between the psychotherapy and control survivor groups might not be due to the psychotherapy, but simply to sex differences—of which we would be totally unaware. It would have been the different treatments that led to the survival of the different patient types, but in the process what became obscured would have been the differential effectiveness of the treatments per se on the clinical measures we are interested in.

PSYCHOTHERAPY "VERSUS" MEDICATION

One further implication of this problem: if different kinds of patients selectively refused to participate in certain long-term treatments, then the possibility must be considered that the wrong question is being raised when we try to compare the relative efficacy of drugs and psychotherapy on a hypothetically homogeneous population. The two preceding papers report on studies which utilized factorial designs, with "medication" as one independent variable and "psychotherapy" as the other. When such factorial designs are used in long-term clinical trials, it might be judicious to view this approach not as the definitive design for examining the separate contributions of drugs and psychotherapy but merely as a starting point in a search for specific patient types suitable for different treatments. For example, not only are investigators and therapists frequently polarized in their attitudes about medication versus psychotherapy but many patients are as well. It does not seem overly unreasonable to suspect that, in some important ways, patients who remain for an extended duration under one kind of regimen may be quite different from those who drop out, and that therefore certain treatment modalities may be intrinsically incapable of comparison within the *same* patient population. If one type of addict refuses to stay in a self-help therapeutic community but will stick with a methadone regimen, then we can best examine methadone's long-term efficacy only in this latter type of population, while the efficacy of the therapeutic community should be evaluated in its own respective population. To attempt to ask whether methadone is "better than" self-help, when different populations are involved, may in the long run turn out to make little sense (unless the assumption is made that patients can be *forced* to remain in certain treatments, in which case it would not be surprising to find that they do not fare very well therapeutically when assigned to an undesired treatment). It may be necessary to ask two separate questions, sequentially considered: (1) what kinds of patients and how many of them will accept (i.e., stick with) a particular treatment modality of specified duration, and (2) for those patients who will accept a generic treatment approach, are some variations more effective than others?

Where does all this leave us, then? It is clear that both of the preceding papers told important stories. Obviously, they differ from each other in so many relevant respects as to make any direct comparison meaningless.

Yet both studies strongly agree in documenting the clinical efficacy of appropriate medication. The "medication believers" will surely obtain much comfort from the impressive antidepressant drug effects reported in these two studies. The "psychotherapy believers" will have to hang in there a while longer to see whether the provocative suggestions from the Weissman et al. study are real or illusory.

NOTES

1. Examination of their Figures 8 and 12 shows this interaction to result from the plausible suggestion that group therapy patients on placebo are indeed improving more than minimal contact placebo patients.

2. Strictly speaking, it is not sufficient to find a nonsignificant treatment effect at the early period and a significant effect later on; a significant treatment-by-time interaction for the same patients is required to support the desired inference.

3. A more sensitive indicator of whether attrition has interfered with the randomization is obtained from the test of *interaction* between survivor status and treatment assignment, a test which quite properly uses *all* subjects in the original sample. Most investigators routinely will look to see if treated and control groups differ within the survivors or within the attritors, and most investigators will make an overall comparison of survivors vs. attritors. The only appropriate test, however, is the simultaneous comparison of survivors and attritors, each stratified by treatment.

4. It has become such common practice now to "adjust" final scores with a pretreatment covariate (usually at least the initial level of the measured variable) that there is a tendency to forget the only valid reason for this adjustment: to increase the sensitivity of the significance tests by reducing the error term and controlling for random, not real, differences between sample means on the covariate.

GENERAL DISCUSSION: I

DR. DONALD KLEIN:* One of the problems in such data analysis is the issue of the difference between clinical significance and statistical significance. When the data is presented in the form of a change in scale scores and statistical significance of that change, it becomes quite difficult to know whether the researchers are talking about a substantial change of the sort that we would be happy with or a statistically significant change that will be of no marked clinical importance.

Let me give an example. In reading your work, it seemed to me that on medication 12 percent relapsed and on placebo 33 percent relapsed. Is that about right?

DR. WEISSMAN: Yes.

DR. KLEIN: That would mean that the actual drug prophylactic effect was only relevant for 20 percent of the people treated, since the difference between placebo relapse and drug relapse was about 20 percent.

If you then prescribe drug prophylaxis for everybody who has had a depression for an eight- or nine-month prophylactic trial, you would be treating four out of five people unnecessarily.

DR. WEISSMAN: Right.

DR. KLEIN: So that certainly fits in very closely with concerns about cost-benefit ratios. We need better predictors of who is actually at risk for relapse. The same argument applies to the psychotherapy issue. If I remember your data correctly, roughly 44 percent of your psychotherapy-treated people show what you consider to be substantial social gains, but in the neighborhood of 25 percent of your minimum contact people show substantial social gains.

DR. GERALD L. KLERMAN:† As one of the coinvestigators, I'd like to respond. I think Dr. Klein's point about the relative benefit of the treatments is very pertinent. Benefit depends on how you look at the results. If you look at these findings from the clinical psychiatric point of view, then the issue of relative benefit and cost is obviously cogent and relevant. You can say, as Dr. Klein does, that the difference between the relapse rate in the "no treatment group" (36 percent) and that in the "treatment group" (13 percent) is only 20 percent and that, therefore, only about one-fifth of the patients benefit. On the other hand, if you look at

*Long Island Jewish-Hillside Medical Center.
†Harvard Medical School.

the relative or proportional reduction in relapse, maintenance therapy reduces the probability of relapse by at least one-half.

As we pointed out in our article in the *American Journal of Psychiatry*,[1] we compared the findings from our study with two other similar studies using similar designs (the British M.R.C. study and the V.A.-N.I.M.H. study). All three studies show that the relapse rate of patients on maintenance tricyclic was cut to at least 50 percent, and perhaps to even one-third of the control group. These studies taken together indicate that there is at least a one-half reduction in the probability of relapse.

Moreover, there is a gradient of response depending on the patient's clinical state. For the group of patients we studied, who are relatively non-bipolar, non-unipolar, neurotic depressions, it could be that time alone may be all that is necessary for most patients given the relative mildness of their illness when compared to the severity of illness of patients in the other samples in the literature. That requires a decision that the clinician and the patient should be prepared to make. But there is now data which can allow the clinician to weigh the relative probabilities of no treatment versus drug treatment.

DR. WEISSMAN: We are in the process of doing a predictor analysis which will examine who benefits most from psychotherapy. This is complicated in a study with many outcomes and predictors, but we will have statistical data on that shortly.

Now, we have done one analysis so far which partially answers your question, and we do have a clinical impression. All patients when they come for treatment for the acute episode do not have social and interpersonal problems. There are some who come because they are depressed and we and they don't know what, if anything, may have precipitated it.

These patients who don't have the salient problems helped by psychotherapy, namely, problems in social adjustment, probably don't need psychotherapy other than a brief rehabilitation period where they might receive help in overcoming the consequences of the illness. On the other hand, patients who have social and interpersonal difficulties could be the candidates for psychotherapy. You would expect the maximum benefit in this group because they have the maximum disorder, and our analysis showed that, as expected.

DR. FRITZ A. FREYHAN:* I have several questions. The study just presented is very impressive because of what appears to be a very precise research design. If, on the other hand, you look into some of the specifics, problems arise. I did not understand, for example, how the diagnosis of depressive neuroses was made. It is quite conceivable that the patient

*Editor-in-Chief, *Comprehensive Psychiatry*.

material included other depressive disorders. If this happens to be the case, it would make a substantial difference regarding the patients' response patterns to drug treatment and psychotherapy.

Another question concerns the choice of the drug. I do not understand why amitriptyline was regarded as the optimal drug for all patients. Amitriptyline is usually the drug of choice for those depressed patients who show prominent symptoms of anxiety and agitation. The drug's sedative effect may well be contraindicated in outpatients who are expected to make a social and occupational adaptation. Thus, while this drug may be beneficial during the initial stage of depression, it loses this advantage when the patient is expected to perform again.

I also have misgivings about comparing the effect of this particular drug to the other mode of treatment designated as psychotherapy. Insofar as psychotherapy is concerned, we need to know what strategies are employed and what the objectives are. The quality and success of the therapy may not depend on "low or high contact" but on the skill of the therapist in identifying treatable psychological problems. In the case of depressive disorders, it is often exceedingly difficult for the therapists, especially non-psychiatric therapists, to distinguish between primary and secondary problems. Moreover, if the depressive phases are cyclic, the patient may get better or worse due to endogenous factors unrelated to treatment.

I could raise additional questions. My main concern is that the study, even though well conceived in principle, cannot really compare the relative merits of complex treatment modalities. I admire the intent and energy which went into the study. I only doubt that the results are as specific as the data seem to imply.

DR. KLERMAN: I think Dr. Freyhan raises relevant issues, but I think we have dealt with all of them in the design and execution of the study.

First of all, in the study of depression we are hard-pressed to find any studies that show any psychotherapy effect, even as modest an effect as occurred in the study that Ms. Weissman reports.

Now as regards the issue of psychopathology, this too is very relevant. We purposely were not looking for patients with classic manic-depressive bipolar illness, nor for a sample of patients with a heavy preponderance of recurrent unipolar or endogenous illnesses. (When the study was designed the unipolar-bipolar distinction was just beginning to emerge in the literature.) We were interested in studying a group of patients who are usually called neurotic or nonpsychotic depressives and for whom outpatient treatment and psychotherapy are usually recommended. The psychiatric textbooks emphasize the classic distinctions between endogenous-reactive and psychotic-neurotic forms of depression, distinctions that emerged in the 1920s and 1930s. The presumption was that if psychotherapy and outpatient treatments were to work, it would be for this group of neurotic or reactive depressives. Therefore, our sample was biased in favor of selecting these relatively milder, ambulatory patients in order to test a psychopathological hypothesis.

Similarly, the design of the psychotherapy was explicated very carefully. As Ms. Weissman has said, we purposely followed Frank's concept, elucidated in the 1950s, that psychotherapy would be most effective for the patient's social effectiveness, personal satisfaction, and interpersonal adjustments. This is why the design contained built-in measures of social adjustment in addition to measures of symptom relief, in order to test the Frank-Hopkins hypothesis about the differential effectiveness of drugs and psychotherapy. Also, in order to describe what psychotherapy did occur, we devised a technique for analyzing the content and process of the psychotherapy.[2] Our data indicate that this type of therapy was supportive; it was directed to the "here and now" interactions of the patients in their current life situations. It did not recover any early childhood experiences. It did not recover unconscious material. It was based on an attempt to clarify patient's manifest behavior in the "here and now."

I think the points that Dr. Freyhan raised are very relevant for evaluating any study of this sort. I think we have dealt with them.

DR. ISAAC MARKS:* Could you put some clinical flesh on the ways in which your patients were better in social adjustment as far as you can judge from clinical impression?

DR. WEISSMAN: To flush out the meaning of the histograms I presented, Dr. Paykel and I have compared the social adjustment of forty patients in this study with forty matched normal controls. We looked at what the impaired social adjustment meant in the family situation and we postulated how psychotherapy might help it. To summarize, the psychotherapy had its major effect in two areas, in reducing interpersonal friction and hostility and in increasing the person's ability to be assertive and to achieve mastery by expressing more directly wishes and needs in the immediate family.

DR. PHILIP MAY:† I must confess I have a little skepticism about the survivor analysis. If you start off with 100 people whom you treated with a certain treatment and then 99 percent of them relapse and you only look at the one who is left, you can quite easily conclude you have had spectacular followup results in that treatment. It seems to me that you had a differential relapse rate in the group of people who were treated with psychotherapy, so you must have wound up with unequal numbers. A much more legitimate analysis would be to take the 40 best people out

*Institute of Psychiatry, London.
†Neuropsychiatric Institute, University of California, Los Angeles.

of the drug group and compare their social adjustment with the 40 people that you had surviving in the psychotherapy group. Or maybe you could have done some correlational analyses with, e.g., social adjustment and then selected your patients for the analysis on that basis. To let patients just drop out is kind of a curious procedure, and you yourself admitted it wasn't entirely correct.

DR. LOTHAR B. KALINOWSKY:* This elaborate study aims at a comparison between psychotherapy and pharmacotherapy in depression. Clinical experience has shown that psychotherapy is effective in neurotic depressions but ineffective or even dangerous in endogenous depressions. This is in accordance with your statement that most of your patients had neurotic depressions. Since this is so, I think you should change the title of your paper to "neurotic depression" rather than referring to depressions in general.

I wonder why you have chosen amitriptyline, a tricyclic antidepressant, when there is general agreement that tricyclics are much more effective in endogenous depression. I think the paper actually supports the need to distinguish very clearly between endogenous and neurotic depressions. They have completely different therapeutic responses to the various treatments we have in psychiatry.

We know from the time before we had any treatment that endogenous depressions usually clear up spontaneously in less than a year. This is overlooked in many studies with perfect methodology, and I think this should also be taken into consideration in a study like this one presented by the authors.

DR. DAVID L. DUNNER:† I would like to make three comments. First, the study was designed to be a prophylactic study in a population which apparently would have a low frequency of recurrence of illness. The results indicate that psychotherapy has little effect as a prophylactic—that is, in preventing relapse or recurrence.

Second, the effects of psychotherapy which were demonstrated were in changes in social adjustment. The question I have is whether these social adjustment effects of psychotherapy have any relation to the fact that the population had depressive illness or whether these same effects could be demonstrated in nondepressives. Is there any particular benefit of psychotherapy in depressives?

The third point concerns our own experiences at the lithium clinic at the New York State Psychiatric Institute, which could be termed a low-contact psychotherapy, high-contact drug clinic. Our patients are seen about 20 to 30 minutes a month, and most of this time is taken up with

*New York Medical College.
†New York State Psychiatric Institute.

rating scales. Our impression has been that most of our patients do quite well without additional psychotherapy. What concerns me is the notion that these patients would benefit further from more intensive psychotherapy—from "coming to grips with their problems." My personal bias is that more intensive psychotherapy may tend to create more problems for these patients than they would otherwise experience.

DR. ROBERT L. SPITZER:* First, let me make a small methodological point. As sophisticated people, we are always making the distinction between clinical and statistical significance in reporting treatment differences. Yet it is very unusual for a research study actually to report the results using statistics which index the magnitude of the treatment differences, rather than just the probability that the differences could be due to chance. It would have been more informative if the treatment differences reported today had been expressed in a statistic which indexed the proportion of improvement scores for which one can account by membership in the various groups. Such statistics are found in an article that I wrote with Jacob Cohen.[3]

Now a more important point in evaluating the results of this study. Here we have a group of subjects who at the start of the study are not that disabled. They are seeing a social worker who by training is focusing her treatment on the specific variable (social adjustment) that is measured by the outcome measure. After seeing the social worker for four and then eight months, the subject reports that yes, in those very areas there has been some improvement. On the other hand, the subjects who are not seeing a social worker do not have the expectation for improvement in social adjustment and then do not report much improvement. The result of the study seems to be that the *self-reports* of social adjustment have changed. There were no independent measures of social adjustment other than the patients' reports.

The whole placebo literature suggests that expectancy or the placebo effect is most prominent when you are dealing with a mild condition. When you are dealing with a severe condition, the placebo effect is wiped out. Perhaps this is an ideal population for the maximization of the placebo effect.

DR. WEISSMAN: I'd like to comment on the important point Dr. Spitzer has made about the objectivity of assessments. We regret that we didn't have raters who were independent of the patients' reports, such as relatives or significant others. We didn't because of the cost and the difficulty we felt there would be in obtaining relatives' cooperation in an outpatient study.

---

*Biometrics Research Unit, New York State Department of Mental Hygiene.

However, we did have raters who were independent of the treatment and were not the therapists. None of the therapists did the ratings of social adjustment, and we did try to systematize the technique by inter-rater reliability studies. One argument against the halo effect in our ratings is the fact that we don't have the improvement on all outcome measures. In fact, we don't have improvement with psychotherapy in areas where we would have expected improvement, that is, dependency, and we don't have a psychotherapy effect after four months.

QUESTION: Does Valium have a depressive effect which perhaps counteracts the anti-anxiety effect in this study?

DR. LIPMAN: We did find a one-week anti-anxiety effect favoring diazepam. One-week drug effects favoring diazepam were also found on the Symptom Checklist factor of Sleep Disturbance and on the Mood Scale factors of Friendliness, Well-Being, Activity, and Carefree. By two weeks, however, these early advantages for diazepam, except for the Sleep Disturbance factor, were no longer present, and diazepam patients were actually doing more poorly than placebo patients on the mood factors Depression and Fatigue. At two weeks, in general, most drug effects favored imipramine, and these were significant on the symptom factors of Depression, Obsessive-Compulsiveness, Interpersonal Sensitivity, and Hostility and the mood factors of Depression and Fatigue.

The diazepam group tended to worsen, relative to their improved status after the placebo-washout period, on most symptom and mood factors. This worsening, however, did not exceed their initial levels of distress upon first entering the study.

The answer to this question, then, is a qualified yes.

DR. KLEIN: I'd like to suggest a hypothesis that there is a real difference between agitation and anxiety, and that this distinction is often not made. The people who suffer from pure anticipatory anxiety, that is, who are looking forward to bad things happening to them, are often not discriminated from people with tension, mild agitation, and often very verbal complaints about how life is treating them. So they end up being considered hostile.

My experience suggests that people who suffer from pure anticipatory anxiety do relatively well on Valium, whereas people who suffer from an agitated reaction do badly on Valium—as a matter of fact, it makes them worse. So I think that probably many of your patients were actually suffering from mild agitated depression. Actually they were screened into the study for depression. Therefore we are not talking about the sort of responsive patients who are screened into a Valium trial for anxiety and don't really have all that much depression.

In studies you yourself have done comparing depressed samples with anxious samples, the depressed patients usually end up with anxiety scores as high or higher than the anxiety samples do, but the anxiety samples don't have high depression scores. There is a real psychopathological difference here, which would account for Valium doing well in anxious samples but not in depression complicated by agitation and miscalled "anxiety." I don't know whether your data allow you to cull out those patients who show agitation rather than anticipatory anxiety; if they do, I suggest you cull out these two groups of patients and analyze them separately.

You did make me happy with your finding about the beneficial imipramine effect on the phobic anxious factor. I'd be very curious to know the distribution of patients along this factor. I would guess that you have a bimodal distribution there, and that the patients who have agoraphobic or phobic anxious syndromes are on the severe end.

This would be the first group to cull out because they confuse the issue by responding well to imipramine. Then look at the remaining sample on the anxiety and agitation measures. I think you will probably be able to find some measures that would specify a mild agitated stage.

In particular, it's been my experience that the kind of agitated depression seen in outpatients results from their being obsessive-compulsive people who got derailed; they have highly cliché-ridden styles of life and something comes along to tip them over. This might also afford you another screen if you have personality or value measures along obsessive lines, associated with manifest precipitating factors.

DR. DUNNER: a comment pertinent to both reports. We have very elegant tools to measure improvement of depressive illness in terms of decreases in depressive symptoms, such as insomnia, inertia, and anorexia. When psychotherapy is compared to anti-depressant drugs, the drugs work better in alleviating these symptoms. I wonder if what we have heard this morning means that the effect of psychotherapy in these illnesses, particularly in depression, is not to treat the depressive state but perhaps to do something else. Do we have a measurement of psychotherapy which will evaluate the effect of psychotherapy independently of the improvement in depressive symptoms? I don't think it is fair to judge the effect of psychotherapy by measuring changes in insomnia or anorexia.

NOTES

1. G. L. Klerman, A. DiMascio, M. Weissman, B. Prusoff, & E. S. Paykel, Treatment of depression by drugs and psychotherapy, *American Journal of Psychiatry*, 1974, **131**, 186–191.

2. Weissman, M., & Klerman, G. L. Psychotherapy with depressed women: an empirical study of content themes and reflection. *British Journal of Psychiatry*, 1973, **123**, 55–61.

3. Common errors in quantitative psychiatric research, *International Journal of Psychiatry*, 1968, **6**, 109–131.

16 COMPARISON OF SHORT-TERM TREATMENT REGIMENS IN PHOBIC PATIENTS: A Preliminary Report

CHARLOTTE M. ZITRIN, DONALD F. KLEIN,
CAROL LINDEMANN, PRISCILLA TOBAK,
MARTIN ROCK, JOEL H. KAPLAN, and VIVIAN H. GANZ

BACKGROUND

The treatment of phobias has remained one of the greatest challenges in the field of psychiatry. Agoraphobia, in particular, has been among the emotional illnesses most refractory to treatment. Until the late 1950s, the principal treatment of phobias consisted of various forms of psychotherapy, including psychoanalysis. In the next few years, two innovative treatment approaches emerged. The first was a behavior modification technique—desensitization in imagination—introduced by Wolpe (1958) and Rachman (1959). Their papers and those that followed reported excellent results. However, they were based upon individual case reports without controls.

It was not until 1966 that a series of prospective studies comparing different treatment modalities in phobic patients appeared. These, by Gelder and Marks and their group (Gelder & Marks, 1966; Gelder, Marks, & Wolff, 1967), showed that desensitization was superior to individual or group psychotherapy and that no symptom substitution occurred. In a crossover study in 1968 (Gelder & Marks, 1968), seven patients previously treated with group psychotherapy for two years, with no improvement, were switched to desensitization and, after four months, showed great improvement. In an ongoing study by Rachman, a compa-

Charlotte M. Zitrin, M.D., Donald F. Klein, M.D., Carol Lindemann, Ph.D., Priscilla Tobak, M.S.W., Martin Rock, B.A., Joel H. Kaplan, M.D., Vivian H. Ganz, M.A., Long Island Jewish-Hillside Medical Center. Reprint requests to Charlotte M. Zitrin, M.D.

This work was supported in part by National Institute of Mental Health grant 23007. Imipramine and matching placebo were kindly supplied by Ciba-Geigy Pharmaceutical Co., Ardsley, N.Y. Sydney Feldman did the statistical analyses.

rison is being made of four types of treatment: psychotherapy, behavior therapy (relaxation and desensitization), relaxation alone, and desensitization alone. Thus far, data obtained on six patients in each group show an overall lead for desensitization on all criteria (Bergin & Garfield, 1971).

The second new treatment approach used drugs. Klein and Fink (1962) reported on the successful use of anti-depressants for panic attacks in agoraphobic patients. However, the patients were reluctant to change their phobic behavior patterns and required much persuasion, direction, and support to do so. Klein (1964) reported a further clinical study of phobic anxious patients, in which twenty-two received imipramine, six received MAO inhibitors, and four received no anti-depressant medication. In all patients given imipramine or MAO inhibitors, the panic attacks were alleviated. Phobic symptoms, however, persisted because of anticipatory anxiety. Supportive therapy was required for this. A double-blind study which followed (Klein, 1967) confirmed the marked superiority of imipramine over placebo.

A retrospective study by Kelly, Guirguis, Frommer, Mitchell-Heggs, and Sargent (1970) showed similar beneficial effects of MAO inhibitors in phobic patients with panic attacks. In a double-blind study of thirty-five nonpsychotic children with school phobia, Gittelman-Klein and Klein (1971) found that, in a six-week period, imipramine was significantly superior to placebo in inducing school return and alleviating subjective distress. Both groups received psychiatric interviewing and social work family counseling.

Solyon, Heseltine, McClure, Solyon, Ledridge, and Steinberg (1973) reported a study comparing behavior therapy to drug therapy. They found a significant decrease in phobias in all groups, with the greatest decrease occurring in those treated with aversion relief. They also found that there was a more rapid effect with phenelzine than with behavior therapy. However, over a two-year followup period, the relapse rate in those treated with the behavior therapies has not exceeded 10 percent, whereas all patients in the phenelzine-treated group who stopped taking the drug relapsed.

Tyrer, Candy, and Kelly (1973) conducted a double-blind control trial of phenelzine and placebo in chronic agoraphobic and socially phobic psychiatric outpatients: they found a significant phenelzine effect at eight weeks but not at four weeks on overall psychiatrists' ratings. Measures of discrete aspects of the syndromes were not as successful in discriminating phenelzine from placebo. Unfortunately, Tyrer et al. did not distinguish in the data analysis between agoraphobia and social phobia. Further, their measures of panics are stated by them to be not entirely satisfactory, since they related only to the three days prior to the evaluation periods and were categorized by very low levels of pathology. They do comment that several patients did report an improvement in unexplained panics.

Lipsedge, Hajioff, Huggins, Napier, Pearce, Pike, and Rich (1973) compared iproniazid with placebo in sixty-one outpatients with severe agoraphobia. In addition, each patient was assigned to methohexitone-assisted systematic desensitization, standard systematic desensitization, or no desensitization. They concluded that iproniazid was superior to placebo and that methohexitone-assisted systematic desensitization was slightly better than the other treatment combinations during an eight-week trial.

We felt that there was a need for a large-scale, controlled, double-blind study of the outpatient treatment of phobias, combining the above-mentioned new treatment approaches. The purpose of the present study was to determine the efficacy of a two-pronged approach combining behavior therapy and imipramine.

Agoraphobic patients seem qualitatively different from other phobic patients in that they present with both spontaneous panic attacks and anticipatory anxiety, each reinforcing the other. In other phobics, spontaneous panic attacks are generally absent, although extreme anxiety may occur in specific phobic situations. Therefore, in our initial design, we planned to divide our patients into "agoraphobic" or "phobic neurosis" categories for treatment purposes. However, we soon found that some patients were not typical of either group, but combined some qualities of each. We finally placed these into a third group which we call "mixed phobic." Our diagnostic criteria for the three groups follow.

AGORAPHOBIA

This term really is a misnomer because the core problem is fear of leaving home. This fear usually is precipitated by spontaneous panic attacks. Typically, these patients fear lack of support and helplessness when panic occurs. The attacks occur without warning and may consist of rapid breathing, palpitations, weakness, dizziness, and fears of death; vomiting, loss of bladder control, loss of rectal control; fainting; and fear of going crazy. As a result, these patients fear going out of the house, especially when alone. They fear going into the street, into crowded places, stores, strange places, cars, trains, buses, planes. Often, they are afraid to be alone, even at home. They are typically dependent, usually female, and frequently give a history of separation anxiety as children.

PHOBIC NEUROSIS

This category consists of specific phobias, like claustrophobia, acrophobia, and fears of animals, insects, darkness, and thunderstorms, and social phobias, such as fear of eating in public, fear of public speaking, fear of meeting people, and fear of name-signing in public. These phobias are distinctly more circumscribed than agoraphobia and less likely to result in phobic generalization. In addition, these patients usually function considerably better than the agoraphobic patient.

MIXED PHOBIC

These patients have characteristics of both phobic neurosis and agoraphobia but are not typical of either. They comprise, for the most part, patients with claustrophobia but no travel restrictions who have spontaneous panic attacks. A small number have travel restrictions and do not appear to have spontaneous panic attacks. This obviously is a heterogeneous group that will require further refinement.

At first, we considered setting up a control group receiving imipramine only. However, there was concern that this group would not have treatment time equivalent to the others, since the patients would be seen only long enough to be given medication and questioned about side effects. We finally resolved this problem by giving this group supportive therapy in addition to imipramine. Thus, our final groups, as reported today, are (1) behavior therapy and imipramine; (2) behavior therapy and placebo; and (3) supportive psychotherapy and imipramine. The patients were randomly assigned to one of the three groups. Groups 1 and 2 are double-blind; Group 3 is single-blind. As a result of this design, we are able to compare first, behavior therapy and supportive therapy, and second, imipramine and placebo. Since we have three diagnostic groups, each divided into three treatment groups, there is a total of nine cells. When the study is complete, there will be 20 patients in each cell, for a total of 180 patients. The present paper is a preliminary report on those patients who have, thus far, either completed treatment or completed half of their treatment sessions.

Our hypotheses are as follows. (1) For agoraphobics, the imipramine will inhibit panic attacks and the behavior therapy will alleviate anticipatory anxiety. Hence, imipramine and behavior therapy combined should be superior to behavior therapy and placebo. (2) For mixed phobic patients, since they have some of the qualities of agoraphobics, the results should be similar to those for agoraphobics, especially if spontaneous panic attacks are present. (3) For phobic neurosis patients who do not experience spontaneous panic attacks, there should be no difference between the imipramine and placebo groups. Therefore, those patients receiving behavior therapy and placebo should do as well as those on behavior therapy and imipramine. (4) With regard to the two psychotherapies, we believe that behavior therapy will be superior to supportive therapy because it is focused more systematically on phobic situations and is more structured toward helping patients to confront those situations.

METHOD

At the onset of treatment, each patient starts with 25 mg. of imipramine or placebo at night. The drug is increased by 25 mg. every second day until the patient is receiving 150 mg. daily. If necessary, further increments, up to a maximum of 300 mg. daily, are given. If the patient reports sudden increase in anxiety, insomnia, or tension, the dose is decreased to the last tolerated one.

Patients receiving behavior therapy are first trained to use a relaxation technique akin to the relaxation of Yoga. Systematic desensitization is carried out while the patient is relaxed. This consists of having the patient imagine phobic situations, starting with the least feared and proceeding in step-wise fashion to the most feared. At times, when possible and indicated, patients are accompanied into phobic situations by a staff member for in vivo desensitization after desensitization in imagination has been accomplished. However, for the most part, patients enter the in vivo situations without accompanying staff personnel, as homework after imaginal desensitization sessions. Patients are requested to practice relaxation several times daily and whenever anxious, tense, or confronting phobic situations. Assertive training, which is similar to supportive therapy but requires a more active role for the therapist, is another important component of the behavior therapy. In addition, general supportive therapy, as detailed below, is given where indicated.

The supportive psychotherapy attempts to help patients to be more rational in relation to phobic situations, to obtain insight, where possible, into the origin of their phobic behavior, and to encourage them to try alternative, more effective means of dealing with phobic and other problem situations. Interpretation, confrontation, and reality testing in an empathic climate are used to help the patient modify pathologic defenses and inappropriate behavior. Therapists may encourage patients to enter phobic situations, but there is no use of relaxation, systematic desensitization, or role playing.

In our view, systematic desensitization and assertive training are extensions of supportive therapy. They differ from the latter, however, in that they focus more systematically on specific problem situations, dealing with them in an ordered fashion based upon their relative severity. In addition, the behavior therapy involves the use of relaxation, the use of role playing during assertive training, and the use of specific assigned tasks as homework.

Each patient is seen for a screening interview to determine acceptability for the project. Thus far, over 300 patients have applied for treatment and 129 have been screened (Table 1). All screening notes are reviewed by two of the investigators (Drs. Zitrin and Klein) separately. If there is any question about suitability, the patient is re-interviewed.

Patients are seen for a total of 26 weekly treatment sessions, each lasting 45 minutes. On admission and at intervals during treatment, the patient is evaluated separately by the therapist and an independent evaluator, both blind to medication (Table 2). The patient also completes several forms (Tables 3 and 4).

At the time of admission, an independent evaluator accompanies the patient on a field visit to determine actual functioning and level of anxiety. This is repeated on completion of treatment. In addition, at the end of treatment, the spouse or a significant other family member is interviewed to get his view of the effect of the therapy.

Followup evaluations are done after three months, six months, one year, two, three, four, and five years.

RESULTS

In this paper, we are reporting on 57 white patients, between twenty-one and forty-five years of age, who have completed at least half of their treatment (13 sessions). This includes 34 patients who have completed the full course of 26 sessions.

Sixty-three percent of the patients are female and 37 percent are male. The mean duration of illness is 8.8 years, with a range of 2 to 37 years. Seventy-five percent have had previous treatment (primarily traditional psychotherapies) with a mean duration of 2.2 years and a range of 3 weeks to 8 years.

The next two tables compare the response to treatment of the three diagnostic groups at the thirteenth session. Table 5 shows the results of imipramine treatment. The agoraphobic and mixed phobic patients

Table 1. Results of Initial Patient Evaluations

Total patients screened	129
Accepted	113
Rejected	16
schizophrenia	7
previous treatment with tricyclic drug	5
severe heart disease	1
below normal I.Q.	1
not phobic	1
not in study's age range	1

Table 2.   Therapist Questionnaires and Evaluations

Onset of treatment
1. Brief Psychiatric Rating Scale (ECDEU)
2. Clinical Global Impression Scale (ECDEU)
3. Hamilton Anxiety Rating Scale
4. Functional Capacity and Subjective Distress on Admission
5. Clinical description of patient

6th, 13th, and 26th sessions
1. Clinical Global Impression Scale (ECDEU)
2. Hamilton Anxiety Rating Scale
3. Goal Attainment of Functional Capacity and Subjective Distress
4. Clinical description of patient

Note: the independent evaluator completes all of the above except for the 6th-session forms.

respond almost identically for all evaluators. There is greater improvement in these groups than in the phobic neurosis group. Note that the patient self-ratings are the most favorable. This is true of all the rating schedules we have tabulated. Usually, as you shall see, the independent evaluator ratings are the least favorable.

In Table 6 there is a similar comparison, this time for the patients on placebo. Again, the agoraphobic and mixed phobic patients respond in the same way, with most patients unimproved in each group. In the phobic neurosis group, more are improved than unimproved by therapist and patient evaluations. Since the agoraphobic and mixed phobic patients appear to be so similar in nature, both characterized by spontaneous panic attacks and responding in the same way to all of the treatment modalities, we decided to group them together in the next four tables.

Table 3.   Patient Questionnaires

Onset of treatment
1. Life History Questionnaire
2. Fear Inventory
3. Agoraphobia Inventory
4. Acute Panic Inventory
5. Taylor Manifest Anxiety Scale
6. Self-Rating Symptom Scale (ECDEU)

6th, 13th, and 26th sessions
1. Agoraphobia Inventory
2. Acute Panic Inventory
3. Taylor Manifest Anxiety Scale
4. Self-Rating Symptom Scale (ECDEU)
5. Fear Inventory (after twenty-six weeks only)

Table 4. The items in this questionnaire refer to things and experiences that may cause fear, nervousness or anxiety. Place a check mark in the column that describes how much it disturbs you.

	None	Very Little	A Little	Some	Much	Very Much	Terror
1. Sharp objects							
2. Being a passenger in a car							
3. Dead people							
4. Suffocating							
5. Failing a test							
6. Being a passenger in an airplane							
7. Worms							
8. Arguing with parents							
9. Rats, mice							
10. Life after death							
11. Hypodermic needles							
12. Roller coasters							
13. Death							
14. Crowded places							
15. Blood							
16. Heights							
17. Being a leader							
18. Swimming alone							
19. Illness							
20. Stores							
21. Illness or injury to loved ones							
22. Driving a car							

Table 5. Comparison of Diagnostic Groups Treated with Imipramine (13th Session)

	Agoraphobia	Mixed Phobic	Phobic Neurosis
Therapist rating			
moderate to marked improvement	8	6	3
minimal to no improvement	5	4	5
Independent evaluator			
moderate to marked improvement	7	6	3
minimal to no improvement	6	4	5
Patient self-evaluation			
moderate to marked improvement	11	9	6
minimal to no improvement	2	1	2

In Table 7 agoraphobic and mixed phobic patients receiving behavior therapy and imipramine are compared to those receiving behavior therapy and placebo at the thirteenth session. Those patients receiving imipramine did significantly better than those on placebo. Again, the patients' ratings are the most favorable. The independent evaluators' ratings are the least favorable.

When all imipramine patients (comprising those treated double-blind in association with behavior therapy and those treated single-blind in association with supportive therapy) are contrasted with the double-blind behavior therapy-placebo patients in Table 8 the same drug effect is found.

Table 6. Comparison of Diagnostic Groups Treated with Placebo (13th Session)

	Agoraphobia	Mixed Phobic	Phobic Neurosis
Therapist rating			
moderate to marked improvement	1	1	7
minimal to no improvement	6	5	4
Independent evaluator			
moderate to marked improvement	1	0	4
minimal to no improvement	7	5	7
Patient self-evaluation			
moderate to marked improvement	2	4	7
minimal to no improvement	6	3	4

Table 7. Agoraphobia and Mixed Phobic Patients: Comparison of Behavior
Therapy-Imipramine and Behavior Therapy-Placebo (13th Session)

	Behavior Therapy-Imipramine	Behavior Therapy-Placebo	t Test	Fisher Exact
Therapist rating				
moderate to marked improvement	9	2		
minimal to no improvement	6	11	$p < .01$[a]	$p = .02$
Independent evaluator				
moderate to marked improvement	8	1		
minimal to no improvement	7	12	$p < .001$	$p = .013$
Patient self-evaluation				
moderate to marked improvement	14	6		
minimal to no improvement	1	9	$p < .01$	$p = .003$

[a]P values are one-tailed here and in the following tables.

Table 9 compares behavior therapy and supportive therapy in imipramine-treated agoraphobic and mixed phobic patients at the thirteenth session. There is no significant difference between these two psychotherapies.

In Table 10 we contrast the agoraphobic-mixed phobic group treated with behavior therapy and placebo with the group treated with supportive therapy and imipramine, at the thirteenth session. Plainly, in such a confounded comparison, the contrast between groups cannot be simply allocated to any one variable. The point of the comparison is to indicate

Table 8. Agoraphobia and Mixed Phobic Patients: Comparison of Imipramine
and Placebo (13th Session)

	Imipramine	Placebo	t Test	Fisher Exact
Therapist rating				
moderate to marked improvement	14	2		
minimal to no improvement	9	11	$p < .01$	$p = .01$
Independent evaluator				
moderate to marked improvement	13	1		
minimal to no improvement	10	12	$p < .001$	$p = .004$
Patient self-evaluation				
moderate to marked improvement	20	6		
minimal to no improvement	3	9	$p < .01$	$p = .004$

Table 9. Agoraphobia and Mixed Phobic Patients: Comparison between Behavior Therapy and Supportive Therapy (13th Session—All Patients on Imipramine)

	Behavior Therapy	Supportive Therapy	t Test	Fisher Exact
Therapist rating				
moderate to marked improvement	9	5		
minimal to no improvement	6	3	n.s.	n.s.
Independent evaluator				
moderate to marked improvement	8	5		
minimal to no improvement	7	3	n.s.	n.s.
Patient self-evaluation				
moderate to marked improvement	14	6		
minimal to no improvement	1	2	n.s.	n.s.

that if behavior therapy is superior to supportive therapy, its superiority is not of a magnitude sufficient to offset the superiority of imipramine to placebo.

In Table 11 phobic neurosis patients receiving behavior therapy with imipramine are compared to those receiving behavior therapy with placebo at the thirteenth session. The conditions are double-blind. In these patients, who do not experience spontaneous panic attacks, there is no statistically significant difference between the imipramine and placebo groups.

Table 10. Agoraphobia and Mixed Phobic Patients: Comparison of Behavior Therapy-Placebo and Supportive Therapy-Imipramine (13th Session)

	Behavior Therapy-Placebo	Supportive Therapy-Imipramine	t Test	Fisher Exact
Therapist rating				
moderate to marked improvement	2	5		
minimal to no improvement	11	3	$p < .05$	$p = .041$
Independent evaluator				
moderate to marked improvement	1	5		
minimal to no improvement	12	3	$p < .01$	$p = .014$
Patient self-evaluation				
moderate to marked improvement	6	6		
minimal to no improvement	9	2	$p < .05$	n.s.

Table 11. Phobic Neurosis Patients: Comparison of Behavior Therapy-Imipramine and Behavior Therapy-Placebo (13th Session)

	Behavior Therapy-Imipramine	Behavior Therapy-Placebo	t Test	Fisher Exact
Therapist rating				
moderate to marked improvement	3	7		
minimal to no improvement	3	4	n.s.	n.s.
Independent evaluator				
moderate to marked improvement	2	4		
minimal to no improvement	4	7	n.s.	n.s.
Patient self-evaluation				
moderate to marked improvement	4	7		
minimal to no improvement	2	4	n.s.	n.s.

Table 12 compares all phobic neurosis patients on imipramine to those on placebo. In these patients, consonant with the double-blind comparisons, there is no significant difference between the drug and placebo groups. Thus, there is no enhancement of therapy by imipramine. There are too few phobic neurosis patients on supportive therapy thus far to make a comparison between this and behavior therapy.

The number of patients who have completed the full course of 26 treatment sessions is too small, when broken down into the different groups, to make statistical analyses similar to those made at the thirteenth session. However, there are some trends which may be seen in Table 13.

Table 12. Phobic Neurosis Patients: Comparison of Imipramine and Placebo
(13th Session)

	Imipramine	Placebo	t Test	Fisher Exact
Therapist rating				
moderate to marked improvement	3	7		
minimal to no improvement	5	4	n.s.	n.s.
Independent evaluator				
moderate to marked improvement	3	4		
minimal to no improvement	5	7	n.s.	n.s.
Patient self-evaluation				
moderate to marked improvement	6	7		
minimal to no improvement	2	4	n.s.	n.s.

Table 13. Comparison of Overall Results (13th and 26th Sessions)

	Sessions Completed	No. of Patients	Marked Improvement	Moderate Improvement	Minimal to no Improvement
			%	%	%
Therapist rating	13	57	0	46	54
	26	34	53	35	12
Independent evaluator	13	56	3	36	61
	26	34	38	35	26
Patient self-evaluation	13	57	14	54	32
	26	34	56	36	9

Here, a comparison is made of treatment results at 13 and 26 weeks. There is a general shift to the left, indicating that significant progress is made in the latter half of the treatment period. At 26 weeks, a relatively small percentage of the patients remains minimally improved or unimproved. If we take the therapist and patient ratings, over 50 percent of the patients are markedly improved at the end of treatment. Another 35 percent are moderately improved. Thus, with all treatment regimens, there is a fairly high successful treatment rate.

Another important finding in this study was the unusual sensitivity to imipramine shown by some of the patients. Although the usual anticholinergic drug effects did not present any special problem, some of the patients were so exquisitely sensitive to the drug that as little as 5 mg. daily produced an immediate excitatory or stimulant effect. Of 38 patients on imipramine, 13, or 34 percent, showed this effect on doses ranging from 5 to 75 mg. per day. The symptoms included insomnia at the onset of treatment (both difficulty in falling asleep and repeated awakening during sleep), jitteriness, and irritability. Almost all were in the agoraphobic-mixed phobic group.

If the dosage is decreased until the symptoms subside, it may be cautiously increased again, as a rule. However, most of these patients remained on relatively small amounts throughout their treatment, if one compares their dosage to that generally used for depressed patients. Nevertheless, their spontaneous panic attacks subsided. This excitatory effect may be the reason why some believe that antidepressants are contraindicated in agoraphobic patients. This may also explain why some patients who have received imipramine report poor results with the drug.

There has been no evidence thus far of symptom substitution.

Two agoraphobic patients successfully treated with imipramine relapsed after the drug was discontinued. They experienced a recurrence of
panic attacks and avoidance behavior.

Four patients who were treatment failures on placebo were placed on
drug only, with subsequent loss of panic attacks and moderate overall
improvement. Two of these were agoraphobic and two mixed phobic.

Fifteen patients who started the treatment program dropped out
(Table 14). Of these, eight refused medication. It is interesting that two of
these were found to be on placebo.

DISCUSSION AND CONCLUSIONS

The preliminary results of this study support several of our working
hypotheses. First, agoraphobic and mixed phobic patients respond
similarly to the different treatment modalities used in this study. Second,
agoraphobic and mixed phobic patients respond much more favorably if
imipramine is part of the treatment regimen. Third, in phobic neurosis
patients, imipramine does not enhance the treatment. Thus, the contrast
in results between the patients with phobic neurosis and the combined
agoraphobic-mixed phobic group is quite striking.

In the agoraphobic-mixed phobic group, there is no significant difference between behavior therapy and supportive psychotherapy at the
thirteenth session, or halfway through treatment. In the phobic neurosis
group, the number in supportive therapy at present is too small to
compare with the behavior therapy group. Therefore, our hypothesis that
behavior therapy in phobic neurosis is superior to supportive therapy is
not subject to analysis as yet.

Table 14.   Patients Stopping Treatment before Completion

Number of patients who have started treatment		77
Number of patients who have dropped out		15
before 5th treatment session	11	
between 5th and 12th sessions	4	
refused medication		8[a]
moved away		1
suicide attempt		1
severe depression		1
marital problems		1
unwilling to comply with program's rules		1
desired therapist change		1
failed to keep appointments—unable to contact		1

[a]Two of these were found to be on placebo.

The principal difference between the agoraphobic and mixed phobic patients on the one hand and the phobic neurosis patients on the other is the existence of spontaneous panic attacks among the former. Therefore, we assume that the effectiveness of the imipramine is due to its effect on these panics. After the attacks subside, the patients seem better able to tolerate and overcome the anticipatory anxiety which leads to avoidance behavior.

For all groups of patients, over 50 percent showed marked improvement and another 35 percent showed moderate improvement at the end of therapy. This represents considerable improvement over the thirteenth session results and must be considered a satisfactory outcome for a brief therapy in patients chronically ill for an average of 8.8 years, most of whom received prior unsuccessful treatment, averaging over 2 years. The rapid elimination of symptoms in these patients did not result in symptom substitution.

Stimulant side effects were troublesome in 34 percent of the patients on imipramine, but these patients showed a beneficial effect, including elimination of spontaneous panic attacks, on small doses of the drug.

It is too early in the followup period to draw any conclusions about relapse rate, but we believe that the followup period is crucial in determining whether the treatment effects for the various groups are permanent or transitory.

It is possible to conceptualize certain psychiatric illnesses (e.g., schizophrenia, recurrent affective disorders, agoraphobia) as consisting of a core phasic disorder complicated by secondary defenses, adaptations, and maladaptations. For instance, endogenous-like depression or psychoses may be secondarily complicated by demoralization, and panic attacks may be complicated by marked travel restrictions. The value of psychotherapy seems most evident in those patients whose core disorder has come under pharmacological control. In patients continually disrupted by their core disorder, psychotherapy is of little or no value (Klein & Davis, 1969). What is not known is why some patients with spontaneous panic attacks develop a phobic orientation and the illnesses of others remain as anxiety neuroses. This requires further investigation.

Although behavior therapy is often conceded to be superior to supportive therapy in the phobic psychoneuroses, its value in agoraphobia is less distinctive. We suggest that the psychoneuroses are not phasic diseases but are dominated by a chronic high level of anticipatory anxiety, controlled by secondary avoidance adaptations. Therefore, in such patients, desensitizing anticipatory anxiety and forcing new adaptations are useful therapeutic procedures. However, similar progress is constantly destroyed by the recurrent panic in agoraphobics, accounting for the low level of success in this group. Indeed, our results thus far indicate that once the panic is under pharmacological control, simple supportive measures may be as valuable as the more elaborate behavior modification procedures. A firm conclusion must await our final figures at the end of treatment.

It would follow, then, that the psychoneurotics should have a relatively low relapse rate but that the agoraphobics should often relapse when medication is discontinued, upon recurrence of their phasic disorder.

Our clinical experience shows that the relapse time is extraordinarily variable. It is not unusual for patients to be symptom-free and to function well for several years and then suddenly to panic and immediately develop travel avoidance. In this case, the primary aversive event appears to be the panic, rather than an external stimulus which elicits an anxiety response. If immediately treated with imipramine, the panics cease and the superstructure of phobic dependent maneuvers does not recur.

Even the successes of behavior therapy with agoraphobics can be understood in the framework of a phasic disorder. Those patients whose panics have spontaneously remitted but who are still dominated by secondary anticipatory anxiety may very well respond to behavior therapy. Actually, in our clinic this group is in the distinct minority thus far.

Procedures such as flooding may also be viewed as methods for concretely and forcibly demonstrating that the reality is less painful than the anticipation, leading to a quick reduction in anticipatory anxiety. We would expect such procedures to be fruitless, however, in the face of recurrent panic. Unfortunately, most studies do not conceptualize the panic as a discrete phenomenon and therefore cannot relate success to the absence of spontaneous panic.

One important diagnostic point is that many patients do not complain of spontaneous panic but only of those circumstances which elicit in them a feeling of being helplessly trapped, e.g., elevators, theaters, tunnels, etc. This makes their illness sound stimulus-bound and similar to the more circumscribed psychoneurotic fears. The examiner must press the patient on whether he ever experiences palpitations, dizziness, dry mouth, etc., for no apparent external reason.

One confusing situation occurs where the patient attributes the panic to an internal thought, in particular about death or cancer. One could hypothesize that the thoughts come *after* the onset of the autonomic discharge rather than before, since these patients will agree that not every thought of cancer leads to a panic. If we find that imipramine blocks these panics, it will be consonant with this hypothesis. Other patients attribute their panics to internal conflicts, but these beliefs are not necessarily diagnostically relevant.

SUMMARY

This is a preliminary report of a double-blind study comparing behavior therapy and imipramine; behavior therapy and placebo; and supportive psychotherapy and imipramine in phobic patients. A total of 57 patients, 63 percent female and 37 percent male, have completed 13 sessions (half of their treatment). This includes 34 patients who have completed the full course of 26 sessions.

The agoraphobic patients, who typically experience spontaneous panic attacks, appear to be qualitatively different, both behaviorally and in their response to treatment, from patients with more circumscribed phobic neurosis. A third group (called "mixed phobic"), with some features of each of the aforementioned groups, reacts to treatment like the agoraphobes and unlike the patients with phobic neurosis. This seems due to the existence of spontaneous panic attacks in the mixed phobic group.

After 13 sessions, the agoraphobic and mixed phobic patients respond much more favorably to imipramine treatment regimens than placebo treatment regimens. In this group there is no apparent difference in outcome between behavior and supportive therapy among patients receiving imipramine.

The phobic neurosis group, after 13 sessions, shows no difference between imipramine and placebo treatment regimens. At present, there are insufficient data to make a comparison between behavior and supportive therapy for this group.

For all treatment regimens, after 26 sessions over 50 percent of the 34 patients are markedly improved, 35 percent are moderately improved, and 15 percent are minimally improved or unimproved.

Four placebo treatment failures are being successfully treated at present with imipramine only. Two agoraphobic patients, successfully treated with imipramine, relapsed when the drug was discontinued. There has been no symptom substitution in any of the groups.

Exquisite sensitivity to imipramine, consisting of immediate insomnia, jitteriness, and irritability, was seen in 34 percent of the patients receiving the drug, almost entirely in the agoraphobic-mixed phobic group. This excitatory effect was managed by prescribing small doses (in some, as little as 5 mg. daily), which, nevertheless, were effective in eliminating panic attacks.

The data indicate that the therapeutic effect of imipramine relates to its elimination of the spontaneous panic attacks. We postulate that agoraphobia, unlike phobic neurosis, has a core phasic disorder—i.e., spontaneous panic attacks—complicated by secondary phobic defenses. As long as this core disorder remains uncontrolled, psychotherapeutic intervention is of little or no value. With imipramine, the core disorder comes under control. This enables the patients to respond to psychotherapy, which reduces the anticipatory anxiety, thus making it possible for them to confront phobic situations.

REFERENCES

Bergin, A. E., & Garfield, S. L. *Handbook of psychotherapy and behavior change*. New York: John Wiley and Sons, 1971.

Gelder, M. G., & Marks, I. M. Severe agoraphobia: a controlled prospective trial of behavior therapy. *British Journal of Psychiatry*, 1966, **112**, 309–320.

Gelder, M. G., & Marks, I. M. Desensitization and phobias: a cross-over study. *British Journal of Psychiatry*, 1968, **114**, 323–328.

Gelder, M. G., Marks, I. M., & Wolff, H. H. Desensitization and psychotherapy in the treatment of phobic states: a controlled inquiry. *British Journal of Psychiatry*, 1967, **113**, 53–73.

Gittelman-Klein, R., & Klein, D. F. Controlled imipramine treatment of school phobia. *Archives of General Psychiatry*, 1971, **25**, 204–207.

Kelly, D., Guirguis, W., Frommer, E., Mitchell-Heggs, N., & Sargent, W. Treatment of phobic states with antidepressants. *British Journal of Psychiatry*, 1970, **116**, 387–398.

Klein, D. F. Delineation of two drug-responsive anxiety syndromes. *Psychopharmacologia*, 1964, **5**, 397–408.

Klein, D. F. Importance of psychiatric diagnosis in prediction of clinical drug effects. *Archives of General Psychiatry*, 1967, **16**, 118–126.

Klein, D. F., & Davis, J. M. *Diagnosis and drug treatment of psychiatric disorders*. Baltimore: Williams & Wilkins, 1969, ch. 13.

Klein, D. F., & Fink, M. Psychiatric reaction patterns to imipramine. *American Journal of Psychiatry*, 1962, **119**, 432–438.

Lipsedge, M. S., Hajioff, J., Huggins, P., Napier, L., Pearce, J., Pike, D. J., & Rich, M. The management of severe agoraphobia: a comparison of iproniazid and systematic desensitization. *Psychopharmacologia*, 1973, **32**, 67–80.

Rachman, S. The treatment of anxiety and phobic reactions by systematic desensitization psychotherapy. *Journal of Abnormal Social Psychology*, 1959, **58**, 250–263.

Solyon, L., Heseltine, G. F. D., McClure, D. J., Solyon, C., Ledridge, B., & Steinberg, G. Behavior therapy versus drug therapy in the treatment of phobic neurosis. *Canadian Psychiatric Association Journal*, 1973, **18**, 25–31.

Tyrer, P., Candy, J., & Kelly, D. A study of the clinical effects of phenelzine and placebo in the treatment of phobic anxiety. *Psychopharmacologia*, 1973, **32**, 237–254.

Wolpe, J. *Psychotherapy by reciprocal inhibition*. Stanford, Calif.: Stanford University Press, 1958.

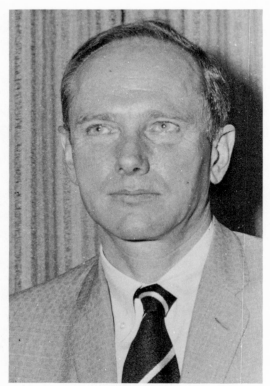

PHILIP R. A. MAY, M.D.
Paul H. Hoch Award Lecturer

Philip May embodies Paul Hoch's character traits—he is gentle, considerate, charming, and highly intelligent; he has a fierce drive to study, to learn, to carry out research, and to contribute to the knowledge of man. Like Hoch, May is respected by his colleagues as an individual inspired by the noblest and most humane traditions of medicine.

Dr. May first came to the United States in 1941 on a fellowship and fell in love with southern California. After earning his M.D. at Stanford in 1944 he returned to England, where he earned an M.B. and did his residency. In 1955 he came back to southern California to teach at U.C.L.A. and to pursue his research interests. He is now Professor of Psychiatry and Clinical Director of the Neuropsychiatric Institute at U.C.L.A. and president of the American College of Neuropsychopharmacology.

Philip May fell in love not only with southern California but with Genevieve Stewart, a psychoanalyst, who became his wife. The Mays live on a bluff in Malibu, and their home has become a center for colleagues, American and foreign, from a diversity of disciplines and walks of life.

Phil May is an outstanding student and researcher, yet he is equally capable as a clinician and administrator. During his administration the Brentwood Veterans Administration Hospital, then an undistinguished institution, became a place of ferment and progress and is now one of the best psychiatric centers in the whole Veterans Administration system. But research is May's greatest involvement; his contributions to evaluation of treatment are well known, especially his classical *Treatment of Schizophrenia*, published in 1968. This definitive comparative analysis of five different therapeutic modalities showed the superiority of ataractic drug therapy and combined drug and psychotherapy, as well as casting doubt on the efficacy of psychotherapy alone. Most notable among his recent works is a remarkable and complete analytical survey of all the significant literature in the field of psychiatric therapy of schizophrenia—a true landmark effort in this field.

The pleasure of his friends and associates at the honor conferred upon Dr. May is increased by their conviction that Paul Hoch, too, would have been delighted at this award.

Milton Greenblatt, M.D.
Past President, American Psychopathological Association

PROLOGUE: PAUL HOCH

Paul Hoch was, to paraphrase Dr. Joseph Zubin, the Churchill of the American Psychopathological Association; a person of extraordinary accomplishments, and an outstanding model to follow for those of us who have had the special opportunity of emigrating from Europe to this country.

Seemingly tireless, meticulous, calm, logical, modest, unbiased, and vastly productive, he was firmly grounded in the best of European medicine and psychiatry as they existed in Hungary, Germany, and Switzerland in the period between World Wars I and II. He came to the United States in 1933, to New York, where he acquired an international reputation, not only as a professor, teacher, and clinical scientist but eventually as a new kind of Commissioner of Mental Hygiene. In this capacity he pioneered in open hospitals, extramural service, patients' rights, and modern treatment programs, tinged always by his special interest in teaching and research.

I am glad that I had the opportunity to see Dr. Hoch in two kinds of action—as what Dr. Fritz Freyhan and Dr. Heinz Lehman call "a statesman and diplomat in the world of psychiatric affairs," who had the quiet ability to defuse the most touchy situation, and as a distinguished lecturer. In these contexts and in his writings he had a remarkable gift for direct and penetrating, no-nonsense observation.

Dr. Henry Brill observed that Paul Hoch was dedicated to improving the lot of the mentally ill and to seeking a solution to the problem of schizophrenia. I would like to share with you a few quotes from his writings (see Lewis & Strahl, 1968) that appeal particularly to me because of my own interests in this field.

On prevention: "prevention is as unclear as the etiology of schizophrenia. I do not know of a single, reliable study showing that we can prevent something when we do not know what it is."

On treatment: "not a single treatment available today, either organic or psychotherapeutic, . . . affects schizophrenia qualitatively. All the treatments we have affect schizophrenia only quantitatively."

On drugs and psychotherapy: "how these two approaches will relate to each other can only be surmised today, but it is possible that psychotherapy will be more effective, more goal-directed, and more economical if ego supportive measures could be relegated to some extent to chemotherapy, which by reducing the emotional intensity of symptoms will permit a less anxiety-ridden psychotherapeutic elucidation of conflicts."

"There is great need for a scientific evaluation of the effectiveness of psychotherapies."

"I believe it will be very important to find out what kind of psychiatric case should be treated with what kind of therapy, instead of using generalizations and bending the therapy to some theoretic principle."

"The increased use of different drugs will necessitate new psychotherapeutic techniques. . . . regardless of how many effective drugs we have in the future . . . many of these patients will always need some psychotherapeutic attention. . . . In a great many patients, drugs relieve . . . distress but the . . . adaptation to the environment which was . . . faulty before he developed the mental disorder remains the same. The drug does not change that. It is here that guidance, support, advice, and even more incisive forms of psychotherapy are indicated."

And finally, a statement that I cherish: "Psychotherapy itself is, of course, a procedure which is as organic as the introduction of a drug, but it is not applied directly to the nervous system. It has to pass through all the filtering and defense mechanisms which shield the organism against external stimulation whereas drugs are introduced directly into the organism."

I would like to think that the research I am about to describe follows in Paul Hoch's path.

Philip R. A. May

17

THE PAUL H. HOCH AWARD LECTURE:
A Followup Study of the Results of Treatment of Schizophrenia

PHILIP R. A. MAY and A. HUSSAIN TUMA

INTRODUCTION

In studying the treatment of mentally ill patients, followup is a platitude in critical discussion, highly recommended, yet seldom accomplished in reality. We hope it will be worthwhile to examine not only the results but also some of the issues that arise as the result of actually doing such a study. A brief resume of the research design will serve as a background for discussing the operational, procedural, and practical problems with which the investigator must deal.

Philip R. A. May, M.D., Chief of Staff for Program Evaluation, Research and Education, Veterans Administration Hospital, Brentwood, California, Professor of Psychiatry, Neuropsychiatric Institute, University of California, Los Angeles.

A. Hussain Tuma, Ph.D., Assistant Chief, Clinical Research Branch, National Institute of Mental Health.

This paper originates in the Schizophrenia Research Project conducted at Camarillo Hospital, Camarillo, California, in collaboration with members of the Los Angeles Psychoanalytic Society. The study was financially supported in part by research grants from the State of California Department of Mental Hygiene, by National Institute of Mental Health Research Grants NIMH-02719, NIMH-04589, and NIMH-19619, and by contract with the Psychopharmacology Research Branch of the National Institute of Mental Health (PH-43-66-49). Camarillo Hospital and the Neuropsychiatric Institute of the University of California at Los Angeles contributed generously in space and timely assistance.

Computing assistance was obtained from the Health Sciences Computing Facility, University of California at Los Angeles, sponsored by National Institutes of Health Special Resources Grant RR-3.

Supplies of trifluoperazine (Stelazine) and chlorpromazine (Thorazine) were donated by Smith, Kline and French Laboratories, Philadelphia, Pennsylvania; supplies of procyclidine (Kemadrin) were donated by Burroughs, Wellcome and Company, Inc., Tuckahoe, New York.

We are indebted to the many who contributed to the work of this project and, in particular relation to this paper, to Wilfrid J. Dixon, Ph.D., Chairman of the Department of Biomathematics and Director of the Health Sciences Computing Facility, University of California at Los Angeles; to Coralee Yale, M.A., Statistician, Health Sciences Computing Facility; to Penelope Potepan, B.A., Research Assistant, Schizophrenic Research Project; to Mrs. Jane Kirksey, Medical Data Processor, Schizophrenia Research Project; and to Mrs. Ada Hirschman, whose volunteer participation eased many troublesome moments.

DESIGN OF THE SCHIZOPHRENIA RESEARCH PROJECT

We selected 288 male and female first admission schizophrenic patients with no significant prior treatment from admissions to Camarillo State Hospital. We wished to study those patients for whom treatment might make the greatest difference between success and failure. Accordingly, using the principle of "triage," patients were excluded if, in clinical judgment, they were considered to have little chance of leaving the hospital in less than two years or if they were already restituting during the initial evaluation period (average 18 days).

It should be noted particularly that we were studying the middle section of the prognostic range. This does provide some rational basis for assuming that the results may be somewhere near the median for the entire prognostic range. However, it is possible that different treatment tactics may be applicable to patients who may perhaps leave the hospital rapidly regardless of the treatment given, or, at the other extreme, to those patients who may perhaps become chronic in any case. One must therefore be cautious in generalizing from the results of this study to the treatment of these other prognostic sectors.

Figure 1 summarizes the overall design of the study. (Complete details are given in May, 1968). After selection and initial evaluation, patients were assigned by a random method to five treatment groups,

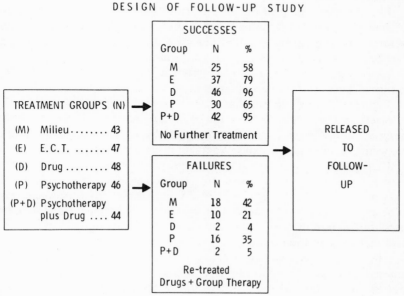

FIG. 1

individual psychotherapy, antipsychotic drug (Stelazine), individual psychotherapy plus antipsychotic drug, electroshock, and milieu, or control (none of the above specific treatments). The five groups were satisfactorily equated in terms of demographic, history, and initial status variables. Therefore, there is no reason to believe that the patients in the five treatment groups were not reasonably homogeneous or did not come from the same population. The groups included some patients who were assaultive, suicidal, mute, or greatly disorganized in their behavior.

Examinations were done before assignment to treatment; at intervals during treatment; at the time of release or termination of treatment; at three and six months after release from the hospital; and every year thereafter and during any subsequent readmission until funds ran out, i.e., a minimum of two years followup and in some cases up to five years.

Evaluation of outcome in the followup phase included a wide range of criteria selected to represent the different vantage points of the clinical psychiatrist, clinical psychologist, social scientist, social worker, patient, and family respondent intimately familiar with the patient. The various measures used covered cognitive, affective, social, occupational, and family adjustment variables. The present paper will focus on only one of the movement criteria, namely, time in hospital, in an effort to illustrate both the importance and complexity of some of the issues involved in conceptualizing and carrying out data analyses in this area. Subsequent publications will present material on the other dimensions of outcome.

For patients in all groups, treatment was continued up to a maximum of one year unless the patient was successfully released from hospital before that. Treatment could be abandoned as a "failure" if the patient had been on the treatment for at least six months and the supervisor and therapist agreed that it had been given a good trial and that further continuation with that particular method was unlikely to succeed.

Figure 1 (*center*) shows that the proportion of patients successfully released as the result of their initial study treatment ranged from 58 percent and 65 percent in the *Milieu* and *Psychotherapy Alone* groups, respectively, to 95 percent and 96 percent in the *Psychotherapy Plus Drug* and *Drug Alone* groups. (See the appendix at the end of the paper for a clarification of technical terms.) ECT (79 percent) was in the middle. As previously reported (May, 1968), there were parallel differences and rank ordering in length of hospital stay, cost of treatment, and clinical condition at termination of treatment, as rated by nursing staff, therapists, and independent interviewers.

The 180 successes were given no further treatment in the hospital and entered the followup study directly. Since it would have been unethical not to give additional treatment to the 48 failures, they were re-treated with antipsychotic drugs and group psychotherapy, a combination that was believed at the time to be the most desirable and practical and potentially effective. All except two of those who had failed to respond to their initial treatment responded to this re-treatment, and eventually all 48 were released into the followup study (Fig. 1 *right*).

If a patient was readmitted to hospital, he was re-treated with his original treatment unless this had been declared a failure: in the latter case he was re-treated with group therapy plus ataraxic drugs (if *that* had already been tried and declared a failure, treatment was chosen by clinical judgment).

Otherwise, once a patient had entered the outpatient followup period, treatment was not controlled: all patients had available to them what was, by then current standards, a fairly good level of outpatient social casework and other clinic treatment. In general (apart from ECT) the original treatment tended to be continued as long as further outpatient treatment was deemed necessary—if it had been successful. However, a substantial number of patients (but by no means all) were given outpatient drug therapy if symptoms recurred.

It must be emphasized that the study was designed to investigate the outcome of hospital treatment only, i.e., to answer the question "what happens in the long run to patients who have been treated in hospital with treatment 'X,' either after they have been successfully treated and discharged, or after treatment 'X' has been discontinued as a failure?"

PRACTICAL PROBLEMS

The design was relatively simple. It was in the execution that one found out why angels fear to tread. The harsh realities of data collection and analysis prompted a thoughtful, even agonizing, reappraisal. As Helen Sargent (1960) delicately observed, "Soon we run into such apparently insurmountable obstacles that it may seem better to switch our interests." An elegant research design may in action prove to be too ambitious to cope with uncontrollable and unpredictable human factors.

Time. The development and execution of a prospective followup study of treatment takes time—three years for the design and pilot stages, five years to follow 228 patients through their treatment in the hospital, plus two additional years of followup in the community. Thus a total of ten years was required for design and data collection alone.

Attrition and Ethics. The longer the followup, the more one's patients scatter over increasingly larger areas. The captive "in-hospital" situation differs fundamentally from community followup, where success depends entirely upon locating the patient and his family, eliciting their interest, and gaining their cooperation. The general trend towards mobility, particularly in urban areas, makes it difficult to maintain contact with any group over an extended period of time. Schizophrenic patients and their families seem to be particularly difficult. Many move around erratically and without notice, leave no address, avoid relatives and research investigators, or are frankly hostile.

Thus a followup study of schizophrenic patients poses massive problems in data collection and record keeping, as well as vexing considerations of ethics and motivation (discussed in detail in May, Tuma, & Kraude, 1965).

Reappraisal. It has gradually been realized, at least by the sophisticated, that a design paradigm of regular evaluation, consistent viewpoint, and zero attrition is unattainable. It is, however, not so well recognized that it is practically impossible to maintain tight controls on treatment, especially outpatient treatment, for a prolonged period of years.

Followups of controlled studies are doomed to depreciate progressively with the passage of time from the end of the controlled treatment period, with much of their discriminating power being eroded by contamination. The progressive effects of aging introduce more and more "noise" into the experiment; so do a multiplicity of environmental changes and experiences. Even more important, there is increasing contamination by newer treatments. Patients who relapse or continue to have symptoms are (necessarily and properly) re-treated with newer and better methods. Since the incidence of re-treatment is likely to be highest in the groups that had the worst showing to start with (particularly any control, no-treatment group), it is inevitable that the longer the followup, the more all treatments approximate the same end result. This artifact must contribute substantially to the familiar "finding," often referred to by the cynical, of superior immediate outcome in the face of insignificant gains in the long run.

It must be concluded that the theoretical paradigm for controlled, long-term followup remains under ordinary circumstances an unattainable ideal. At best we may hope to get a reasonable estimate of what happens to our patients. It is unlikely that we ever will obtain a finely accurate and complete picture.

Followup studies induce a degree of humility. They also lead one to question what may be called the "followup dogma." To speak against followup studies is akin to blasphemy, but what do they accomplish? The notion that knowledge of the "natural history" of the disease, regardless of treatment and other circumstances, can be attained is a figment of the imagination (Lewis, 1936). As for studies of treatment outcome, there must be grave doubt whether followup longer than two to five years has any value, except as a piece of history. The results of such studies should be treated with reserve unless the investigator demonstrated followup of a complete sample and unless the criteria are clearly such as to be unresponsive to variation in social attitudes or to more recently developed methods of treatment. On the other hand, short-term, immediate outcome, now viewed somewhat as second best, would seem to be a legitimate field of interest, susceptible to study with a reasonable degree of accuracy.

PROBLEMS IN DATA ANALYSIS

Figure 2 shows that 100 percent of the patients were followed for two years after first admission (except for one patient who departed to

NUMBERS AND PERCENTAGES OF PATIENTS FOLLOWED-UP

A. FROM DATE OF FIRST ADMISSION

Rx SUCCESSES

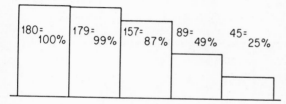

Rx FAILURES

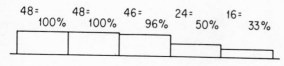

ALL PATIENTS

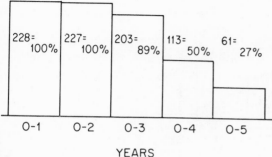

FIG. 2

Mexico early in the study, before we had established procedures to follow up persons in that country). Three-, four-, and five-year followup was 89 percent, 50 percent and 27 percent, respectively, including approximately equal proportions of successes and failures.

Figure 3 shows followup from the date of first release: 100 percent for the first two years, and 70 percent, 38 percent, and 11 percent for three, four, and five years, respectively.

Figures 1, 2, and 3 illustrate three major complications in analysis of studies that follow up the results of a particular treatment or treatments.

Choice of Baseline. Wherever the hospital treatment period can vary in length among patients (almost invariably the case), meaningful interpre-

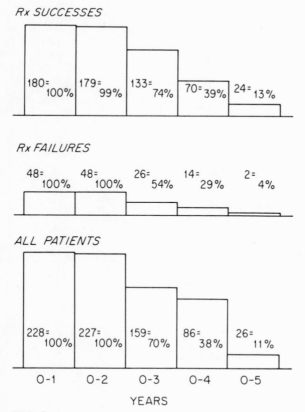

NUMBERS AND PERCENTAGES OF PATIENTS FOLLOWED-UP

B.   FROM DATE OF FIRST RELEASE

Rx SUCCESSES

180= 100%   179= 99%   133= 74%   70= 39%   24= 13%

Rx FAILURES

48= 100%   48= 100%   26= 54%   14= 29%   2= 4%

ALL PATIENTS

228= 100%   227= 100%   159= 70%   86= 38%   26= 11%

0-1   0-2   0-3   0-4   0-5

YEARS

FIG. 3

tation requires that data be analysed from two different baselines; as a cohort from date of first admission and as a cohort from first release or termination of treatment.

Stratification between Successes and Failures. Wherever treatment failures are re-treated with some treatment other than the original experimental treatment (usually the case, for ethical reasons), it is highly desirable to analyze the data for successes and failures separately. If re-treatment is the same for all failures (as in the present study), it is legitimate to combine the two in a third analysis. Thus, even in the absence of sample attrition (see below), six separate analyses may be required for each variable under study (two baselines × three stratifications).

Sample Attrition. If there has been substantial sample loss at any particular followup point, the possibility that the later samples are biased must be seriously considered.

In the present study, the one- and two-year samples are firm at 100 percent, and probably most clinical investigators would accept the three-year samples (89 percent from first admission and 70 percent from first release), particularly since the proportionate representation of successes and failures has been reasonably maintained and the reason for loss was non-selective (cutoff of funds) rather than selective difficulty in tracing patients.

The four- and five-year followup samples, however, show a serious diminution in sample size (N = 113, or 50 percent, at four years from admission; N = 86, or 38 percent, at four years from release; N = 61, or 27 percent, at five years from admission; N = 26, or 11 percent, at five years from release). Although, in general, there does not seem to be selective loss from failures or successes, a wise and conservative approach would require that the four- and five-year data be treated with considerable reserve.

Yet, even so, most investigators would wish to analyze these data. Commentary on the in-hospital analysis has included the speculation that the two psychotherapy groups might develop long-term advantages in followup (e.g., Feinsilver & Gunderson, 1971). Under the circumstances, one cannot afford to throw away information that might be potentially useful as a source for speculation. And in any case, an objective research analysis of a small number of cases may be (in the value judgment of the authors) more valuable than an equal number of the subjective case reports that already abound in the literature.

The problem, of course, is how to estimate or adjust for the potential bias. Our approach (suggested by Dr. Wilfrid J. Dixon), described in a later section, is "Reverse Cohort Analysis." This procedure requires a series of analyses for each time period for which the N is questionable. Hence, if the effect of sample attrition at three, four, and five years is to be investigated, a total of 18 analyses could be required for each variable (2 baselines × 3 stratifications × 3 reverse cohorts)!

It can therefore be seen that adequate analysis of followup data poses a formidable logistic problem in data analysis.

OUTCOME CRITERIA

The outcome variables examined in this paper are the number of days in hospital over cumulative periods of 1, 2, 3, 4, and 5 years from first admission and from first release (stay). In general, length of stay is a crude, but nevertheless major, global measure of outcome. It represents the net result of the varying assessments of the patient, his family, the hospital staff, and the community concerning the amount of time that the patient was in such a (sick) mental state that he needed to be in the special environment of the hospital, rather than in the community. It must be conceded that the length of stay is susceptible to changes in administrative policy; to the whims of relatives, patient and staff alike; and to the vagaries of placement opportunities in the community. Nevertheless, it is a commonly used criterion that has a certain degree of face validity.

ANALYSES

The length-of-stay data for the five treatment groups were compared by Duncan Multiple Range Tests for the significance of differences among the means (Duncan, 1955, 1957). A three-way analysis of variance, excluding the ECT group, examined the effects of *Sex, Drug, Psychotherapy*, and *Drug-Psychotherapy Interaction*.

Computations were made of the amount of variance accounted for by these various effects, and of the effect-size ratios (Cohen, 1969). Where the design is non-orthogonal due to unequal cell size, and particularly when the number of cases is small, there is a confounding of effects, i.e., "double-counting." In such situations (e.g., in the five-year data), the total amount of "variance accounted for" may exceed 100 percent, so in such cases the computations must be treated with reserve and taken only as a rough guide, rather than as a precise estimate.

Having given due and important weight to the caveats and qualifications outlined above, the data may now be considered.

HOSPITAL STAY RESULTS

Days-in-hospital is a much more satisfactory and sensitive index of health status than number of readmissions, since a high readmission rate may indicate that borderline patients are being successfully maintained in the community with the support of frequent, brief, readmission. Long periods of hospital stay, on the other hand, are an unequivocal indication of treatment difficulty.

Hospital Stay from Date of First Admission. *All patients.* Over the first three years after admission, the mean *Stay* was significantly ($D < .01$, see appendix for clarification) greater in the *Psychotherapy Alone* and *Milieu* groups than in the other three treatments, with *Psychotherapy Alone* consistently the greatest.

Three-way analysis of variance indicates a negative (but not statistically significant) effect from *Psychotherapy* ($-.6810$ at one year, $-.3011$ at two years, $-.3914$ at three years) and a significant, or extremely significant, positive effect from *Drug* ($+.0000$ at one year, $+.0390$ at two years, $+.0001$ at three years). *Interaction* was positive, but clearly not significant ($-.9292$, $+.8837$, and $+.4790$ at one, two, and three years, respectively).

Successes only. Considering only the successes, *Psychotherapy Alone* had the longest mean *Stay* over the first three years. *Milieu* was intermediate; the other three treatment groups had the shortest *Stay*, with little difference between them.

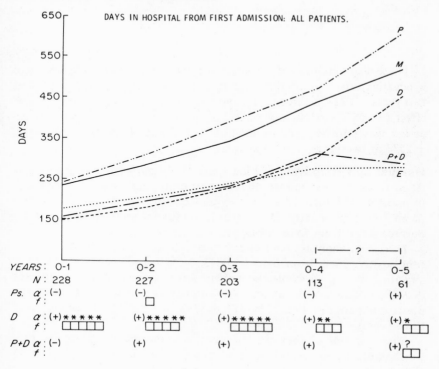

FIG. 4

SYMBOLS FOR EFFECT SIZE RATIOS (f), SIGNIFICANCE LEVELS (α)
AND DIRECTIONAL SIGNS

(f)

Little or none	< .009	
Trace	.010-.034	▦
Small	.035-.074	□
Modest	.075-.199	▭▭
Medium	.200-.374	▭▭▭
Large	.375-.549	▭▭▭▭
Very large	.550 +	▭▭▭▭▭

(α)

Direct. ⎧ Positive effect   (+)
Signs ⎨ Negative effect   (−)
      ⎩ Analysis not valid ( )

Not significant	> .30	
Questionable	.30-.20	?
Approaching signif.	.20-.0501	*
Significant	.05-.0101	**
Highly signif.	.0100-.0011	***
Very highly signif.	.0010-.0002	****
Extremely signif.	< .0002	*****

FIG. 5

Three-way analysis of variance indicated that *Psychotherapy* had a negative effect (borderline significant: −.1947 at one year; −.0734 at two years; −.0728 at three years) and that *Drug* had a significant positive effect (+.0087, +.0168, and +.0252 at one, two, and three years). *Interaction* was positive, tending towards significance (+.4178 at one year, +.2537 at two years, +.0914 at three years).

Hospital Stay from Date of First Release. *All patients.* When *Stay* was dated from the first release, the differences among the groups were less prominent, although here also *Psychotherapy Alone* had the longest mean *Stay*, significantly (D < .05) different (at one and two years, but not at three years) from *Drug Alone* at the other extreme.

Three-way analysis of variance indicates a significant or nearly significant positive effect from *Drug* (+.0673, +.0000, and +.0511 at one, two, and three years). *Psychotherapy* effect was negative, but not significant (−.2428, −.3020, −.6636 at one, two, and three years). *Interaction* was positive but not significant (+.7312, +.8193, and +.4100, at one, two, and three years).

Successes only. When the successes are considered separately, *Psychotherapy Alone* had the longest mean *Stay*, but not significantly so (D > .05), with little difference among the other four groups.

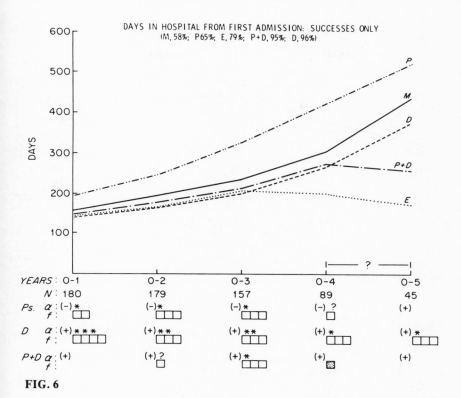

FIG. 6

Three-way analysis of variance indicates that *Psychotherapy* had a negative effect (borderline: –.1666, –.1359, and –.2200 at one, two, and three years). *Drug* had a positive effect (nonsignificant or borderline: +.1464, +.3263, and +.2135 at one, two, and three years). *Interaction* was positive, generally borderline significant (+.5941, +.1086, +.1703 at one, two, and three years).

Hospital Stay: Summary. It may be concluded that the *Psychotherapy Alone* patients had the longest followup *Stay*, regardless of the baseline chosen for analysis and whether or not analysis was restricted to the successes.

Drug had a highly significant effect on initial *Stay*, and this effect persisted over the first three years. Further, there was a (significant or nearly so) effect from having had drug therapy that was additional after discharge to outpatient status. By comparison, the effect of having received *Psychotherapy* was negative (but not statistically significant).

When the successes alone are considered, the negative effect from having received *Psychotherapy* becomes somewhat more prominent

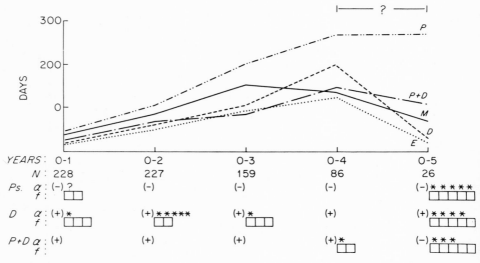

DAYS IN HOSPITAL AFTER FIRST RELEASE: ALL PATIENTS.

FIG. 7

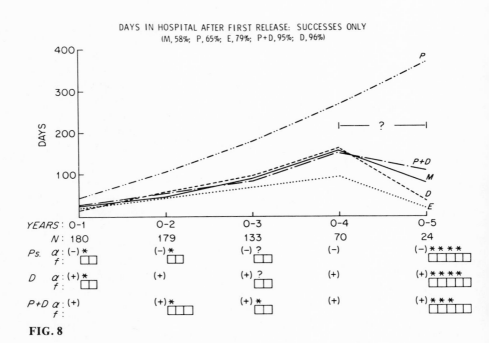

DAYS IN HOSPITAL AFTER FIRST RELEASE: SUCCESSES ONLY
(M, 58%; P, 65%; E, 79%; P+D, 95%; D, 96%)

FIG. 8

(borderline significant), considered either from admission or from release. Although the positive effect of drug treatment remains significant when *Stay* is dated from first admission, *Drug* effect is reduced from significant to borderline when *Stay* is dated from first release. The same trends tend to continue into the fourth and fifth years. The five-year plots are, however, markedly out of line, as will be discussed below. This was resolved by Reverse Cohort Analysis.

FOUR- AND FIVE-YEAR RESULTS: REVERSE COHORT ANALYSIS

The plots of mean stay for the different treatment groups (Figs. 4–8) strongly suggest that the trends established in the first three years from admission and release persist into the fourth and fifth followup years. These samples, however, show a serious diminution in N, which, as previously discussed, introduces a problem of potential bias. For example, the out-of-line changes in mean *Stay* among the groups in the fifth year could merely reflect changes in sample composition, rather than true change in status of the groups.

Diminishing N also complicates comparative interpretation of significance level data, for, as sample size diminishes, a difference must be larger to be declared significant. Thus a given difference between groups might be declared to be statistically insignificant in these later years purely as a function of sample size and degrees of freedom.

The technique of Reverse Cohort Analysis aims to mitigate these problems and to allow for a more meaningful interpretation of such data. Figure 9 depicts three-, four-, and five-year Reverse Cohort Analyses. In the five-year analysis, for example, the outcome course of those who were followed for five years from admission, the "Five-Year Reverse Cohort," is traced back by analyzing the results *for this group only* at four, three, two, and one years. Similarly, outcome for the "Four-Year Reverse Cohort" is traced back by analyzing their results at three, two, and one years; likewise, the "Three-Year Reverse Cohort" is traced back by analysis of their data at one and two years.

This technique has two important effects. First, for any given Reverse Cohort, the N remains the same at all time points: hence the results for statistical significance and effect size are strictly comparable at different time points. Second, it is possible to compare the courses of the three-, four-, and five-year Reverse Cohorts over time, looking for differences that might indicate sample bias in one or more of the cohorts. (When so doing, it must be vigilantly kept in mind that differences in significance levels *between* reverse cohorts may be attributable purely to differences in sample size.[1])

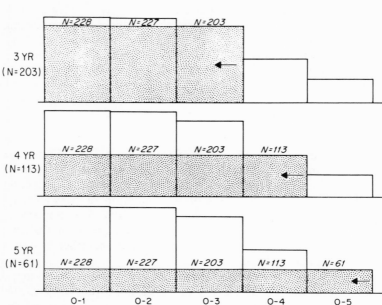

FIG. 9

Obviously, Reverse Cohort Analysis cannot make a silk purse out of a sow's ear. It can, however, provide important additional information, as we will now see.

Days in Hospital from First Admission. *All patients.* Figure 10 shows that mean *Stay* for *Psychotherapy Alone* and *Milieu* in the five-year reverse cohort was consistently longer over the entire five-year period than in the other three treatment groups.

Figures 11 and 12 show that this applies also to four- and three-year reverse cohorts. Further, the rank order, values, and spacing of the five treatment groups are similar in the different reverse cohorts at comparable points in time; i.e., the data from the three reverse cohorts are generally consistent at any one point in time.

The only inconsistency is a modest one. The mean values for *Drug Alone* in the five-year cohort are closer to *Psychotherapy Alone* and to *Milieu* than are the *Drug Alone* values in the other cohorts. This suggests that, compared to the other, larger cohorts, perhaps the cohort followed into the fifth year may have contained a higher proportion of patients who did not do so well on drugs.

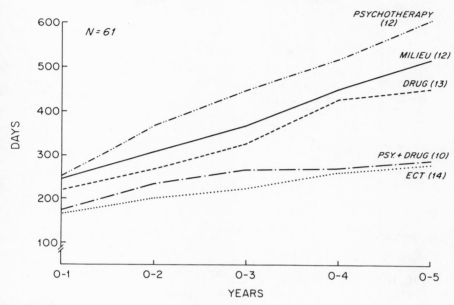

REVERSE COHORT ANALYSIS: PATIENTS FOLLOWED 5 YEARS.
DAYS IN HOSPITAL FROM FIRST ADMISSION: ALL PATIENTS.

FIG. 10

Figure 13 plots the significance levels for *Drug, Psychotherapy,* and *Interaction* effects over time for the different reverse cohorts. The *Psychotherapy* effect is seen to be consistently negative, but not significant. The *Drug* effect is consistently positive, but of diminished (borderline) significance throughout the entire course of the five-year cohort. This supports the interpretation that the (smaller) five-year cohort contained a higher proportion of patients who did poorly after having received initial treatment with drug therapy. The *Interaction* effect is consistently positive (but nonsignificant) in all cohorts.[2] Note also that the ECT group did as well as *Drug Alone* and *Psychotherapy plus Drug.*

Successes only. Figures 14–16 show that the same general picture pertains if only the successes are considered. *Psychotherapy Alone* and *Milieu* were consistently worse in all three reverse cohorts at all points in time. In the successes, however, *Milieu* in the five-year reverse cohort is somewhat out of line with the other two cohorts, although it is in the same rank order. The implication is that the five-year reverse cohort from release may have contained a somewhat disproportionate number of failures on *Milieu.*

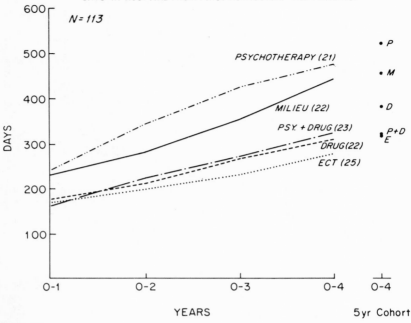

FIG. 11

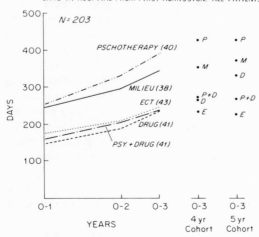

FIG. 12

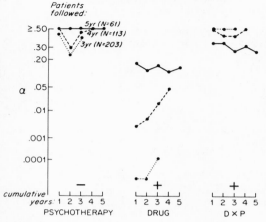

REVERSE COHORT ANALYSIS: DAYS IN HOSPITAL FROM FIRST ADMISSION.

DIRECTION & SIGNIFICANCE LEVELS FOR PSYCHOTHERAPY, DRUG & INTERACTION EFFECTS. ALL PATIENTS.

FIG. 13

REVERSE COHORT ANALYSIS: PATIENTS FOLLOWED 5 YEARS.

DAYS IN HOSPITAL FROM FIRST ADMISSION: SUCCESSES ONLY.

(M, 58%; P, 65%; E, 79%; P+D, 95%; D, 96%)

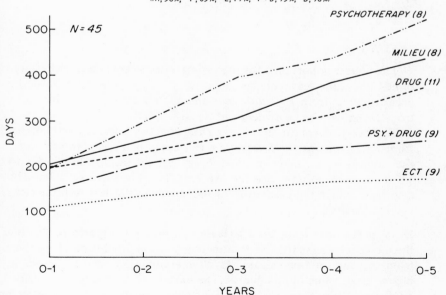

FIG. 14

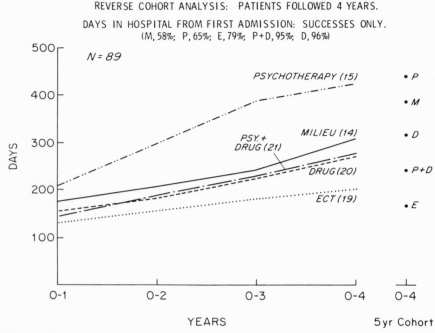

REVERSE COHORT ANALYSIS: PATIENTS FOLLOWED 4 YEARS.
DAYS IN HOSPITAL FROM FIRST ADMISSION: SUCCESSES ONLY.
(M, 58%; P, 65%; E, 79%; P+D, 95%; D, 96%)

FIG. 15

The reverse cohort data for the various effects show that, for the larger three- and four-year cohorts, there is a fairly consistent borderline negative effect from *Psychotherapy* and a fairly consistent positive effect from *Drug*, with some evidence of positive *Interaction*.

The five-year cohort shows less *Drug* effect (borderline) and no effect from *Psychotherapy* or *Interaction*: this could be at least in part due to the reduced N, but taken in conjunction with the mean values in Figures 14–16 the implication is that the five-year cohort of successes is biased by disproportionate representation of patients who did less well on *Drugs* and on *Milieu*.

Days in Hospital from First Release. *All patients.* Figures 18–20 show the mean values for the five treatment groups, plotted in reverse cohorts from the date of first release. *Psychotherapy Alone* had a consistently higher mean value in all cohorts. The deviatingly low values for *Milieu*, *ECT*, and *Drug Alone* in the five-year cohort suggest that this particular cohort of patients followed up from release has been biased by the inclu-

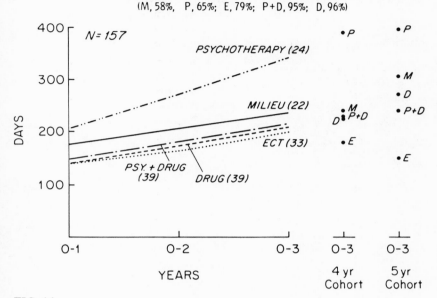

FIG. 16

sion of a disproportionate number of patients who did relatively well after having received these particular treatments.

Figure 21 confirms this suspicion, showing marked differences in *Psychotherapy*, *Drug*, and *Interaction* effects between the five-year and the other two cohorts and (much less prominently) between the three- and four-year cohorts.

The largest (three-year) cohort shows a consistently negative and nonsignificant effect from having received *Psychotherapy*, a borderline to significant positive effect from *Drug*, and little *Interaction* effect. The five-year cohort shows a progressively increasing and significant negative effect from *Psychotherapy* and a progressively increasing significant positive effect from *Drug* and *Interaction*. A preliminary speculation would be that the five-year cohort from release (in contrast to the five-year cohort from admission) is biased by containing a disproportionate representation of psychotherapy failures and of drug responders, i.e., there may have been a bias against drug therapy and in favor of psychotherapy in the data for patients who were followed up for the longest time after admission.

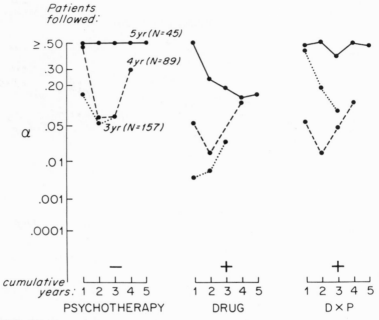

REVERSE COHORT ANALYSIS: DAYS IN HOSPITAL FROM FIRST ADMISSION.
DIRECTION & SIGNIFICANCE LEVELS FOR PSYCHOTHERAPY, DRUG &
INTERACTION EFFECTS. SUCCESSES ONLY.
(M, 58%; P65%; E, 79%; P+D, 95%; D, 96%)

FIG. 17

Successes only. Figures 22–24 show means for the successes only. Again, *Psychotherapy Alone* did consistently worse, with little to choose between the other groups. Here, also, the data suggest that the five-year cohort data are out of line, being deviantly low for *Milieu*, *ECT*, and *Drug Alone.*

Figure 25 shows the data for the various effects. In the largest (three-year) cohort there is a fairly consistent indication of borderline negative effect from *Psychotherapy* and borderline positive effects from *Drug* and *Interaction.* The five-year cohort shows increasing effects in the same direction but of dramatically greater magnitude.

A preliminary speculation is that the five-year cohort data from release (but not from admission) for *Drug Alone*, *Milieu*, and *ECT* contain disproportionate numbers of patients who did well after having received these treatments; i.e., there may have been a bias against *Psychotherapy*

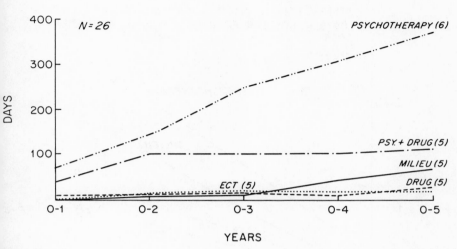

FIG. 18

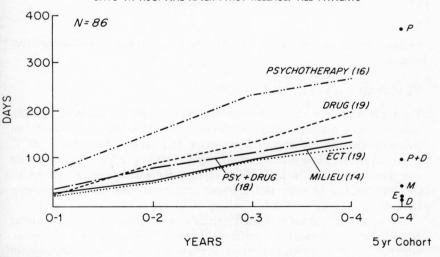

FIG. 19

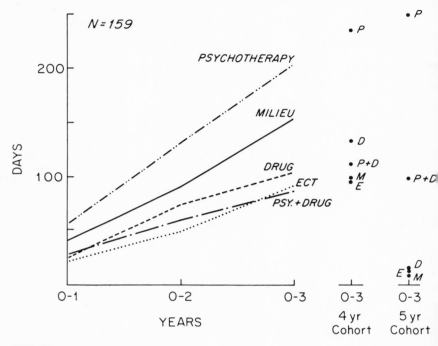

REVERSE COHORT ANALYSIS: PATIENTS FOLLOWED 3 YEARS.
DAYS IN HOSPITAL AFTER FIRST RELEASE: ALL PATIENTS.

FIG. 20

in the data for patients who were followed up for the longest time after release.

SUMMARY AND CONCLUSIONS

The main finding in the movement data reported here is that patients who were initially treated with *Psychotherapy Alone* fared less well on followup than those who received other treatments, particularly *ECT*, *Drug Alone*, or *Drug plus Psychotherapy*. This applied whether followup was dated from admission or from release and whether one considers all patients treated or only those whose treatment was declared to be a success.

By contrast, patients treated initially with drugs, with or without psychotherapy, showed a significant decrease in time spent in hospital, whether this is dated from time of admission or from time of release. In fact, patients treated initially with *Drugs* show a trend towards spending

REVERSE COHORT ANALYSIS: DAYS IN HOSPITAL FROM FIRST RELEASE.

DIRECTION & SIGNIFICANCE LEVELS FOR PSYCHOTHERAPY, DRUG & INTERACTION EFFECTS. ALL PATIENTS.

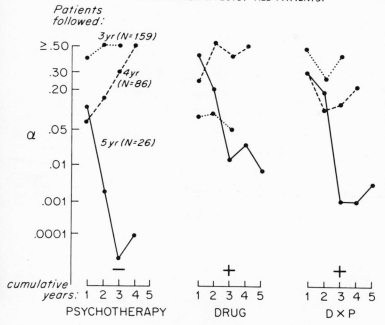

FIG. 21

less time in hospital after their release, although reduction in frequency of readmissions is questionable. Thus there may be perhaps a post-hospital advantage to patients who receive drugs during their first admission —over and beyond the in-hospital advantages of speedier release, lessened cost, and better global condition at time of release.

Drug effect is less marked where analysis is confined only to those patients when treatment was declared to be a success. It must be remembered, however, that 95 to 96 percent of the *Drug Alone* and *Drug plus Psychotherapy* patients were successfully released, compared with 58 percent of *Milieu*, 65 percent of *Psychotherapy Alone*, and 79 percent of *ECT*.

These findings can be taken as beyond reasonable doubt for the first three years of followup. The Reverse Cohort Analyses indicate that the trends probably continue into the fourth and fifth years from admission and into the fourth year from release. The reverse cohort data from the

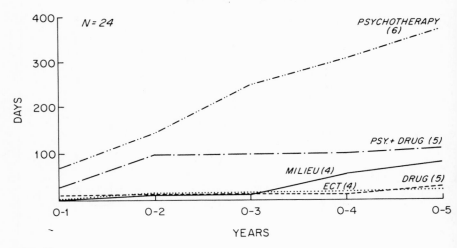

FIG. 22

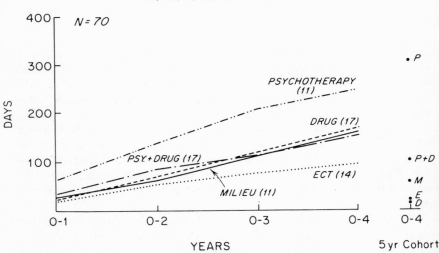

FIG. 23

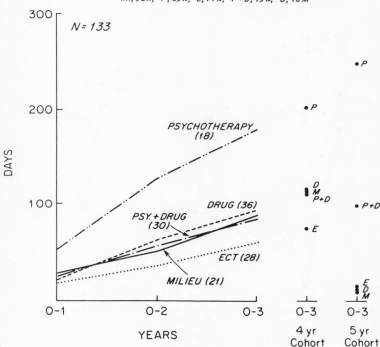

REVERSE COHORT ANALYSIS: PATIENTS FOLLOWED 3 YEARS.

DAYS IN HOSPITAL AFTER FIRST RELEASE: SUCCESSES ONLY
(M, 58%;   P, 65%;   E, 79%;   P+D, 95%;   D, 96%)

FIG. 24

fifth year from release are in the same direction, but there is reason to believe that they may be biased.

Patients treated with ECT seem to do about as well as (even better than) those who received drug therapy. (The investigators are reluctant to accept the glib hypothesis that this represents conscious avoidance of the hospital because of fear of treatment: unconscious fear cannot, of course, be excluded.)

Other project data must be examined in depth before we come to any definitive conclusions, especially in the case of psychotherapy and ECT. Nevertheless, it does seem that the results of this followup study should have an important impact. It seems in particular that certain widely held beliefs are not sustained; i.e., it was not true that drug-treated patients relapsed rapidly or more frequently than non-drug-treated patients. On the contrary, the initial advantages of drug treatment seem to be sustained for at least two to five years.

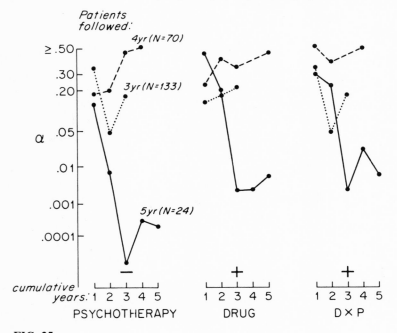

REVERSE COHORT ANALYSIS: DAYS IN HOSPITAL FROM FIRST RELEASE.
DIRECTION & SIGNIFICANCE LEVELS FOR PSYCHOTHERAPY, DRUG &
INTERACTION EFFECTS. SUCCESSES ONLY.

(M, 58%; P65%; E, 79%; P+D, 95%; D, 96%)

FIG. 25

Considering that the patients in this study were not given significant maintenance therapy after they left the hospital, the results are impressive. There even seems to be some extra secondary advantage to having had drug therapy that accrues to the patient after his release. One might speculate that this is due to avoidance of the secondary social disarticulation and institutionalism that accompany prolonged hospital stay. This may account also for the trend toward apparently adverse effects from psychotherapy—it may be that it is the prolonged hospital stay itself that is noxious, rather than the psychotherapy received there. It may also be that drug-treated patients are more cooperative with subsequent treatment, particularly with drug therapy; it could also be that psychotherapy-treated patients are (unwittingly perhaps) influenced toward resistance to drug therapy. Light may be shed on this subject by subsequent analysis of additional data from the project.

APPENDIX:
List of Conventional Terms, Abbreviations, and Notations

To avoid long-winded repetition in the text, the following phrases, terms, and notations have been used.

SIGNIFICANCE LEVELS

Where the actual level was determined, the (two-tailed) significance level (p) is given in parentheses to four significant figures (e.g., .0050). In addition to this more precise reporting, in order to speak distinctly to the clinician, we have used certain terms in the text as conventional designations for specified ranges of significance:

not significant	$p > .30$
questionable significance	$p = .30-.20$
approaching significance	$p = .20-.0501$
significant	$p = .05-.0101$
highly significant	$p = .0100-.0011$
very highly significant	$p = .0010-.0002$
extremely significant	$p < .0002$

If only the larger limit was determined, that value is given (e.g., $< .05$).

If a significance level is derived from a Duncan New Multiple Range test, it is preceded by the notation "D" (e.g., $D < .05$). (In this case, however, this is a "protection level," not a significance level.)

TREATMENTS, TREATMENT EFFECTS, AND TREATMENT GROUPS

The five treatment groups are identified as follows:

Milieu (M): the patient group treated with milieu care only.

Drug Alone (D): the patient group treated with milieu care and ataraxic drug.

ECT (E): the patient group treated with milieu care and electroconvulsive therapy.

Psychotherapy Alone (P): the patient group treated with milieu care and individual psychotherapy.

Psychotherapy plus Drug (P + D): the patient group treated with milieu care, individual psychotherapy, and ataraxic drug.

Specific treatment effects separated by analysis of variance are identified as follows:

Drug: the effect of ataraxic drug.

Psychotherapy: the effect of individual psychotherapy.

The following terms are used to refer to the respective methods of treatment (as distinguished from the patient groups or the specific treatment effects):

Ataraxic Drugs

Individual Psychotherapy

Electroconvulsive Therapy (or ECT)

Milieu Therapy: a general approach to treatment that includes nursing, occupational therapy, industrial therapy, rehabilitation, social casework, and supportive care.

The combination of Individual Psychotherapy and Ataraxic Drugs.

NOTES

1. A possible solution to this problem might be comparison with an equal number of cases randomly selected from the cohorts with larger Ns. Comparison with the mean of a number of such random samples would be preferable, if technically feasible.

2. As discussed previously, one cannot be confident that the diminished significance is not a function of the diminished N.

REFERENCES

Cohen, J. *Statistical power analysis for the behavioral sciences.* New York: Academic Press, 1969.

Duncan, D. B. Multiple range and multiple F tests. *Biometrics,* 1955, **11,** 1–42.

Duncan, D. B. Multiple range tests for correlated and heteroscedastic means. *Biometrics,* 1957, **13,** 164–176.

Feinsilver, D. B., & Gunderson, J. G. Psychotherapy for schizophrenics—is it indicated? A review of the relevant literature. *Schizophrenia Bulletin,* 1971, **6,** 11–23.

Lewis, A. Manic depressive psychoses. *Journal of Mental Science,* 1936, **82,** 488–557.

Lewis, N. D. C., & Strahl, M. O. The complete psychiatrist: the achievements of Paul Hoch. Albany, N.Y.: State University of New York Press, 1968.

May, P. R. A. *Treatment of schizophrenia.* New York: Science House, 1968.

May, P. R. A., Tuma, A. H., & Kraude, W. Community follow-up of treatment of schizophrenia—issues and problems. *American Journal of Orthopsychiatry,* 1965, **35,** 754–763.

Sargent, H. D. Methodological problems of follow-up studies in psychotherapy research. *American Journal of Orthopsychiatry,* 1960, **30,** 495–506.

18 SOCIOTHERAPY AND THE PREVENTION OF RELAPSE AMONG SCHIZOPHRENIC PATIENTS: An Artifact of Drug?

GERARD E. HOGARTY, RICHARD ULRICH,
SOLOMON GOLDBERG, and NINA SCHOOLER

Recently we presented data which indicated that maintenance chemotherapy to a very large extent, and a sociotherapy to a lesser degree, forestalled relapse among schizophrenic patients in aftercare (Hogarty & Goldberg, 1973; Hogarty, Goldberg, Schooler, & Ulrich, 1974). A review of these preliminary findings (Mosher, Gunderson, & Buchsbaum, 1973) has raised a legitimate question regarding the independence of treatment effects, namely, that "it is possible that the real contribution of major role therapy (our sociotherapy) was in encouraging the discharged patients to continue taking their medications regularly." The question asked is whether the strong prophylactic effect of drug and the identifiable but less pronounced effect of sociotherapy are truly "additive," as claimed, or whether the urging and reinforcement embodied in social casework simply assure that sociotherapy patients take their medication more faithfully than non-sociotherapy patients and consequently relapse less quickly.

Our data could not absolutely disprove the hypothesis that some relationship exists between drug taking, sociotherapy utilization, and relapse. Only a study which assures compliance with drug (e.g., one which employs injectable long-acting phenothiazine) and absolutely guarantees stratification of the non-drug intervention could yield a definitive answer. Still, available data have enabled us to ask a series of questions related to

Gerard E. Hogarty, M.S.W., and Richard F. Ulrich, B.S., University of Pittsburgh School of Medicine.

Solomon Goldberg, Ph.D., and Nina Schooler, Ph.D., Psychopharmacology Research Branch, National Institute of Mental Health.

This work was supported by National Institute of Mental Health Grants MH15829 and MH15830.

the hypothesis. The results are sufficiently equivocal as to cast doubt upon the supposition that a simple and direct relationship between drug taking and sociotherapy utilization fully explains the modest prophylactic effect of sociotherapy. Before presenting these findings, a brief overview of the study design and major results is appropriate.

METHOD AND EARLIER RESULTS

The rationale for the study developed from a recognition that relapse among discharged schizophrenic patients continued to be a serious public health problem and that levels of adjustment and performance among non-relapsed patients are poor. The few controlled studies of drug and placebo among discharged schizophrenics testify to the prophylactic property of maintenance phenothiazine treatment, but little information was available regarding the magnitude of the drug vs. placebo difference (Hogarty & Goldberg, 1973). We wished to ascertain whether the difference in effect between the two was large enough to have real clinical impact or whether it was only of modest size but statistically significant. Regarding the sociotherapies, evidence could be found both to support and to reject their effectiveness in preventing relapse or enhancing role performance (Hogarty & Goldberg, 1973). At no time had a long-term controlled aftercare study of both drug and sociotherapy been undertaken with discharged schizophrenics.

Following discharge from three Maryland state hospitals, schizophrenic patients from Baltimore were randomly assigned at clinic intake to Major Role Therapy (MRT), a combination of intensive social casework and vocational rehabilitation counseling. All patients were stabilized on chlorpromazine for two months and then randomly assigned to identical-looking tablets of chlorpromazine (Thorazine) or placebo. The study required 120 patients at each of three clinics. Patients stratified by sex were randomly assigned to all possible combinations of drug-placebo and MRT–non-MRT, creating the following four treatment groups: drug alone, drug and MRT, placebo alone, and placebo and MRT. Although the goal for total sample size was only 360, 374 patients actually were studied. The study was conducted at three clinics for two purposes; to obtain a sizable sample within a reasonable amount of time and to enable us to examine the consistency of results across facilities.

To be eligible for the study, patients were obliged to meet the following criteria: within age group eighteen to fifty-five; primary hospital diagnosis of schizophrenia confirmed by the research psychiatrist; current hospitalization of less than two years; no evidence of organic brain syndrome; intelligence quotient above 70; no history of unmanageable drinking or drug abuse; no history of serious suicidal or homicidal behavior during drug-free intervals; history of having taken phenothiazine as an inpatient and no medical contraindications for chlorpromazine therapy; residence within commuting distance of the clinic; availability of a "significant other" for rating purposes and supervision of medication; appearance at the clinic within twenty-one days of discharge; and no use of an ataractic other than study medication during the course of investigation.

The minimal dose of coded study medication (chlorpromazine or placebo) was 100 mg. a day. At clinic intake, the average chlorpromazine dose, or its equivalent, was 280 ± 145 mgs. per day. At the point of random assignment, (two months) an average chlorpromazine dose of 265 ± 135 mgs. per day was prescribed. Drug survivors averaged 270 ± 140 mgs. per day throughout the two years of study, and placebo survivors averaged 275 ± 190 mgs. per day. Drug relapsers in the first and second year averaged 295 ± 180 mgs. and 245 ± 130 mgs. per day, respectively; placebo relapsers in the first and second year averaged 330 ± 200 mgs. per day and 265 ± 130 mgs. per day, respectively.

MRT was administered by M.S.W. social workers, with an average of nearly seven years of experience (the range was five to ten years), most of whom were graduates of more functional (Rankian) schools of social work. MRT was viewed as a psychosocial problem solving method designed to respond to the interpersonal, personal, social, and rehabilitative needs of study patients and their families. An effort was made to avoid a therapeutic relationship with non-MRT patients and merely to evaluate their needs. When indicated, non-MRT patients were referred to other community resources, but these referrals were not routinely followed through. MRT attempted an approximate solution of practical problems, which frequently included situational crises. The primary goal toward which social workers were directed was the resolution of personal and/or environmental problems that directly affected the patient's performance as a homemaker or as a real or potential wage-earner. Otherwise, therapeutic objectives ranged from improving the quality of interpersonal relationships and ameliorating social isolation to the rudiments of self-care, financial assistance, and medication taking. Principles of practice included acceptance, clarification, material and emotional support, and appropriate assurance.

MRT and non-MRT patients were prepared for the study in the same way, and both groups were urged to take medication and to keep scheduled clinic appointments. These efforts to ensure adherence to the study design by non-MRT patients act to blur the distinction between the two treatments. They might better be labeled "high" and "low" sociotherapy. This ambiguity represents an unavoidable defect in the controlled study of the psychotherapies, one that has the effect of weakening tests of comparative efficacy. It further acts to obscure the relationship between drug compliance, sociotherapy utilization, and relapse, as mentioned above.

Findings related to relapse and adjustment were observed to replicate across the three independent clinics. Regarding tenure, drug was superior to placebo in forestalling relapse over the two-year study. Only 48 percent of drug patients but 80 percent of placebo patients relapsed. A variety of nonspecific and situational factors probably influenced relapse on drug, particularly the sex of the patient. Females on drug remained significantly longer in the community than drug-assigned males. Black females relapsed less quickly than others in the first year following discharge, as did all females on MRT (Hogarty et al., 1974).

Our sociotherapy had no effect on forestalling relapse over the entire course of the study but did appear to lower relapse for those patients able to survive the first six months in the community following discharge. In the period between 7 and 24 months, 44.3 percent of MRT patients and 57.8 percent of non-MRT patients relapsed ($p = .05$). In that the difference between drug and placebo was not significantly greater under the MRT condition, the effects of drug and of MRT were judged to be additive. However, a larger number of MRT survivors were found among drug-assigned patients, although no significant interaction was observed.

The challenge of the question at hand, therefore, will be to determine whether this modest effect of MRT, particularly among drug patients, is an artifact of the drug itself.

Elsewhere, we observed that neither drug nor sociotherapy in themselves influenced the adjustment of survivors throughout the study (Hogarty, Goldberg, & Schooler, 1974). At 18 and 24 months a pattern of effects was observed: among drug-assigned patients those receiving MRT adjusted better, and among the few placebo survivors those not receiving MRT adjusted better. Because placebo itself was not an effective treatment (80 percent relapsed), the better adjustment which characterized the few placebo-alone survivors was of theoretical interest only and would be of practical importance only in the event that accurate prediction becomes possible. Further, females on the active treatments (drug or MRT) appeared to adjust better than males on the active treatments. On the inactive treatments (placebo and non-MRT), males adjusted better. In the absence of clear main effects on adjustment for either drug or MRT, the issue regarding the independence of the sociotherapy effect is addressed directly to its prophylactic action. By definition, the effect of sociotherapy on adjustment is interactive with the effect of drug.

RESULTS

Our approach to the issue of whether or not the prophylactic effect of sociotherapy, observed between 7 and 24 months, is truly independent of drug involves a series of questions regarding dose level, regularity of medication taking, and the relationship between sociotherapy utilization and drug utilization. Compliance with both drug and sociotherapy was recorded by research social workers on a five-point scale which ranged from taking as prescribed (1) to not taking as prescribed (5). Most variance could be saved by simply dichotomizing the scales into "taking"–"not-taking" categories.

Drug Dose. First, the superiority of MRT, particularly among drug-treated patients, could simply reflect more appropriate drug dosage levels for this group. However, MRT survivors, on the average, were prescribed somewhat less medication (257 ± 100 mgs. per day) than non-MRT survivors (295 ± 100 mgs. per day). MRT relapsers did receive slightly (but not significantly) more medication than non-MRT relapsers (285 vs 260 mgs. per day), but the difference does not support the hypothesis.

Regularity of Medication Taking. For the most part, when a patient relapsed, he or his family reported that medication was not being taken as prescribed. Thus, the question of whether medication taking was more regular among MRT patients could be approached by examining only the medication-taking records of each patient while he remained (non-relapsed) in the community. At one year, an approximately equal number of MRT and non-MRT patients are non-relapsed and surviving in the community. Table 1 summarizes all the "non-relapsed" records regarding medication taking for this group throughout the study. Over all, there is an equivalency of medication taking among MRT and non-MRT patients. MRT patients did have a slightly better record of medication taking, but this is due to the MRT-placebo group. These one-year survivors on placebo and MRT continue to have lapses in medication taking in the second year, however, at a rate equal to that of placebo-alone patients. Thus, the evidence does not indicate greater regularity in medication taking among eventual MRT survivors.

Prevention of Drug Non-Compliance. A direct approach to the question of MRT's independence is to ask whether MRT is more likely than non-

Table 1. Medication-Taking Records[a] of One-Year Survivors

	Taking	Not Taking
Drug + MRT (N = 63)	228	35
Drug alone (N = 61)	220	36
Placebo + MRT (N = 29)	84	22
Placebo alone (N = 20)	61	20

[a]Sum of available ratings from months 1, 2, 6, 12, and 18.

MRT to prevent a lapse in medication taking *at any time*. If the hypothesis is true that sociotherapy is simply an artifact of drug taking, then one would expect to find more MRT than non-MRT patients surviving the entire two years of study without a single lapse in medication taking. Table 2 indicates that both in absolute numbers and in percentages more non-MRT patients survived without a single lapse in drug taking than did MRT patients: only 57 percent of the drug + MRT survivors did so as compared with 80 percent of the drug-alone survivors. Similarly, only 30 percent of the placebo + MRT patients survived without a single instance of drug non-compliance, as compared with 58 percent of the placebo-alone patients. Even if "missing data" cases are considered as not having complied with medication, only 46 percent of MRT cases survive without a lapse in medication taking, as compared with 63 percent of non-MRT. Thus, the ability to survive for two years without a single incident of medication non-compliance is more characteristic of non-MRT survivors.

Relationship between Medication Taking and Sociotherapy Utilization. A less direct approach to the issue of MRT independence involves a possible correlation between sociotherapy utilization and drug taking. The implication exists that a greater relationship between drug and casework utilization among MRT patients would account for the reduction in relapse in this group. Obviously, there is more useful variance for correlating drug taking and sociotherapy utilization among MRT patients, who had a greater range of services and opportunities for participation available to them than did non-MRT patients. Still, among relapsed patients, the average correlation between sociotherapy utilization and medication taking was .35, with a slight advantage for the non-MRT patients. The picture changes, however, for survivors.

Table 3 indicates that over time, particularly at the end of the second year, a relationship between casework utilization and medication taking is

Table 2. Lapses in Medication Taking for Two-Year Survivors

	No Lapses[a]		One or more Lapses[a]		Missing Cases
	N	%	N	%	N
Drug + MRT	26	57	20	43	(4)
Drug alone	28	80	7	20	(7)
Placebo + MRT	3	30	7	70	(3)
Placebo alone	7	58	5	42	(1)

[a]"Lapses" includes cases with no more than one missing data point.

Table 3. Correlations between Drug and Sociotherapy Utilization for Two-Year Survivors

	Study Month		
	2	12	24
Drug + MRT (N = 45)	.22	.44	.46
Drug alone (N = 35)	.22	.26	.11
Placebo + MRT (N = 13)	.42	.17	.67
Placebo alone (N = 12)	.00	.23	−.32
All MRT (N = 58)	.14	.33	.43
All non-MRT (N = 47)	.19	.26	−.03

observed. The importance of this relationship is further defined in the light of related information on drug taking and casework utilization which characterizes survivors throughout their entire course of treatment. Table 4 suggests that over the two years of study there is a distinct tendency not to take medication as faithfully among drug and placebo survivors, while MRT and non-MRT patients both tend to increase their utilization of available casework services. In view of these tendencies, the positive correlation noted in Table 3 indicates a particularly meaningful relationship between medication and sociotherapy compliance in the MRT group that could negate the independence of sociotherapy as a

Table 4. Medication-Taking (Drug or Placebo) and Casework Utilization (MRT or Non-MRT) Histories of Two-Year Survivors

	Intake	Treatment Month					
		1	2	6	12	18	24
Drug							
Cases taking	74	69	71	67	61	56	55
Cases not taking	4	7	4	5	14	18	20
Placebo							
Cases taking	19	17	20	18	16	11	10
Cases not taking	3	5	2	4	4	8	11
MRT							
Cases using	—	35	39	39	40	41	40
Cases not using	—	17	16	14	13	11	13
Non-MRT							
Cases using	—	19	20	24	24	24	29
Cases not using	—	26	25	18	19	18	13

factor in preventing relapse. However, closer inspection of the types of variation that occur in medication taking among MRT and non-MRT survivors provide the most feasible explanation of the MRT effect yet offered.

Variations in Drug Taking. As an introduction, it should be noted that about 85 percent of all survivors either had no lapse in drug taking or quit once and never resumed. Table 5 summarizes all types of drug non-compliance at all periods for survivors throughout the two years of study. First, there are more instances when patients switched from "taking" drugs as prescribed to "not taking" among MRT patients (26 instances) than among non-MRT patients (10 instances). Within the 26 instances of non-compliance among MRT recipients, there are 17 instances (involving 13 patients) where medication was resumed after once having been discontinued, but only 3 such instances (2 patients) within the non-MRT group. Of the 13 MRT patients returning to medication after a period of non-compliance, 10 are chlorpromazine-treated patients and only 3 are on placebo.

COMMENT

Our results do not negate the role of sociotherapy in urging greater compliance with prescribed medication. At the same time, they do not fully support the argument that the modest prophylactic effect of sociotherapy is wholly an artifact of chlorpromazine. Aside from a positive relationship between sociotherapy utilization and drug taking observed at the end of the second study year, the course of patients over the entire study indicates that MRT does not contribute to higher and perhaps more appropriate levels of drug dose, nor does it induce greater overall regularity in medication taking throughout the two years. In fact, more

Table 5. Variations in the Instances of Medication Non-Compliance among Two-Year Survivors

Type of Variation between Consecutive Ratings	Drug		Placebo		Total	
	MRT	Non-MRT	MRT	Non-MRT	MRT	Non-MRT
Taking to not taking	20	7	6	3	26	10
Not taking to taking	13[a]	2[b]	4[c]	1	17	3
Not taking to not taking	15	15	11	5	26	20

[a]Represents 10 patients.
[b]Represents 1 patient.
[c]Represents 3 patients.

non-MRT patients than MRT patients survive without a single lapse in medication taking. Rather, there is nothing in the data inconsistent with the notion that MRT, in its own right, sustains some patients during a temporary lapse in medication taking who in all probability would have relapsed otherwise. The numbers involved are small, yet they are adequate to account for the modest prophylactic effect of MRT reported earlier. Clearly, it is the strength of active medication that is primarily responsible for preventing relapse among discharged schizophrenic patients; the influence of social casework is also seen in those patients able to return to active medication. At the same time there is evidence that non-drug intervention has at least a temporary sustaining power which is independent of pill taking *per se*. This conclusion is supported by data that indicate a 42 percent increase in direct contacts among MRT recipients over the course of the study and by recent evidence that 8 MRT survivors received intensive contact (more than ten contacts per month during one or more study months), whereas only one non-MRT patient received such service, and this at his own initiation.

In the future, studies which assure drug compliance (i.e., those employing long-acting phenothiazines) and a more refined separation of sociotherapy and non-sociotherapy intervention should yield a more definitive answer regarding the specific nature of the effect of sociotherapy on maintenance of medication among schizophrenic patients in aftercare.

REFERENCES

Hogarty, G., & Goldberg, S. Drug and sociotherapy in the aftercare of schizophrenic patients: one year relapse rates. *Archives of General Psychiatry*, 1973, **28**, 54–64.

Hogarty, G., Goldberg, S., & Schooler, N. Drug and sociotherapy in the aftercare of schizophrenic patients: Adjustment of nonrelapsed patients. *Archives of General Psychiatry*, 1974, **31**, 609–618.

Hogarty, G., Goldberg, S., Schooler, N., & Ulrich, R. Drug and sociotherapy in the aftercare of schizophrenic patients: two year relapse rates. *Archives of General Psychiatry*, 1974, **31**, 603–608.

Mosher, L. R., Gunderson, J. G., & Buchsbaum, S. Special report: schizophrenia, 1972. *Schizophrenia Bulletin*, 1973, **7**, 42.

19

DISCUSSION:
Sources of Variance in
Studies of Drugs and
Other Therapies

RICHARD I. SHADER

Dr. May in his paper has highlighted some of the problems in carrying out longitudinal research, and special emphasis should be placed upon the issues of long-term funding, the time involved on the part of investigators who must remain together over the years, and the very thorny issue that one loses control over treatment assignments during followup. This loss of control over treatment assignments over an extended period of time is also reflected in the fact that many events both related and unrelated to the experimental design may occur during the period of time from the inception of an experiment to the final assessment, and that each of these events as well as alterations in treatment become important sources of variance that may contribute to differences in outcome among study groups. It would seem unlikely, then, with such powerful intervening variables, that differences among initial treatments would remain over time. Indeed, it would seem likely that differences would wash out. Such an expectation would argue against feeling that many predictions would stand up over time. Nevertheless, Dr. May and his colleagues made some important predictions which did stand up over time, and I think it would be useful to highlight some of these because they are truly unique in studies of this type.

First of all, the principle of triage was used. Patients from the middle section of the prognostic range were selected in order to include patients who would be likely to have the opportunity to leave the hospital within two years and to exclude those patients who were likely to show some

Richard I. Shader, M.D., Associate Professor of Psychiatry, Harvard Medical School; Director, Psychopharmacology Research Laboratory, Harvard Medical School and Massachusetts Mental Health Center; Director of Clinical Psychiatry, Massachusetts Mental Health Center.

From the Psychopharmacology Research Laboratory at Harvard Medical School and the Massachusetts Mental Health Center. The work was supported in part by U.S. Public Health Service Grants MH12279 and FRO-5555.

immediate reintegration following hospitalization or those who would be likely to require chronic, unremitting, hospital-based care. Those of you who are familiar with the literature on the natural history of schizophrenia, whether this literature is from the nineteenth century or from the twentieth century after the introduction of psychopharmacological agents, are probably aware that, in general, prediction of recovery is a difficult art at best. About 20 to 30 percent of persons who enter hospitals diagnosed as having something that we call schizophrenia restitute fairly promptly and have no further episodes. 40 to 60 percent show a phasic or intermittent course; another 20 to 30 percent generally go on to become chronic patients. It is therefore interesting to note that 180 of the 228 patients recovered sufficiently to be discharged despite the varying treatment regimens that were employed in this study. This left 48 patients who looked as though they were not recovering.

The authors of the study believed that the most desirable and practical treatment available was a combination of group therapy and antipsychotic medication, and this combination was then given to this group of 48 treatment failures. Here we notice a significant thing, namely, that 46 of the 48 treatment failures responded to this new intervention—a striking prediction-response finding. In other words, it was predicted that group therapy and antipsychotic medication would be effective, and 96 percent of patients who had not responded to other treatments were able to recover enough to leave the hospital. Over all, then, 226 patients at this point had responded to treatment out of the original 228, which again is a striking confirmation of a prediction, namely, that patients were selected in order to yield a sample which would be expected to leave the hospital within two years. I personally find these two predictions and their subsequent confirmation to be most unusual in research of this type, and it would encourage me to always say "yes" to Dr. May if he were to invite me to go to the horse races with him. I would like to make two other points about this excellent paper.

I think it would be important to understand a bit more about the method of reverse cohort analysis. While Dr. May's presentation makes it clear that the reverse cohort permits us to study a group which has been constructed in order to minimize the potential bias introduced by attrition in the sample size over time, it is not clear to me whether an evaluation was then done to see whether the reverse cohort was significantly different from the original entire sample from which it was drawn. In other words, if, as shown in Figure 8, 61 patients survived five years and one traces that cohort of 61 patients back over the five-year period to examine them at admission, do the 61 patients in the cohort appear to reveal no differences at base line from the remaining 167 patients who made up the original sample? While it is true that the whole is usually made up of the sum of its parts, it is often true in research that the parts do not reflect the whole when one tries to generalize from one of the parts.

This is particularly important when we pay attention to the next finding, perhaps the most crucial observation in Dr. May's material. We notice in the overwhelming majority of analyses that the cohort which originally received electroconvulsive therapy does the best at followup. They have the fewest days in hospital from first admission. This is clearly observed in Figure 13 (for successes only) and again in Figure 17 (for all patients). One hypothesis which could be generated from it is that ECT, which initially led to a small number of days in hospital, had profound long-term consequences even though it was not usually given as an intervening treatment. It suggests that if patients are given ECT and reintegrate rapidly and therefore have brief initial hospitalizations, this rapid pulling together helps patients to remain out of the hospital over the subsequent years. Perhaps the reduced time spent in an acute psychosis is terribly important. This would argue against positions taken by some psychotherapists that the patient must stay with the psychosis in order to understand the illness and fully recover. It is important to note also in Figure 17 that patients receiving psychotherapy alone have the longest number of days in hospital after first release.

A number of other questions should be raised, and I propose to highlight them but not to go into any detail. I've emphasized the sources of variance introduced by the many intervening events and treatments which occur after entrance into the followup phase. Equally important is the question of homogeneity in the sample. Dr. Paul Hoch's interest in sub-groups of schizophrenic patients might have led him to raise this point. It might be reasonable to wonder whether any of the patients in this group were pseudoneurotic schizophrenics. Do treatment results apply equally to all diagnostic sub-groups within this entity we call schizophrenia? How much variance is there within the treatments themselves? Are all doses equally appropriate across groups? How similar are therapists? Can we deal with psychotherapy as a homogeneous variable? In our own studies of acute schizophrenia, we have found that therapist type can account for some of the range in improvement scores (Shader, Grinspoon, Harmatz, & Ewalt, 1971).

I would like to move on now to the excellent paper which comes from Dr. Zitrin working with Dr. Donald Klein and colleagues on the problem of treating phobic patients. In this study we have three treatment groups: behavior therapy and imipramine, behavior therapy and placebo, and supportive psychotherapy and imipramine. A prediction or hypothesis is put forward that imipramine and behavior therapy combined should be superior to behavior therapy and placebo for agoraphobic patients. I am sure that Dr. Zitrin and her colleagues have considered this point, but it is generally agreed that anticipatory anxiety is also well treated by the use of anti-anxiety agents from the benzodiazepine class, and one might wonder why a treatment cell utilizing drugs of this class is not also included. Certainly this could be the basis of another study.

Let us look at some sources of variance within this design. First of all, we are told that patients who were assigned to behavior therapy were at times, when possible and indicated, accompanied into phobic situations by staff members. This suggests that for some patients this form of desensitization was done and for other patients it was not done—again we are dealing with a source of variance, making this a non-uniform treatment. Let us examine the definition of supportive psychotherapy. It attempts to help patients to obtain insight and to encourage them to try alternative means of dealing with their phobic problems. Interpretation, confrontation, and reality testing in an empathic climate are used to help the patient modify pathologic defenses and inappropriate behavior. Therapists may encourage patients to enter phobic situations. I would like to make two points here. First, insight, interpretation, confrontation, reality testing, and working through by examining the conditions under which phobic experiences are felt is by no means a simple supportive therapy. Indeed, it doesn't seem in some respects too different from classical psychotherapy. Going back to phobic material in supportive psychotherapy is really a form of working through which is in most instances a form of desensitization, even though it may be less efficient than that which is done in behavior therapy. It would seem to me then that with enough time one would expect these treatments to yield equal results, although they might not do so in the beginning. I personally would expect the differences to wash out by two years. (However, I don't expect my predictions to have the same likelihood of coming to fruition as those of Dr. May.)

It is also important to note in patient selection that 75 percent had had previous psychotherapy, suggesting that this treatment by and large was not successful; if it were, the patients would not be coming back again. This biases the design against psychotherapy because we are including patients for whom it has not worked well in the past. By contrast, patients are excluded if they have had prior treatment with tricyclic antidepressants. This eliminates the possibility of including people who by prior history have been failures with tricyclics. While the numbers are small, in any larger study this could lead to significant confounding of the data because the biases in favor of drug and against psychotherapy could be antagonistic in the same cell.

A few other points can also be made about this study in a brief way. It is unclear to me from the data analyses presented in the tables whether the interpretation of the results takes note that multiple comparisons have been made and whether, accordingly, adjustments have been made in the probability levels to take the multiple comparisons into account. I, too, have had Dr. Zitrin's experience of finding patients who are unusually sensitive to imipramine. In my experience these have usually been women, and I have wondered whether or not this sensitivity to imipramine might be the result of some interaction with oral contraceptives. Dr. Arthur Prange at Chapel Hill has alerted the scientific community to possible interactions between estrogens and tricyclic antidepressants (Prange, Wilson, & Alltop, 1971). This brings up another point about this study as well as the study by May and colleagues. It is striking to me that the sex of the therapists is not mentioned, and analyses are not done which might examine the interaction of sex of the therapist with sex of the patient. This point will also come up later in the discussion of the paper by Hogarty.

I am intrigued also by the issue of symptom substitution. In my own clinical experience this is a very complicated issue. I believe that fears and phobias often develop in conflict situations, and that if one approaches a patient in active conflict with the intention of symptom removal, the removal of the symptom without any attention to the underlying conflict will be followed in many instances by symptom substitution. However, many patients who come for treatment of fears and phobias have had these symptoms for long periods of time—they no longer appear to be associated with any active conflict and are, indeed, more like habits. When these habitual fears which are not maintained by any current conflict situation are removed by treatment, it is my impression that symptom substitution does not occur. It would seem important, then, to know something about the nature and function of the phobia in the patient's life and also to examine for symptom substitution not only while the patient is still in treatment (and in a therapeutic relationship) but also after the discontinuation of therapy to see what happens at that time. This brings up another source of variance, namely, that phobias are not all one thing. Clearly there are fears of dangers in the environment which come from actual negative experience with the environment. There are those fears and phobias which represent displacements from feared objects. There are even more complicated phobias which involve projection and then displacement, and obviously if we go to classical psychoanalytical literature other elements, such as regression, can also enter into the understanding of the symptom formation.

Let me make one last comment on this paper in the spirit of inquiry. In my experience patients with fears and panics often have increased heart action and may have premature contractions and palpitations. How often might these be increased by imipramine?

Let us move on now to the excellent paper by Hogarty and colleagues. This paper crystallizes even more clearly for me some of the issues that have to do with sources of variance when we look at psychotherapy and at the diagnosis of schizophrenia. In the introductory remarks the properties of urging and reinforcement are mentioned as part of social casework, and later major role therapy (MRT) is defined as a psychosocial problem-solving method designed to respond to the interpersonal, personal, social, and rehabilitative needs of patients and their families. The primary goal is the resolution of personal and/or environmental problems that directly affect the patient's performance as a homemaker or as a real or potential wage-earner. Principles of practice include acceptance, clarification, material and emotional support, and appropriate assurance. Again this is a very powerful form of psychotherapy, perhaps not dissimilar to Zitrin's "supportive psychotherapy"—and I would be willing to speculate that it is not too different from May's therapists' approach to the schizophrenic patient which is called "individual psychotherapy." We may wonder about the diagnosis of schizophrenia. Were there any symptom criteria which were uniformly applied? Did the same research psychiatrist confirm the diagnosis in all 374 patients? If so, this was a monumental effort.

I mentioned earlier a concern with the sex of the therapists, and the question of same- versus opposite-sex pairings of therapist with patient. Mr. Hogarty has indicated that the majority of his social workers were male. It is mentioned that the sex of the patient influenced relapse on drug. Females on MRT relapsed less quickly on drug. I would wonder whether this would have been the same with female therapists. On the other hand the main effect from MRT might have been more pronounced with female therapists. How good are male therapists in giving "vocational rehabilitational counseling" to women whose primary vocational role is homemaker?

One last comment concerns the hypothesis that more appropriate dosage levels would presumably be higher drug doses (e.g., "MRT relapsers did receive slightly [but not significantly] more medication than the non-MRT relapsers . . . but the difference does not support the hypothesis"). Isn't it equally possible that even "slightly higher" doses might put a few patients over the border into a drug dosage which sedates the patient or produces enough motor slowing to interfere with vocational performance? In my own clinical and research experience with the aftercare of chronic schizophrenic patients, too much drug can be just as improper as too little.

It should be obvious that it would be impossible to control for the various sources of variance in these studies. In my view, finding the truth in such scientific inquiry really means conducting a series of studies, each of which is an approximation. The sum of an infinite series of approximations is the best we can do in our search for truth. I, for one, would be willing to accept a good study, supported by two sound replications. I hope that the excellent work which has been presented to us today will be replicated by others so that we can adopt these findings in our pursuit of better clinical care.

REFERENCES

Prange, A. J., Jr., Wilson, I. C., & Alltop, L. B. The effect of estrogen on imipramine response in depressed women. Paper presented at the Fifth World Congress of Psychiatry, Mexico City, 1971.

Shader, R. I., Grinspoon, L., Harmatz, J. S., & Ewalt, J. R. The therapist variable. *American Journal of Psychiatry*, 1971, **127**, 49–52.

GENERAL DISCUSSION:II

DR. LEON SALZMAN:* I'd like to discuss the problem of clinical categories with the understanding that I am simply conveying some of my own concerns about this kind of research without coming up with any answers.

Now, what happens in this type of research is that we have more and more attempts to refine the clinical descriptions of the phenomena without even approaching a minimum definition of the phenomena. And we have the most exquisite testing, statistical correlations, and cross-correlations on phenomena that haven't been clearly defined.

Dr. Shader touched on this, and I am inclined to agree with him except that, curiously enough, even in his attempt at clarification we run into the same problem. For example, he wants to distinguish phobias by calling one an avoidance type and the other a displacement type. This creates new problems with few benefits, particularly since classically the displacement maneuver has generally been classified as an obsessional defense, not as a phobia. But avoidance is typically a phobic defense. This may be playing the same semantic game in which this paper gets involved while trying to distinguish phobic neuroses, agoraphobias, and mixed phobias, as if these were distinguishable qualitative responses to anxiety, producing valid separate disorders.

Now there is some value, I think, in selecting target problems and symptoms and defining and specifying those drugs which are useful for certain behavioral manifestations. Clearly there's been an enormous payoff to this approach, and there is no doubt any more that we have a whole assortment of drugs that are useful in dealing with certain behavioral problems, all related ultimately to anxiety. My point is this: should we spend our time designing more and more research which still uses hazy and ill-defined categories presumed to represent classifications of separate and distinguishable disease entities? This was the tendency in our earlier classification systems before we recognized that a great many presumed separate illnesses were merely variations of a more inclusive disease category. We seem to be getting back to this earlier period at which our ignorance prevented us from distinguishing a symptom from the disease itself. Refinement of our observational skills does not justify categorizing, and in fact is bringing us back a hundred years to the more inclusive kinds

*Albert Einstein College of Medicine.

of disorders. We are now breaking them down into an enormous number of related disorders, each having a slightly different manifestation or slightly different response to anxiety, as though they were different disorders, and then coming up with a lot of very interesting data about each of these symptoms in regard to a battery of different drugs.

I believe we have spent enough time devoting so much of our talent to discovering the specific drug for a particular phenomenological change. We should try rather to define the clinical entities in a way that would enable us to investigate and perhaps discover what constitutes the core of phobia, which is what this paper is trying to achieve. "Phobia" is a generic word for an avoidance technique, and avoidance in the face of anxiety and anticipatory anxiety is present in every phobia, sometimes more and sometimes less.

These are quantitative issues and not qualitative ones, and we get sidetracked when we think of the phobias as different disorders. I believe that the same problems arise with depression. We hear about "tension depressions" and "retarded depressions" as though they are different phenomena.

The response to drugs for the present is so specific that Dr. Shader suggests that perhaps the best definition of phobia is something Tofranil will alter. This brings us away from clinical physiological mechanisms to some mechanical determinations far removed from the concepts of a dynamic psychology based on reactive and adaptive tendencies of an organism. If in fact it is true that Tofranil is specific for phobias, we might define it in this manner. However, even limited clinical experience would reveal this to be an error; in fact, you have heard that Tofranil is good for other disorders and modalities of behavior which respond equally well to no treatment at all. The behavioral therapists claim about 80 percent success with desensitization alone. The drug people would get about 80 percent success without behavioral therapy.

I think that I have made my point: I think that the kind of research that combines outmoded clinical categories and definitions with the most sophisticated mathematical methods will not move us any closer to understanding such phenomena.

DR. JOSEPH ZUBIN:* Regarding the paper by Zitrin et al. I think we all ought to remember that science can only approximate clinical reality but can never displace it, no matter how far our knowledge advances. We will always be left with some hiatus between the true living entity and our attempt to measure and conceptualize it. So I think we ought to be tolerant of the shortcomings of this paper, and despite them forge ahead to get closer and closer to the true situation.

*Biometrics Research Unit, New York State Department of Mental Hygiene.

I would like to point out two virtues. First, the authors have revived a concept that goes all the way back to Adolf Meyer, namely, that there is a distinction between a focal or core disorder and the illness it gives rise to. The illness is defined as the response of the organism to the core disorder which the organism is suffering from. No two illnesses are ever the same because although the same core condition may be involved each illness is seen not in its basic core form but in the effect of the core disorder upon the organism, which varies in personality and in the situational condition in which it dwells. For this reason no two tubercular patients who have the identical lesion have the same illness. They have the same focal disorder, but the response to it may be in one case a galloping tuberculosis leading to death and in the other a short episode from which recovery quickly occurs.

So it seems to me that reviving this distinction between focal disorder and illness in psychopathology is a very important thing not only in the case of the paper we have here today, but in the case of our entire approach in the psychological-psychiatric domain. It suggests the reason why it is so difficult to diagnose schizophrenia. The difficulty is not caused by the fact that there is no core disorder—although a core disorder has yet to be demonstrated—but by the fact that the disorder develops in people who have different personalities and so the picture is different. The disorder hits different organisms in a variety of ways.

The second virtue of this paper, I believe, is that the authors believe that imipramine is a necessary prerequisite for psychotherapy. It seems to me that this is another example of a good sound psychophysiological approach to a disorder: it looks upon an emotion or emotional disorder as composed of two components, cognitive and physiological. The one way that you can really overcome the combination of a physiological and a cognitive deviation is somehow or other to extinguish one in the presence of the other.

If you cut off the physiological response through imipramine and then present therapeutically the anxieties which are present and talk about them in the absence of the reinforcing physiological component, eventually even the cognitive element in the disorder will disappear. So I think these two virtues of this study certainly make it deserve our full attention.

DR. ISAAC MARKS:* I'd like to address myself to several issues. First, diagnosis. I'd like to support Dr. Klein's division of the disorders into agoraphobia and others, and this is based upon empirical data, not just upon clinical impression. These data show that you get certain kinds of phobias much more than others, and that only the cluster of phobias found with agoraphobia is commonly associated with spontaneous panic

*Institute of Psychiatry, London.

attacks. Other phobias, especially specific ones, only rarely have panics striking out of the blue. The data are collected in my book, *Fears and Phobias* (1969). Other studies also support this sort of division. We don't know much about the classification of the phobic disorders beyond this. We can question whether agoraphobia consists of a number of sub-entities. But I think it is useful to differentiate between agoraphobics and specific phobics.

Now, the other point concerns the importance of the panic attacks, which is one of the key issues in this study. The clinical impression patients often give us is that the panics are important. Some people talk about these as "conditioning experiences"; Freud and Breuer in their 1892 paper spoke about these intense affective experiences having lasting consequences.

But whether we can regard these as core phenomena, I think we just don't know. We need more data. The problem is that the condition we can call "panic phobic" states or "agoraphobic syndrome" has had at least twenty different labels attached to the various aspects of its Protean manifestations, and one is always tempted to latch onto one small aspect anywhere from A, B, C, or D onward as the core. I, like you, and others who have published on the subject, have had agoraphobic patients who reveal exposure fantasies, but one cannot conclude from this that exhibitionist fantasies are at the heart of agoraphobia—they could simply be an epiphenomenon in a small minority. It is similarly hard to accept panics as the core feature of agoraphobia, as we often see agoraphobics without panics.

What I think we need to have in studies of this kind is more process analysis and predictive correlations of features present at the start with subsequent outcome. It is not enough just to present the outcome data as such. It is also necessary to look at the individual scales and how they change over time during and after treatment. And this can be done with this study: look at the measurement of anticipatory anxiety; look at the measurement of phobic avoidance; look at the measurement of mood changes; see how they curve in time in the drug groups, in the placebo groups, during supportive behavior therapy, and so on. Then I think you will begin to understand where the locus of change may be. That will give us some clue to what is changing first. And I think the virtue of this type of study is that it lends itself to answering these questions.

Another point is that behavior therapy is not behavior therapy is not behavior therapy. Essentially this study was looking at desensitization in fantasy, which is a different approach entirely from desensitization or exposure in vivo. There is good evidence to show that exposure in vivo is much more potent than exposure in fantasy. In other words, one needs to specify the psychological maneuvers in more detail for meaningful conclusions to be drawn. It is interesting that the outmoded procedure of desensitization in fantasy seems to have an effect. The next step would be to try the combination of drugs with prolonged exposure in vivo.

Lastly, the question of the sex of the therapist. There have been several studies in which the sex of the therapist was correlated with the sex of the patient and with outcome, and the results were negative.

DR. ZITRIN: I agree with Dr. Shader and the others who pointed out the importance of determining the etiological factors where possible. As I said at the outset, this is a preliminary paper. We have been gathering extensive historical data on all of our patients, including detailed developmental histories. We hope that we will get some answers eventually from the data that we have collected both at the beginning, when we screened the patients, and as various facts emerge during the course of treatment.

I can say that in most of our patients who were adults when the phobias began, there was a fairly discrete precipitating factor. I can't say anything more about the etiological factors at the present time.

With regard to psychotherapy versus behavior therapy, first let me point out that this was not a psychoanalytically oriented insight therapy. What I said was that occasionally insight was obtained by a patient. This was not sought in the way it is in a more prolonged psychoanalytically oriented psychotherapy. But occasionally we did find that it was easily available to the patient; perhaps it was preconscious, perhaps it had been uncovered in previous treatment, But that was certainly not the primary focus of the supportive psychotherapy.

The in vivo desensitization was of rare occurrence. But since it did occur on rare occasions, I thought we should mention it. I thought I clarified the point by saying that for the most part this was not done, but that the patients were given homework assignments which included in vivo desensitization on their own without the presence of personnel from the clinic.

A question was raised about the relationship of the excitation effect to oral contraceptives. We are obtaining on each patient a history of whether or not she has received in the past or is presently receiving oral contraceptives. I do know that a few of the patients who showed excitatory effects were not on oral contraceptives. I can't give you detailed figures. Also some of the patients who showed these effects were men.

I certainly agree that we have to look at the process notes and examine those very carefully. And, as I mentioned, we have many questionnaires that are completed by the patient, the therapist, and the independent evaluator during the course of this study, in addition to very detailed process notes. We hope to get some data from those sources.

I also want to point out that although the desensitization in fantasy did not seem to be effective in the agoraphobic-mixed phobic group, it was effective in the more focal phobic neuroses. In the latter group we found that imipramine did not enhance the effect of the behavior therapy.

All of these patients showed avoidance behavior except for patients who had cancer phobias, and which involved thoughts of having cancer. And what these patients did, of course, was to constantly run to the doctors and get all kinds of tests to be sure that they didn't have cancer.

The question was asked whether improvement included improvement in avoidance. Yes, it did. As part of the design the patients go on a field visit with an independent evaluator before treatment begins and after termination of treatment, and their avoidance behavior is detailed at both of those times. In addition, there is an interview with the spouse or a significant other family member at termination of treatment, and the independent evaluator determines from these other family members the avoidance behavior of the patient. So we do not rely only on the patient's report to the therapist.

I wonder if Dr. Klein could tell us whether the patients dropped, that is, not considered for treatment, had previous tricyclics, and whether he could also comment on the use of amitriptyline.

DR. KLEIN: What we would have liked, actually, is for the patients to have had neither previous psychotherapy nor previous drug treatment. However, we wouldn't have had a study since three-quarters of the patients had had previous psychotherapy, and that's that. We held, at least, to the medication aspect.

We are not trying to make a case of imipramine against psychotherapy; comparative strengths are not the issue. The major issue is what particular sub-group imipramine works on and what particular sub-group psychotherapy works on.

I'd like to make one theoretical point. The most interesting thing to me in this paper was that imipramine didn't work in the non-agoraphobic-phobic neuroses. It is no news to me it worked on agoraphobics; this was pointed out thirteen years ago, and we since have done double-blinds showing it. What we are interested in doing is showing that the effect of imipramine on phobics is not a broad symptomatic general effect against anxiety, but rather is very specific to the effects within a syndrome.

In other words, we were out to show that this was not, as Dr. Salzman would have it, a quantitative business, but indeed a qualitative business. That is the core of our particular presentation. I am afraid we just didn't get through there.

DR. FRITZ A. FREYHAN:* Dr. Shader referred to the World Health Organization statistics regarding the outcome of schizophrenic disorders. According to these statistics about one-third of schizophrenic patients

*Editor-in-Chief, *Comprehensive Psychiatry*.

have a good prognosis; for one-third the prognosis is poor; and one-third fluctuate in terms of morbidity. We must remember that the identical statistical breakdown was first observed by Eugene Bleuler. The difference in prognosis was a major reason for Bleuler to change the diagnostic term from "dementia praecox" to the "group of schizophrenias." Bleuler published these findings in 1911.

DR. ZUBIN: I might remind Dr. Freyhan that Manfred Bleuler's book, which was published recently, has a better outcome than one-third–one-third–one-third, which means something has happened to change outcome. By the way, I believe that in this country I was the first to point out this one-third–one-third–one-third ratio, and I attributed it at that time to a theorem of human judgment. If you are not certain how to classify, you put one-third in one category, one-third in the opposite category, and one-third in the middle. Today we push the middle third out into the community; that is why we have only one-third left.

I want to make some comments on Dr. May's paper. First of all, there were two striking things that he brought out. One, that ECT is still good for schizophrenics, which is something I hadn't realized. In fact, it seems to be the best thing for schizophrenics, better than any of the other treatments. And secondly, his attempt at presenting curves of release working backward from the date of release rather than forward from the date of admission is an interesting idea.

In regard to the first point, is it possible that we have succeeded in reducing a British-trained psychiatrist's acumen in distinguishing between schizophrenia and depression? Is it possible that those schizophrenics who benefitted from ECT were really suffering from affective disorders? I should think with his British training Dr. May would have certainly detected the differences. But maybe we have spoiled him in the last ten or fifteen years he's been with us, so that he has adopted the loose American diagnosis of schizophrenia which includes many affective disorders.

Regarding the second point, granted that backward analysis is very interesting and certainly summarizes the data in a very fine fashion, it might be that now, knowing what is going on in the data, we could perhaps use an index, something like the outcome index that Burdock et al. developed some time ago. In this index we take P, the proportion of time out of the hospital, multiply it by r, the number of releases, divided by a, the number of admissions. The number of releases r, is raised to the third power, while the number of admissions is raised to the fifth power. And when you do that, you find that the patients distribute themselves as follows in accordance with this index.

One group of people comes in and gets out and stays out; one group comes in and stays in for a long, long time. The first one has an index of near 1, the second index near 0, and there is an oscillating group in the middle with an index somewhere between .20 and .50. Maybe Dr. May would also get three cohorts, a group that gets in briefly and gets out and stays out; a group that comes in and stays in most of the time during followup; then a group of oscillators in between.

DR. HEINZ LEHMANN:* Like Dr. Shader and Dr. Zubin, I am quite surprised and rather stunned by the ECT figures. Somehow I must have missed them, Dr. May, in your previous publications. Anyway, I wasn't aware of them. Now, what I would like to know is: precisely how did you treat them, how many ECT's did they get, and also how long did they stay in the hospital? What the two treatments—drug and ECT and drug and psychotherapy—had in common is that psychopathology is very quickly extinguished, in comparison to the time lag with milieu therapy and psychotherapy alone.

Not all the patients were hospitalized, but perhaps it is just as important—maybe more important—that they remain longer in a world of their own, in a pathological state. We do know from clinical experience that the more often a schizophrenic patient relapses, the worse are his chances of remaining really well afterward and also the more he will deteriorate. Usually, after the third relapse there is some definite personality degradation.

Therefore it is important to prevent relapses so that the patient won't have to go back to the hospital and will have a chance to remain as well as possible. Now, ECT relapses tend to be quite frequent, and I wonder if you had any particular technique for making sure that patients wouldn't relapse. Did you keep them long enough in the hospital after the ECT was terminated or did you give them several courses? I should like to have some more details on this.

DR. FREYHAN: One brief comment on the efficacy of ECT. It is, of course, true that this treatment proved very successful for selected groups of schizophrenic patients. We published some studies on this topic based on long-term evaluations at the Delaware State Hospital. What was not practiced prior to drug treatment was maintenance treatment. There have been and there continue to be advocates of ECT maintenance treatment for recurrent depression. I am unaware of any systematic studies on ECT maintenance treatment for schizophrenic patients. At any event, the literature has never been specific on the symptomatologies in schizophrenic disorders which should be regarded as indications for ECT. Nearly all references pertain to the conventional subgroups, linking therapeutic responses with catatonic, paranoid, or hebephrenic types.

*Douglas Hospital, Montreal.

DR. MAY: First, I have to admit that it wasn't me who did the predicting. I had teams of two psychoanalysts who interviewed the patients together, and they did the predicting.

About the electroshock business; it was done in what I would consider to be a pretty decent style. That is we did it under anesthesia using pentathol with anectine. So I just cannot buy the notion that these patients stayed out of the hospital because they were afraid of it. They may have had unconscious fears, but we did our very best to do it in a reasonable fashion.

Did we study other criteria? Yes, indeed, of course. If I had shown you the other criteria, we'd be here until the end of the month, twenty-four analyses for each one. Some of them I haven't analyzed yet. A lot of these data are in my office awaiting analysis. Amongst other things, I went over each patient's clinical course as plotted on the chart and made my own personal rating of how well I thought that patient had done. So I have ratings that range all the way from something as subjective as that down to the real ratings of people who actually saw the patients.

Length of stay is a terribly interesting thing. I think it is better than readmission rate. Frequent readmissions can merely indicate that you are maintaining marginal patients very nicely by floating them in and out of the hospital for a few days at a time. So a high readmission rate may not mean very much. But overall length of stay in a hospital is a very good, crude index of how a patient was doing according to a vector. It is the net result of the opinions of many: his family, significant others, and the people who are giving the treatment.

Essentially you can see length of stay as the vector result of three impinging forces. It is, of course true that length of stay is susceptible to the whims of the therapist, to the whims of the family, and to the whims of the patient. It is also susceptible to the availability of placement facilities in a community. So I don't think it is an infallible criterion. But if you look at it the other way, I find it very difficult to accept being in the hospital as much of a criterion of health. It is very difficult for me to believe that if somebody stays in a hospital a long time, that is a good thing. I haven't seen many patients who I thought were in good shape who stayed in the hospital for a length of time. Yes, I have sometimes seen people who stayed in a hospital for a week or two unnecessarily, but I haven't seen very many people in good shape who stayed much longer than that.

The fact that all patients were in the same kind of geographic area, at least when they were first discharged, evens things out among treatments. Whatever the policy of the hospital, whatever the whims of the staff in this respect, whatever the facilities were, at least these were probably fairly randomly distributed amongst treatment groups. That is how I feel about length of stay.

Concerning how long the electroshock patients stayed in the hospital on their first admission, this group was down at the bottom with the drug and psychotherapy plus drug groups. They were all discharged fairly rapidly. The difference between the three groups was not statistically significant. The psychotherapy and milieu groups stayed by far the longest. The problem is one of how you count the length of stay for somebody who fails. If you add that in, the electroshock group was right in the middle because it had a higher number of failures. And so in point of fact if you took the failures into account, then the electroshock group was in the middle. In terms of the clinical judgments of outcome by nurses, therapists, and psychoanalysts, even in terms of cost of treatment, electroshock was somewhere in the middle. And the interesting thing to me was that males did badly and females did well, and I am hard put to explain that. I have done all sorts of funny little analyses since then trying to figure out why.

On the subject of psychotherapy, I was asked if the length of stay data were affected by the small number of patients. No, it wasn't. Every time we do an analysis we use a statistical technique we call Winsorizing, which enables you to pay less attention to extreme cases. We used three stages of Winsorizing: In the first stage you pay a little less attention to the extreme cases; in the second stage you pay even less; and in the third stage you almost ignore them. When we did that, the only evident change was that the significance of the effects we found became greater. The negative effect from psychotherapy was greater and the drug effect was greater. In other words, extreme cases merely confuse the issue. If you are considering the usual case, the situation is more drastic than I depicted here. I think this is really understandable when you think about how data are distributed. You have a general effect from something, and then you have extreme cases which come in and add noise to the data. That is essentially what we found there.

DR. ZUBIN: I'd like to ask Gerry Hogarty about the astounding finding that some patients in the major role therapy group did worse. I wonder whether it is possible that there was too much elevation of expectation induced as a result of the major role therapy in people who couldn't stand the additional stimulus that the social worker gave them to look forward to a better life. Is that one of the reasons?

MR. HOGARTY: Dr. Zubin asks whether psychotherapy by itself is bad for you. Well, according to our criteria of tenure and adjustment, indeed it is. Patients relapsed just as often on our form of psychotherapy alone as they did on placebo alone: 80 percent of the time. We can hardly recommend psychotherapy itself as a means of forestalling relapse among schizophrenic patients until we are able to identify those who cannot survive without drug.

The other side of the question concerns adjustment. If the patient is lucky enough to survive on psychotherapy alone, will it enhance his adjustment? The answer is no! Drs. Goldberg and Schooler, with whom I worked closely on this study, suggested that we might have greater confidence ultimately in our drug comparisons than in our placebo comparisons because of the fact that selection factors would less likely be operating in the larger drug groups than in the smaller placebo groups. Thus, for patients able to survive on psychotherapy (and placebo), indeed their adjustment is worse than those surviving on placebo alone. But it might be that patients who survive on psychotherapy are a select group as compared to those who survive on placebo alone. Only time will tell. At this point, age, sex, and initial level of disturbance do not account for the differences between placebo and psychotherapy plus placebo. The thrust of our recommendation is, of course, that if you took those patients on placebo and psychotherapy and provided them with drug, in all probability their adjustment would have been better than it would on drug alone. We are not recommending psychotherapy alone as a strategy for managing schizophrenic patients after discharge. However, in combination with drug, there are distinct and obvious effects on adjustment and behavior.

DR. ALFRED S. FRIEDMAN:* Mr. Hogarty comments in his paper that females on drug treatment do better on followup than males. Is this also true when you look at the whole sample?

MR. HOGARTY: Well, the women did relapse less frequently than men. In terms of survivors, the ladies did better on either drug or MRT when there are these effects.

DR. FRIEDMAN: This reminds me of a new finding that we have in a study of three hundred families with a schizophrenic offspring. While the schizophrenic daughters were equal in amount of hospitalization and degree of psychopathology to the schizophrenic sons, both parents of the female schizophrenics showed psychopathology more than the parents of male schizophrenics. There are suggestions in the literature that mothers of female schizophrenics show more psychopathology. But our new finding is that the fathers of the female schizophrenics also show more psychopathology. This made us wonder whether at least these younger female schizophrenics may be less vulnerable than males to a relapse, to a schizophrenic episode, or to being hospitalized or rehospitalized. In other words, does it take a worse home situation and more psychopathology in the parents to bring this about?

*Philadelphia Psychiatric Center.

MR. HOGARTY: Dr. Friedman raises a very interesting point. As is customarily found in studies of schizophrenia, most male patients are single and large numbers of them continue to live with parents. Conversely, female patients are no longer living at home, are frequently married, and are less likely to be involved with parents. If parents' psychopathology is an important variable, it is more likely to influence the tenure and adjustment of male patients than female patients simply because more parents are directly involved with such patients. This phenomenon would be worth exploring further.

A question was raised concerning stress and its interaction with treatment. The British have accumulated evidence to indicate that maintenance chemotherapy tends to serve as a good buffer against environmental stress. Whether psychotherapy has its own ability to insulate patients against stress I don't know. What is suggested by our results is that stress may interact with treatment and perhaps sex and race as well, at least with certain sub-groups of schizophrenic patients. I would single out the black patients in our study, for example, with regard to relapse. It seems that blacks had a more variable response to treatment, both good and bad, according to sex. My guess is that we might see something of the same thing when we look at adjustment data by race. This indicates to me that there may be external environmental factors that operate differentially in different sub-groups of schizophrenic patients. I am not suggesting that these factors operate differently etiologically, but that they may operate precipitously for different individuals. If this is true, syndromes of schizophrenic behavior might subtly differ with social class, ethnic origin, or culture and may reflect the effects of stress from goal striving and deprivation, as described by Parker. If this is true, recommended treatment strategies will ultimately have to differ along class, ethnic, or cultural lines rather than being blanket and uniform. This is especially true of somatic treatment, as we now see. I think that is the message we get today from therapists who work with minority groups, and I think there is a ripple in our early results that suggests a certain validity to the claim.

Publications of the American Psychopathological Association

Vol. I   (32nd Meeting):   *Trends of mental disease.* Joseph Zubin (Introduction), 1945.*

Vol. II   (34th Meeting):   *Current therapies of personality disorders.* Bernard Glueck (Ed.), 1946.

Vol. III   (36th Meeting):   *Epilepsy.* Paul H. Hoch and Robert P. Knight (Eds.), 1947.

Vol. IV   (37th Meeting):   *Failures in psychiatric treatment.* Paul H. Hoch (Ed.), 1948.

Vol. V   (38th Meeting):   *Psychosexual development in health and disease.* Paul H. Hoch and Joseph Zubin (Eds.), 1949.

Vol. IV   (39th Meeting):   *Anxiety.* Paul H. Hoch and Joseph Zubin (Eds.), 1950.

Vol. VII   (40th Meeting):   *Relation of psychological tests to psychiatry.* Paul H. Hoch and Joseph Zubin (Eds.), 1951.

Vol. VIII (41st Meeting):   *Current problems in psychiatric diagnosis.* Paul H. Hoch and Joseph Zubin (Eds.), 1953.

Vol. IX   (42nd Meeting):   *Depression.* Paul H. Hoch and Joseph Zubin (Eds.), 1954.

Vol. X   (43rd Meeting):   *Psychiatry and the law.* Paul H. Hoch and Joseph Zubin (Eds.), 1955.

Vol. XI   (44th Meeting):   *Psychopathology of childhood.* Paul H. Hoch and Joseph Zubin (Eds.), 1955.

Vol. XII   (45th Meeting):   *Experimental psychopathology.* Paul H. Hoch and Joseph Zubin (Eds.), 1957.

Vol. XIII (46th Meeting):   *Psychopathology of communication.* Paul H. Hoch and Joseph Zubin (Eds.), 1958.

Vol. XIV   (47th Meeting):   *Problems of addiction and habituation.* Paul H. Hoch and Joseph Zubin (Eds.), 1958.

Vol. XV   (48th Meeting):   *Current approaches to psychoanalysis.* Paul H. Hoch and Joseph Zubin (Eds.), 1960.

Vol. XVI   (49th Meeting):   *Comparative epidemiology of the mental disorders.* Paul H. Hoch and Joseph Zubin (Eds.), 1961.

Vol. XVII (50th Meeting):   *Psychopathology of aging.* Paul H. Hoch and Joseph Zubin (Eds.), 1961.

Vol. XVIII (51st Meeting):   *The future of psychiatry.* Paul H. Hoch and Joseph Zubin (Eds.), 1962.

Vol. XIX   (52nd Meeting):   *The evaluation of psychiatric treatment.* Paul H. Hoch and Joseph Zubin (Eds.), 1964.

*This volume was published by King's Crown Press (Columbia University). Volumes II through XXVI were published by Grune & Stratton. Volumes XXVII through XXIX were published by The Johns Hopkins University Press.

Vol. XX	(53rd Meeting):	*Psychopathology of perception.* Paul H. Hoch and Joseph Zubin (Eds.), 1965.
Vol. XXI	(54th Meeting):	*Psychopathology of schizophrenia.* Paul H. Hoch and Joseph Zubin (Eds.), 1966.
Vol. XXII	(55th Meeting):	*Comparative psychopathology—Animal and human.* Joseph Zubin and Howard F. Hunt (Eds.), 1967.
Vol. XXIII	(56th Meeting):	*Psychopathology of mental development.* Joseph Zubin and George A. Jervis (Eds.), 1968.
Vol. XXIV	(57th Meeting):	*Social psychiatry.* Joseph Zubin and Fritz A. Freyhan (Eds.), 1968.
Vol. XXV	(58th Meeting):	*Neurobiological aspects of psychopathology.* Joseph Zubin and Charles Shagass (Eds.), 1969.
Vol. XXVI	(59th Meeting):	*The psychopathology of adolescence.* Joseph Zubin and Alfred M. Freedman (Eds.), 1970.
Vol. XXVII	(60th Meeting):	*Disorders of mood.* Joseph Zubin and Fritz A. Freyhan (Eds.), 1972.
Vol. XXVIII	(61st Meeting):	*Contemporary sexual behavior: critical issues in the 1970s.* Joseph Zubin and John Money (Eds.), 1973.
Vol. XXIX	(62nd Meeting):	*Psychopathology and psychopharmacology.* Jonathan O. Cole, Alfred M. Freedman, and Arnold J. Friedhoff (Eds.), 1973.
Vol. XXX	(63rd Meeting):	*Genetic research in psychiatry.* Ronald R. Fieve, David Rosenthal, and Henry Brill (Eds.), 1975.

Also published under Association auspices: *Field studies in the mental disorders.* Joseph Zubin (Ed.), 1961.

This book was composed in Times Roman text and display type by Jones Composition Company. It was printed on 60-lb. Warren 1854 regular paper and bound in Columbia Fictionette by Universal Lithographers, Inc.

Library of Congress Cataloging in Publication Data

American Psychopathological Association.
    Evaluation of psychological therapies.

        1. Psychotherapy—Evaluation—Congresses.
I. Spitzer, Robert L.   II. Klein, Donald F.,
1928-   III. Title.
RC480.A53 1975   616.8'914   75-11360
ISBN 0-8018-1721-8